A Textbook of Orthodontics

DENTAL HANDBOOKS

Child Management in Dentistry (Second Edition)
G.Z. Wright, P.E. Starkey and D.E. Gardner

Complete Dentures
J.A. Hobkirk

Dental Care for Handicapped Patients
B. Hunter

Dental Treatment of the Elderly
J.F. Bates, D. Adams and G.D. Stafford

Endodontics in Clinical Practice (Third Edition)
F.J. Harty

Essentials of Dental Caries: The Disease and its Management
E.A.M. Kidd and S. Joyston-Bechal

General Anaesthesia and Sedation in Dentistry (Second Edition)
C.M. Hill and P.J. Morris

A Guide to Dental Radiography (Third Edition)
Rita A. Mason

Killey and Kay's Outline of Oral Surgery
Part 1 (Second Edition)
G.R. Seward, M. Harris and D.A. McGowan

Local Anaesthesia in Dentistry (Third Edition)
G.L. Howe

An Outline of Oral Surgery Part 2
H.C. Killey, G.R. Seward and L.W. Kay

Outline of Periodontics (Second Edition)
J.D. Manson and B.M. Eley

Paediatric Operative Dentistry (Third Edition)
D.B. Kennedy

The Psychology of Dental Care (Second Edition)
G.G. Kent and A.S. Blinkhorn

Silver Amalgam in Clinical Practice (Third Edition)
I.D. Gainsford and S.M. Dunne

A Textbook of Orthodontics

Second edition

W. J. B. Houston
PhD, FDS RCS (Edin), DOrth RCS (Eng)
Late Professor of Orthodontics
United Medical and Dental Schools of Guy's and St Thomas Hospitals, London

C. D. Stephens
MDS, FDS RCS (Edin), FDS MOrth RCS (Eng)
Professor of Child Dental Health
University of Bristol

W. J. Tulley
PhD, BDS, FDS, DOrth RCS (Eng)
Emeritus Professor of Orthodontics
United Medical and Dental Schools of Guy's and St Thomas Hospitals, London

With contributions by

M. E. Foster, MB, ChB, MScD, FDS FFD
Consultant Oral Surgeon
North Manchester General Hospital
Crumpsall, Manchester

M. Mars BDS, FDS RCPS, FDS DOrth RCS
Consultant Orthodontist
The Hospital for Sick Children, Great Ormond Street, London

D. Poswillo DDS, DSc, MDhc, FDS, FIBiol, FRCPath
Professor of Dental Surgery
United Medical and Dental Schools of Guy's and St Thomas Hospitals, London

Wright

Wright
An imprint of Butterworth-Heinemann Ltd
Linacre House, Jordan Hill, Oxford OX2 8DP

℞ A member of the Reed Elsevier group

OXFORD   LONDON   BOSTON
MUNICH   NEW DELHI   SINGAPORE   SYDNEY
TOKYO   TORONTO   WELLINGTON

First published 1986
Reprinted 1989
Second edition 1992
Reprinted 1993

British Library Cataloguing in Publication Data
Houston, W. J. B.
   A Textbook of Orthodontics. – 2Rev. ed
   I. Title   II. Stephens, C. D.
   III. Tulley, W. J.
   617.6

ISBN 0 7236 0986 1

Library of Congress Cataloguing in Publication Data
Houston, W. J. B.
   A textbook of orthodontics/W. J. B. Houston, C. D. Stephens, W. J.
   Tulley; with contributions by M. E. Foster, M. Mars, D. Poswillo. –
   2nd ed.
   Includes bibliographical references and index.
   ISBN 0 7236 0986 1
   1. Orthodontics.   I. Stephens, C. D.   II. Tulley, W. J. (Walter
   Jack)   III. Title.   IV. Series.
   [DNLM: 1. Orthodontics.   WU 400 H843t]
   RK521.H68   1992
   617.6'43 – dc20   92–8127
                                                          CIP

Typeset by Cambridge Composing (UK) Ltd, Cambridge
Printed in Great Britain by Redwood Books, Trowbridge, Wiltshire

Dedication

Bill Houston's tragic death in early August 1991 was a great loss to all who knew him and who had benefited from his kindly advice and his inspired teaching.

Bill qualified in 1960 and his progress was rapid. He was appointed to the Chair of Orthodontics at the Royal Dental Hospital at the age of thirty-six and during the next seventeen years made a major contribution to teaching and research, both there and later as Professor and Head of the Department of Children's Dentistry and Orthodontics at Guy's Hospital Dental School.

Among his many achievements he had been Dean of the Royal Hospital Dental School, Editor of the *British* and the *European Journals of Orthodontics*, and Secretary and later President of the European Orthodontic Society. He was the first to introduce the changes which led to a dramatic improvement in the standards of postgraduate orthodontic training in the UK in the 1970s. At the time of his death he was actively involved with his European colleagues in drawing together recommendations with the objective of harmonizing future standards of postgraduate orthodontic training in Europe.

Bill was a very private person who had many friends, but few who would regard themselves as close to a man who had the energies and abilities to excel in such diverse interests. Those who thought they knew him were frequently astonished to find another facet of his life revealed to them. He was widely read, and enjoyed many outdoor activities including sailing, orienteering, hill walking and climbing. He was a member of the Swiss Alpine Club and it was in the Alps which he so loved that he met his untimely death.

CDS/WJT

Contents

Preface   ix

1   The scope of orthodontic practice   1
2   The normal development of oral function   14
3   Development of the occlusion   28
4   The classification of occlusion and malocclusion   42
5   Examination of the patient   54
6   Cephalometric analysis   80
7   Facial growth   119
8   Treatment planning   141
9   Local factors and early treatment   166
10 Class I malocclusions   205
11 Class II, division 1 malocclusions   223
12 Class II, division 2 malocclusions   241
13 Class III malocclusions   257
14 Tooth movement   266
15 Removable appliances   277
16 Fixed appliances   302
17 Functional appliances   323
18 Stability and retention   346
19 Oral surgery for orthodontic patients
    David Poswillo and Murray Foster   357
20 Clefts of the lip and palate
    Michael Mars   388

Index   403

Preface

It is 5 years since this book appeared as the successor to the *Manual of Practical Orthodontics*. Inevitably, in an era that has shown an increasing pace in technological development, this period has seen a great number of changes in clinical orthodontic practice. For example, bonded brackets are now used routinely on anterior teeth, and ceramic brackets and superelastic wires have become commonplace.

Within the UK the same period has also seen several significant political changes, most of which have yet to have their full effect on the practice of orthodontics. The first was the publication of the Report of the Committee of Enquiry into Unnecessary Dentistry (the Schanshieff Report), which in 1986 commented on the place of orthodontic treatment within a publicly funded health care service. The second was the acceptance by the specialty that a 3-year postgraduate training period should be adopted for orthodontics in the UK, and the third is the current proposal before the General Dental Council that there should be an orthodontic specialist register.

There is now increasing acceptance that not all malocclusions should be treated, especially as part of state-funded health care, and that specialist skills are necessary if the more complex malocclusions are to be treated successfully. The work of Shaw *et al.* (1991) has shown that a significant proportion of orthodontic treatment carried out by simple removable-appliance treatment produces very limited occlusal benefit, and the study of Gravely (1990) demonstrated that the level of patient satisfaction is much higher when fixed orthodontic appliances have been used (see Chapters 1 and 4).

The move to establish a specialist register is perhaps a recognition by a majority of the dental profession that specialist orthodontic skills are needed, as well as a wish that those with specialist skills be identifiable to the public. It is, however, also tacit acceptance that the undergraduate curriculum cannot prepare the graduate for independent practice of dentistry in all its aspects.

It seems likely that future orthodontic practice in the UK will see a higher proportion of treatment being undertaken by specialists using fixed appliances and that the role, and therefore the training, of the undergraduate will be focused on recognition and referral rather than treatment planning and execution. However, there is no immediate prospect of more specialist orthodontists being trained and hence the practitioner (particularly the general practitioner with additional training) will continue to play a key role in the provision for orthodontic treatment for the time being.

In the light of these developments it is not surprising that there have been significant changes to *A Textbook of Orthodontics*. Our aim has still been to provide a basic text for the undergraduate and a primer for the postgraduate. We are, however, convinced of the need for continuing education for the general practitioner and we hope that the book will also prove suitable for those now running extended general-practitioner training courses in orthodontics.

We have strengthened the text in many ways. There are over 130 new illustrations. We have enlarged the introductory chapter on the scope of orthodontic treatment to include a section on the use of indices. The chapter on case assessment has been entirely rewritten and we have restructured the chapters on treatment planning and early treatment. Professor David Poswillo with Mr Murray Foster has updated Chapter 19, and Mr Michael Mars has contributed a new Chapter 20. To cater for the postgraduate we have tried to provide up-to-date references and, where appropriate, have indicated further reading.

Once again we are indebted to all our friends and colleagues for their encouragement and help. It is impossible to mention everyone by name, but we particularly wish to acknowledge the contributions made by the following:

Mrs Mary Calvert
Miss Sue Farrant
Mr Nigel Harradine
Mr Ian Hathorn
Mr Des McElRoy
Mr Bob Mordecai
Mrs Kathy Postlethwaite
Mr Allan Thom
Miss Cheryl Tracey
Mr David Ramsay
Mr Steve Richmond
Mr Laurence Usiskin

WJBH
CDS
WJT

References

Gravely, J. F. (1990) A study of need and demand for orthodontic treatment in two contrasting National Health Service regions. *British Journal of Orthodontics*, **17**, 287–292

Shaw, W. C., Richmond, S., O'Brien, K. D., Brook, P. and Stephens, C. D. (1991) Quality control in orthodontics: indices of treatment need and treatment standards. *British Dental Journal*, **170**, 107–112

Chapter 1

The scope of orthodontic practice

Introduction

Orthodontics is the branch of dentistry concerned with growth of the face, development of the occlusion and the prevention and correction of occlusal anomalies. Thus the study of orthodontics includes factors such as variations in facial development and growth, and in orofacial function, that may influence occlusal development; and also the effects of occlusal variations on facial appearance and on the health and function of the masticatory system.

Orthodontic practice

Clinical orthodontics is increasingly becoming the province of the specialist. Although modern materials and components have in many respects simplified the use of orthodontic appliances, patients quite justifiably are expecting a higher quality of result. This is not only technically demanding, but treatment must be based upon a thorough understanding of the aetiology of malocclusion, of facial growth and occlusal development, and of the problems of long-term occlusal stability. In many mild malocclusions it is quite easy by using directly bonded, fixed appliances to expand the arches and to obtain what seems superficially to be a satisfactory alignment of the teeth. However, unless treatment has been planned and executed with a profound understanding of orthodontic diagnosis and treatment planning, the result may be unstable even in the short term, and the treatment may well turn out to be deleterious to the patient. Great harm may be done by incompetent orthodontic treatment. Not only may the result be unsatisfactory from an aesthetic and functional viewpoint, but the prospects of subsequent orthodontic correction may have been prejudiced. Patient cooperation is often undermined, and correction of a badly treated malocclusion, particularly where extractions have been undertaken, can be very much more difficult than would have been the case in the absence of previous treatment. It is essential that the practitioner appreciates this, not only when tempted to commence treatment in the belief that if it does not turn out well it can be sorted out later by a specialist, but also when patient cooperation is in doubt. Treatment that has to be abandoned because of poor patient cooperation is almost always a disaster for oral health, particularly when extractions have been undertaken; and in the great majority of these cases the patient would have been very much better off without any intervention.

The place of orthodontics in general dental practice

General dental practitioners have the responsibility of monitoring the dental status of their child patients and so it is important for them to have a thorough understanding of occlusal development, of the factors that may influence it, and of the indications for treatment and its timing. A number of common simple occlusal problems can be treated with removable appliances and these should be within the scope of the general practitioner with the appropriate skills and training. However, it is important for practitioners to appreciate the limitations of their own experience and of the appliances they are competent to use. What seems superficially to be a simple irregularity may in reality be much more complex, and ill-advised attempts to treat such problems with extractions and removable appliances may only make things much worse.

General dental practioners have the responsibility for referring their patients, adults as well as children, for specialist advice and treatment. The referring practitioner will continue to look after the general dental care of these patients, and must have enough understanding of fixed orthodontic appliances to be able to supervise oral health and to provide routine dental care where necessary. Clearly, while appliances are in place, the person providing the orthodontic treatment should also monitor oral health, give oral hygiene instruction and refer the patient back for routine care as necessary. On completion of appliance treatment, the orthodontist should supervise the occlusion at least until it has fully settled. There should be agreement between the specialist and general practitioner as to who will be responsible for supervision of the longer-term occlusal changes, including eruption of third molars; and for maintenance of any appliances used for long-term retention.

Unfortunately, not all specialists will consistently provide a reasonable standard of orthodontic care, and the general practitioner must have enough expertise to know what standard of result can reasonably be expected for each patient, taking account of the limitations that may be imposed by the quality of the dentition, skeletal and soft tissue relationships, and patient compliance. The general practitioner is not acting responsibly if he or she continues to refer patients to a specialist who does not provide an acceptable level of care.

Occlusal variation

Central to the study of orthodontics is occlusal variation, and so it is convenient to start with the concept of ideal occlusion. Ideal occlusion in man is seldom if ever found: it is hypothetical concept based upon the anatomy of the teeth and is useful as a benchmark by which occlusal irregularities and treatment objectives can be judged. While all the possible approximal and occlusal contacts required to satisfy ideal occlusion can be described in detail, this would be of limited value from a clinical point of view and it is enough to specify a number of general principles.

Ideal occlusion in the permanent dentition (Fig. 1.1).

1 Each arch is regular with the teeth at ideal mesoiodistal and bucco-lingual inclinations and the correct approximal relationship at each interdental contact area. In particular:
  a The size of the teeth must be coordinated: a mismatch of tooth size between upper and lower arches invariably causes irregularity. The most obvious problems are peg-shaped upper lateral incisors or unusually large upper central incisors, but more subtle mismatch in incisor size is not uncommon.
  b A number of different arch forms are compatible with ideal occlusion, but they must be symmetrical, and the upper and lower arch forms must be coordinated.
  c All teeth must be angulated slightly mesially.
  d The buccal surfaces of the incisors are labially inclined, but from the canines posteriorly the buccal surfaces are progressively more lingually inclined.
2 The arch relationships are such that each lower tooth (except the central incisor) contacts the corresponding upper tooth and the tooth anterior to it (Fig. 1.1). The upper arch overlaps the lower anteriorly and laterally. In particular:

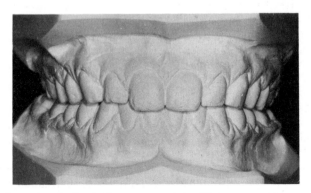

Figure 1.1 Normal occlusion in the permanent dentition.

  a Labial segments – the lower incisor edges occlude with the cingulum plateaux of the upper incisors and their inclinations are such that the overjet is 2–3 mm and the overbite is between one-third and one-half of the height of the lower incisor crowns. The midlines coincide. The occlusal plane is only slightly curved.
  b Buccal segments – both anteroposteriorly and transversly the upper and lower teeth have the correct intercuspal relationships. In particular, note that the upper canine occludes in the embrasure

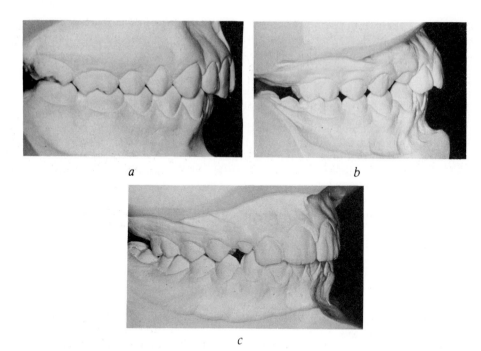

a   *b*

c

Figure 1.2 (a) A Class I buccal segment relationship. There is full intercuspation of all the buccal teeth. Note that the distobuccal cusp of the upper first permanent molar occludes with the embrasure distal to the lower molar. In this case the anterior buccal cusp of the upper first permanent molar occludes with the buccal groove of the lower molar, but in some cases, it lies behind the groove. (b) A pseudo Class I molar relationship. The anterior buccal cusp of the upper first permanent molar occludes with the buccal groove of the lower molar. However the upper first permanent molar does not occlude with the lower second permanent molar. Note that this molar relationship does not allow a correct intercuspation of the premolars and canines, and that the buccal segment relationship is fundamentally Class II. (c) When the occlusion in (b) is viewed obliquely, as is normally done when examining the occlusion in the mouth, the buccal segment relationship appears to be Class I.

between the lower canine and first premolar, and that the disto-buccal cusp of the upper molar occludes fully in the embrasure distal to the lower first permanent molar. The mesiobuccal cusp may not occlude directly with the anterior buccal groove of the lower first permanent molar as described by Angle but slightly distal to it (see Fig. 1.2).

3 When the teeth are in maximum intercuspation, the mandible is in a position of centric relation, i.e. both mandibular condyles are in symmetrical retruded unstrained positions in the glenoid fossae.

4 During mandibular excursions, functional relationships are correct. In particular, during lateral excursions there should be either group function or a cuspid rise on the working side with no occlusal contact on the contralateral side (see Fig. 1.3); and in protrusion the occlusion should be on the incisor teeth but not on the molars.

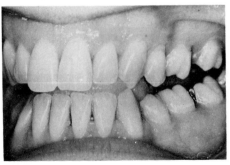
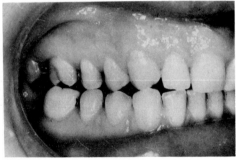

a   *b*

Figure 1.3 In the lateral excursion there should be either (a) cuspid rise where only the canine teeth on the working side are in contact, or (b) group function where most of the teeth on the working side are in contact. Note that the teeth on the non-working side should be out of contact.

Andrews (1972) pointed out that it is the inclination of the crown not of the long axis that is important, and summarized the requirements of an ideal occlusion as 'six keys' which should also be treatment objectives:

I   Correct molar relationships.
II   Correct crown angulation (mesiodistal tip).
III   Correct crown inclination (buccolingual inclination).
IV   Absence of rotations.
V   Tight approximal contacts.
VI   Flat occlusal plane.

Normal occlusion (Fig. 1.1)

This term encompasses minor deviations from the ideal that do not constitute aesthetic or functional problems. It is not possible to specify precisely the limits of normal occlusion and so there can be disagreement even between experienced clinicians about the categorization of borderline cases. For example, a minor irregularity of the lower incisors might be considered acceptable by one but not by another. Where there is no evidence that an irregularity is or could be disadvantageous to the patient, the occlusion should be classified as normal.

Malocclusion

Appreciable deviations from the ideal that may be considered aesthetically or functionally unsatisfactory are called malocclusions. However prevalent malocclusion may be (Table 1.1) it is important not to equate the possession of a malocclusion with the need for treatment. A malocclusion that is considered to be unsightly by one patient may be acceptable to another, depending upon other facial features, personality and attitudes.

Table 1.1 Prevalence of malocclusion (per cent)

	Gardiner (1956) 5–15 yr	Todd (1975) 11–12 yr	Foster and Day (1974) 11–12 yr
Class I (including normal)	65.7	63.0	44.3
Class II			
division 1	3.0 ⎫	18.5 ⎫	27.2 ⎫
division 2	0.8 ⎬ 8.1	4.5 ⎬ 33.5	17.7 ⎬ 52.2
indefinite	4.3 ⎭	10.5 ⎭	7.3 ⎭
Class III	0.4	3.0	3.5
Some treatment required	74.2	41.5	59.9

A potentially traumatic occlusal relationship merits treatment in the well-motivated patient but may be best left alone in the patient with a neglected mouth.

Indications for orthodontic treatment

Aesthetic criteria

By far the most common reason for a patient to seek orthodontic treatment is dissatisfaction with the appearance of the teeth. Facial appearance can be very important to an individual's self-image, well-being and success in society. Dental iregularities can be facially handicapping and thus merit orthodontic treatment on these grounds alone. The social acceptability of a particular occlusion depends not only on the arrangement of the teeth but on other facial features such as nose, lips and cheeks, on the personality of the patient, and on the attitudes of the society in which they live.

Children with malocclusions are more susceptible to teasing by their peers (Shaw, Meek and Jones, 1980), and attractive children are often considered by adults to be more intelligent (Shaw, 1981). An increasing number of adults seek orthodontic treatment, clearly because they believe that an improvement in dentofacial appearance would improve their social relationships or employment prospects. Where the dental practitioner considers that orthodontic treatment is justified on aesthetic grounds, the possibilities of treatment should be pointed out, but it should not be pressed on the patient. Judgement is required where the patient is a child who at that time is not concerned by their malocclusion, but who could reasonably be expected to become so later. Many malocclusions, particularly Class II arch relationships, are more readily treated while the face is still growing, and this should be pointed out to parents and child. If the parents are concerned and the child is compliant, it is appropriate to proceed with treatment; but if the parents are not interested or child is not likely to cooperate, treatment should definitely not be started. It is preferable to be faced with an untreated malocclusion than a treatment failure in an adult who later seeks treatment.

As aesthetic benefit is such an important aspect of orthodontic treatment, it is essential to plan treatment to maximize this. Too often treatment is planned and success is judged from plaster models of the occlusion without taking account of the facial appearance. In many minor malocclusions, dentofacial relationships are good and treatment must be planned so as not to prejudice dentofacial aesthetics, for example by excessive retraction of upper and lower incisors following injudicious extraction of first premolars. Where there are severe skeletal malrelationships, it may well be best to plan a combined orthodontic and surgical approach, and expert advice must be sought. It is in the moderately severe Class II malocclusions which are still within the scope of orthodontic appliance correction that the greatest care must be taken not to plan occlusal improvement at the expense of facial attractiveness. Even if the incisor relationships could be corrected by movement of the upper incisors alone, this may not give an attractive result if it would lead to their being too far back in the face. It is the relationship of the upper incisors to the upper lip that is particularly important (Lo and Hunter, 1982): they should support the lip at an appropriate angle to the base of the nose (Fig. 1.4) and the incisor edges should lie about 2 mm below the upper lip at rest. If the incisors are retracted too far or hang down below the upper lip the facial appearance will not be good (see Fig. 11.14).

The optimal aesthetic result may not be stable: for example in a Class II occlusion, proclination of the lower incisors may be required if the upper incisors are not to be retracted beyond the aesthetic ideal. This presents the clinician with a difficult decision as to whether it is better to compromise on aesthetics or on stability with resort to permanent retention (see Chapter 18). The general dental practitioner should not embark on treatment that is not expected to be stable.

Functional criteria

Orthodontic treatment has often been recommended on the grounds that malocclusion may be detrimental to dental health. However, there is little evidence for this belief (Shaw, Addy and Ray, 1980). Three aspects of oral disease have to be considered: caries and periodontal disease; traumatic occlusion; and craniomandibular disorders.

Caries and periodontal disease

It might be expected that dental irregularity would be associated with caries and periodontal disease. However, the relationship is not simple. Indeed many of the earlier studies found no relationship between malocclusion and caries or periodontal disease because they used crude general indices of malocclusion and of the disease process, which could hardly be expected to reveal an association, even if it did exist: any association must be specifically between local irregularity and disease at that site (Ramfjord and Ash, 1981). More refined studies investigating

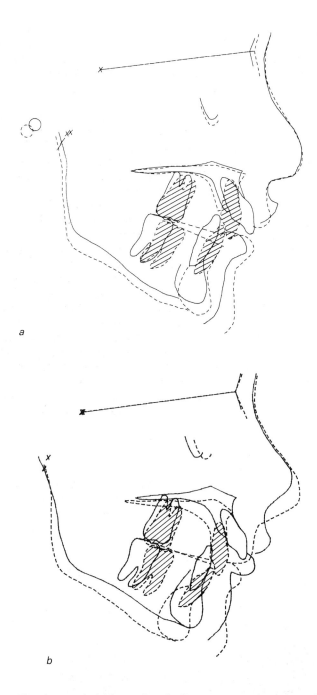

Figure 1.4 The changes in labionasal angle that may accompany retraction of the upper incisors. The effects are rather unpredictable because the effects of growth may be superimposed on those of treatment. (a) The change is favourable as the pretreatment nasolabial angle was quite acute; (b) an unfavourable increase in an already obtuse angle.

these relationships found that where plaque control is excellent, dental irregularity is not associated with dental disease, but where oral hygiene is mediocre, gingivitis and caries tend to be found at areas of irregularity because plaque is allowed to accumulate there (Addy *et al.*, 1988). Where oral hygiene is poor, plaque formation is generalized and so the association disappears.

This makes it difficult to advocate orthodontic alignment of irregular teeth on the grounds of reducing caries or inflammatory periodontal disease, particularly when orthodontic appliance wear is itself associated with an increased risk of caries and gingivitis (Ingervall, 1962; Zachrisson and Zachrisson, 1972). When appliances are in place, plaque control is more difficult. Unless scrupulous attention is given to oral hygiene and preventive measures such as fluoride mouth rinses, there is the real risk of caries around bonded attachments. Early caries also occurs under orthodontic bands if the cement leaches out and this is not rectified speedily. An increase in gingival inflammation is very common while orthodontic appliances are in place, but this is usually transient and clears up rapidly when the appliances are discontinued, provided that oral hygiene is good. A minor loss of up to 1 mm of alveolar crestal bone can occur during a course of orthodontic treatment (Zachrisson and Alnaes, 1974), even in patients with excellent plaque control. If oral hygiene is poor when appliances are in place, there is a serious risk to oral health in terms of caries and periodontal disease and treatment may have to be discontinued. In the patient with pre-existing periodontal disease, the risks of further damage during appliance wear are appreciable: appliances must not be fitted until the periodontal condition is stabilized, and plaque control must be meticulous.

Traumatic occlusion

A number of occlusal irregularities, such as instanding upper incisors or labial crowding of a lower incisor, can be associated with periodontal damage in an appreciable proportion of cases with these conditions (Fig. 1.5). They clearly require orthodontic intervention as a matter of urgency.

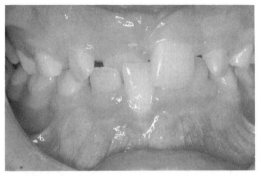

Figure 1.5 A traumatic relationship with gingival recession at one lower incisor. The reverse overjet must be corrected urgently.

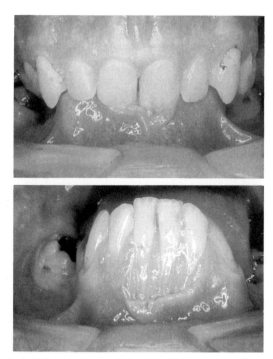

Figure 1.6 Periodontal trauma produced by loss of posterior teeth. This patient, who was in his mid-20s, had lost his permanent first and second molars as a teenager.

Periodontal trauma may also be found in association with a very deep overbite, particularly where posterior tooth support has been lost (Fig. 1.6). If plaque control is excellent, periodontal damage may not occur, even if the lower incisors occlude on the gingiva palatal to the upper incisors. However, this cannot be guaranteed. Because deep overbites are very difficult to correct in adults and are potentially traumatic, there is a good case for advising treatment in the mixed or early permanent dentition.

Craniomandibular disorders

Craniomandibular disorders involve pain or tenderness in the muscles of mastication and temporomandibular joints. It is important to distinguish pathological disorders involving the temporomandibular joints, such as clicking and locking, which may be of traumatic or degenerative origin, from pain and tenderness in the muscles of mastication or region of the joint, which often arise as a result of a combination of occlusal dysfunction and psychological stress. Pathological disorders of the joints need to be investigated thoroughly and treatment will usually involve occlusal rehabilitation, muscle exercises and possibly even surgery.

The majority of patients suffering from pain in the masticatory muscles or tenderness of the temporomandibular joints do not have pathological changes in the joints. Gnathologists place great emphasis on a number of aspects of occlusal function as being necessary for a healthy masticatory system. The position of maximum occlusion should be a position of centric relation: both condyles should be in retruded, unstrained positions in their fossae. A position of maximum occlusion up to 2 mm anterior to the most posterior mandibular position is satisfactory, but lateral or anteroposterior displacements of the mandible are not acceptable. In lateral excursions, it is considered that there should be either group function or a canine-protected occlusion on the working side, and there should be no non-working side occlusal contacts. In protrusion, incisal guidance should disclude the buccal occlusion.

However the relationship between occlusal irregularities and muscle/ joint pain is not simple (McLoughlin, 1988). The majority of people adapt to occlusal malfunction with little trouble; and many of the patients who suffer pain are under some form of psychological stress.

Extensive surveys (Möhlin, 1983; Möhlin and Thilander, 1984) have found little evidence of any general association between malocclusion and craniomandibular disorder. Weak associations are found between lack of incisal guidance and craniomandibular disorder, but the relationship is not strong enough to be of clinical predictive value. Craniomandibular disorder is common, even in children (Möhlin, Pilley and Shaw, 1991). Recent serial surveys (Heikinheimo et al., 1990) have shown that although the prevalence of this disorder remains fairly constant with age, the individuals involved vary, and there does not seem to be any clear association between occlusal features and the onset of, or relief from, pain. Thus surveys give little guidance as to which malocclusions if any should be treated in order to avoid the risk of craniomandibular disorder. The question of orthodontic treatment to improve occlusal function should be considered from two viewpoints: the individual who has no complaint of craniomandibular disorder; and the patient who presents with dysfunction and pain.

The general practitioner will see many patients with occlusal malfunction but who experience no muscle or joint pain. In some of these, tenderness in some of the muscles may be elicited on palpation, but it should be remembered that these signs may be transient. Mandibular displacements, associated with anterior and lateral crossbites, lead to muscular dysfunction, which can be recorded electromyographically (Troelstrud and Møller, 1970) and which give rise to facial pain in certain cases. Thus, early correction of these malocclusions is indicated. Apart from functional mandibular displacements, it is questionable whether other occlusal irregularities can be considered by themselves to justify orthodontic treatment purely on functional grounds: the association between such irregularities and craniomandibular disorders is weak; and orthodontic correction provides no assurance that the individual will not later develop craniomandibular problems anyway.

On the other hand, if orthodontic treatment is to be undertaken for other reasons, usually aesthetic, it is essential that occlusal malfunctions are not introduced; and if fixed appliances are to be used, pre-existing occlusal malfunctions should be dealt with. The tooth movements most likely to introduce occlusal malfunction are buccal tipping of upper molars when the palatal cusps will drop and be liable to create non-working side contacts; and a step relation between lower first and second molars when the latter have not been included in a fixed appliance that altered the occlusal plane.

There is much controversy over the management of patients who present with functional craniomandibular disorders. Some authorities believe that occlusal malfunction is a key factor that requires correction, while others consider that the main problem is psychological stress leading to clenching (Reynders, 1990). In many individuals, both factors are present.

One of the difficulties in evaluating the effectiveness of different approaches to treatment is that frequently the pain is transitory, and whatever approach is adopted appears to work, at least for a time, though recurrence is common. An appropriate strategy in the management of these patients is to deal with both psychological stress and occlusal dysfunction, giving priority to whatever factor seems to predominate in that patient. Few dental practitioners have the training to provide psychological counselling and it may be appropriate to refer the patient to their general medical practitioner or to a specialist clinic. When a patient is suffering from craniomandibular pain, it is often very difficult to examine occlusal function adequately, or even to be able to identify centric relation with confidence. Fitting an occlusal splint, with all round, even occlusion of the teeth, will often relieve the symptoms rapidly and, by removing occlusal feedback, allows the patient to adopt a position of centric relation. It is then possible to identify the nature of any occlusal malfunction and to decide whether this should be corrected by orthodontic tooth movement or by occlusal adjustment and rehabilitation. In general, major tooth malpositions should be corrected orthodontically, although this is not always simple, for example when a molar has overerupted. Minor occlusal interferences in adults should be dealt with by reshaping, although this is best deferred until any orthodontic treatment is complete. In children, it is generally wise to avoid occlusal equilibration until facial growth is complete because occlusal changes occurring with facial growth may make previous adjustments inappropriate. Patients who have had occlusal malfunctions corrected may enjoy permanent relief from craniomandibular problems, but many will have periodic recurrences, often related to episodes of psychological stress.

References

Addy, M., Griffiths, G. S., Dummer, P. M. H., Kingdon, A., Hicks, R. and Hunter, M. L. (1988) The association between tooth irregularities and plaque accumulation, gingivitis, and caries in 11–12 year old children. *European Journal of Orthodontics*, **10**, 76–83

Andrews, L. F. (1972) The six keys to normal occlusion. *American Journal of Orthodontics*, **62**, 296–310

Egermark-Eriksson, I., Carlsson, G. E., Magnusson, T. and Thilander, B. (1990) A longitudinal study on malocclusion in relation to signs and symptoms of craniomandibular disorders in children and adolescents. *European Journal of Orthodontics*, **12**, 399–407

Foster, T. D. and Day, A. J. W. (1974) A survey of malocclusion and the need for orthodontic treatment in a Shropshire school population. *British Journal of Orthodontics*, **1**, 73–78

Gardiner, J. (1956) A survey of malocclusion and some aetiological factors in 1000 Sheffield schoolchildren. *Dental Practitioner*, **6**, 187–198

Heikinheimo, K., Salmi, K., Myllarniemi, S. and Kirveskari, P. (1990). A longitudinal study of occlusal interferences and signs of craniomandibular disorder at the ages of 12 and 15 years. *European Journal of Orthodontics*, **12**, 190–197

Ingervall, B. (1962) The influence of orthodontic appliances on caries frequency. *Odontologisk Revy*, **13**, 175–190

Lo, F. D. and Hunter, W. S. (1982) Changes in the nasolabial angle related to maxillary incisor retraction. *American Journal of Orthodontics*, **82**, 384–391

McLoughlin, R. P. (1988) Malocclusion and the temporomandibular joint – a historical perspective. *Angle Orthodontist*, **58**, 185–191

Möhlin, B. (1983) Prevalence of mandibular dysfunction and relation between malocclusion and mandibular dysfunction in a group of women in Sweden. *European Journal of Orthodontics*, **5**, 115–123

Möhlin, B., Pilley, J. R. and Shaw, W. C. (1991) A survey of craniomandibular disorders in 1000 12-year-olds. Study design and baseline data in a follow-up study. *American Journal of Orthodontics and Dentofacial Orthopedics*, **91**, 193–199

Möhlin, B. and Thilander, B. (1984). The importance of the relationship between malocclusion and mandibular dysfunction and some clinical application in adults. *European Journal of Orthodontics*, **6**, 192–204

Ramfjord, S. P. and Ash, M. M. (1981) Significance of occlusion in the etiology and treatment of early, moderate and advanced periodontitis. *Journal of Periodontology*, **52**, 511–517

Reynders, R. M. (1990) Orthodontics and temporomandibular disorders: a review of the literature 1966–1988. *American Journal of Orthodontics and Dentofacial Orthopedics*, **97**, 463–471

Shaw, W. C. (1981) The influence of children's dentofacial appearance on their social attractiveness as judged by peers and lay adults. *American Journal of Orthodontics*, **79**, 399–415

Shaw, W. C., Addy, M. and Ray, C. (1980) Dental and social effects of malocclusion and effectiveness of orthodontic treatment – a review. *Community Dentistry and Oral Epidemiology*, **8**, 36–45

Shaw, W. C., Meek, S. C. and Jones, D. S. (1980) Nicknames, teasing, harrassment and the salience of dental features among school children. *British Journal of Orthodontics*, **7**, 75–80.

Todd, J. E. (1975) *Children's Dental Health in England and Wales, 1973*, HMSO, London

Troelstrud, B. and Møller, E. (1970) Electromyography of the temporalis and masseter muscles in children with unilateral crossbite. *Scandinavian Journal of Dental Research*, **78**, 425–430

Zachrisson, B. U. and Alnaes, L. (1974) Periodontal condition in orthodontically treated and untreated individuals. II. Alveolar bone loss: radiographic findings. *Angle Orthodontist*, **44**, 48–55

Zachrisson, S. and Zachrisson, B. U. (1972) Gingival condition associated with orthodontic treatment. *Angle Orthodontist*, **42**, 26–34

Chapter 2

The normal development of oral function

The mouth performs a wide range of functions and recent research has highlighted the complexity of these even in the newborn. In textbooks describing the detailed physiology and anatomy of the mouth there is little reference to the development of the various oral functions as the child grows and matures. Dental practitioners need to know something of these milestones in development if they are to appreciate where oral function deviates from the norm to the point of being a problem in the treatment of a malocclusion.

Oral and related functions are discussed here under eight headings: (1) breathing – airway maintenance and mandibular posture; (2) mechanisms of obtaining an anterior oral seal; (3) digit sucking; (4) feeding – suckle feeding, spoon feeding, mastication, swallowing; (5) speech; (6) facial expression; (7) mandibular positions and paths of closure; (8) occlusal function.

Breathing – airway maintenance and mandibular posture

The newborn infant is essentially a nasal breather. The lips may be just together or slightly parted. The upper lip and facial musculature are rather flaccid and immobile compared with the more active lower lip. Breathing is evoked spontaneously at birth and, if the infant is to survive, a posture of the mandible and hyoid bone must be established to ensure that the airway is maintained well before full development of the reflexes that enable the child to orientate its head in space. Some children born with so-called micrognathia may not, in fact, have a very small mandible, but the reflex mechanism required to establish this essential postural position is immature and the tongue can fall back and obstruct the airway if the child is not carefully nursed and safeguarded.

The laryngeal skeleton is high in the neck and there is a close relationship between the dorsum of the tongue, the soft palate and the epiglottis. The infant's tongue fills most of the mouth and is in contact laterally with the cheeks and anteriorly with the lower lip. The tongue is blunt and the tip develops later, coincident with the need for increasing mobility. The tongue has a strong sensory affinity for the lower lip – if the lip is drawn forwards, the tongue follows. As the child grows, the laryngeal skeleton descends in the neck and, although the

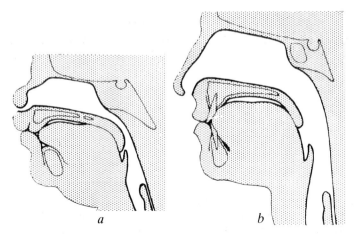

Figure 2.1 Sagittal section of the head of an infant compared with that of an adult showing how the epiglottis descends relative to the soft palate with growth. Note the posterior oral seal between tongue and soft palate.

tongue remains in contact with the soft palate, the glottic opening is no longer in close proximity to the uvula (Fig. 2.1).

The mandible takes up a definite postural position in relation to the maxilla in the first 6 months of life, as the child gains control over the muscles supporting its head and back and sits up. The gum pads at this stage are separated widely at rest. With eruption of deciduous teeth and development of the alveolar processes, the space between the jaws is taken up until the teeth come to lie 2–3 mm apart when the mandible is in the rest position (Thompson and Brodie, 1946).

Mandibular posture changes with the position of the head, and the true resting posture should be examined when the subject is looking straight ahead while sitting or standing upright. Movements of the mandible are described as starting from the 'rest position' and closure from rest into a fully occluded position of the teeth should be a simple hinge movement.

The facial and lingual musculature take no active part in normal breathing. The lips should be together at rest without conscious contraction of the orbicular sphincter, and the tongue and soft palate are in contact. Many children have lips that are too short or flaccid to achieve lip seal without conscious effort (Fig. 2.2), but they do not necessarily breathe through the mouth, as contact of the tongue and palate forms a secondary sphincter, which closes off the airway (Fig. 2.1), and there may also be an adaptive anterior oral seal.

The term 'lip incompetence' is used to describe lips that are anatomically too short to effect a seal without circumoral contraction when the mandible is in the rest position. In cases where a patient is a true mouth breather, the lips may not be 'incompetent' but merely habitually held apart. When nasal obstruction is relieved, a lip seal may or may not be established immediately (Gwynne-Evans, 1951).

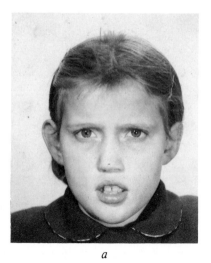 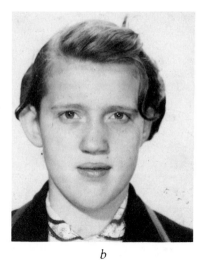

a   *b*

Figure 2.2 (a) This patient has incompetent lips which are habitually parted. She does not mouth breathe because there is an adaptive anterior oral seal and the posterior oral seal is patent. (b) This girl has a Class II skeletal pattern and incompetent lips but postures the mandible forwards to obtain a lip seal.

Where the lips are separated by the incisor teeth, but will come together at rest when the dental interference is removed, they may be described as 'potentially competent' (Fig. 2.3). Approximately 50 per cent of English children at the age of 11 years have some degree of lip incompetence.

Where there is partial or total nasal obstruction, mouth breathing becomes necessary. If the mandible and tongue were merely lowered in

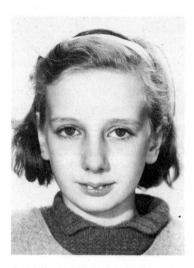

Figure 2.3 The lips are potentially competent, being separated by the teeth. When the overjet is reduced, a lip seal will be obtained.

order to allow this, the tongue would in fact encroach on the pharyngeal airspace. What in fact happens is that the cranium rotates posteriorly to a small extent (Vig, Showfety and Phillips, 1980) while the mandible remains more or less in the same position in space. In effect, relative to the cranium, the mandible rotates posteriorly. Thus the oral airway is established without compromising the pharyngeal airway. These changes affect the position of muscular balance on the dental arches: because the tongue lies at a lower level, the upper arch tends to be narrow; and the lower lip drops relative to the upper incisors, which tend to be proclined. Quite dramatic malocclusions occur in monkeys when the nasal airway is blocked (Harvold, Chierici and Vargervik, 1972) but in children with chronic nasal obstruction it has been found that there are only minor changes in the occlusion and these can be reversed when the obstruction is relieved (Linder-Aronson, 1970). There seems to be little effect on facial growth. In fact, chronic nasal obstruction is not very common and most children with habitually parted lips breathe through their noses. An adaptive anterior oral seal is formed between tongue and lower lip and there is usually a posterior seal between tongue and soft palate. Too much importance has been attached to mouth breathing as an aetiological factor in maldevelopment of the face and occlusion (Fig. 2.4).

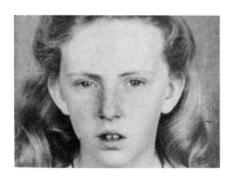 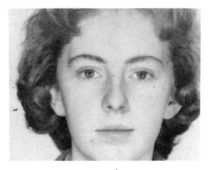

a   *b*

Figure 2.4 (a) A patient with so-called adenoidal facies; in fact she does not breathe through her mouth. (b) With increasing age, the facial musculature has matured and there is a habitual lip seal.

Mechanisms of obtaining an anterior oral seal

Most adults and many children maintain a lip seal with little or no circumoral contraction. Habitually parted lips are more common in young children than in adults. This may be due in part to differential growth in lip length and lower facial height, but can also be attributed to a greater self-awareness in adults, who achieve a lip seal as a matter of habit even though some muscular effort is required.

Where the lips are parted, either because they are too short or because the incisal overjet is large, an adaptive oral seal will usually be produced by contact of the lower lip with the tongue or with the mucosa palatal to the upper incisors. In some cases with an increased overjet, the mandible is postured forwards to facilitate a lip seal (see Fig. 2.2) (Ballard, 1955; 1962).

Digit sucking

Sucking of a finger or thumb is very common in the infant, who appears to derive comfort and pleasure from the habit. It is of little importance at this age and its role in the aetiology of malocclusion has been overemphasized in the past.

Although the deciduous dental arches may be malformed by persistent sucking, reflecting the way in which the force is exerted, many children give up the habit before the eruption of permanent teeth – and many habits do not have the intensity or duration to cause malformation. Sucking habits are only one of the factors that may deflect the permanent incisors from their path of eruption (Fig. 2.5). It is better to regard sucking habits as a normal feature of infant behaviour, certainly up to the age of 3 years.

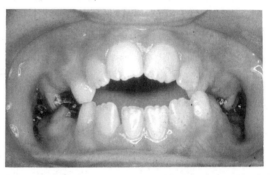

Figure 2.5 There is an anterior open bite and the overjet is increased as a result of digit-sucking habit.

Dummy sucking

Many parents provide young infants with a 'dummy' to suck, which can be very effective in calming them. In some children, dummy sucking is continued until school age (Larsson, 1985; 1986). However, it is very rare for this habit to persist beyond this time, and it is rarely replaced by a digit-sucking habit. Dummy sucking can produce a malocclusion in the deciduous dentition but the effects are not as marked as with digit sucking (Larsson, 1986; 1987), and there is rarely an effect on the permanent dentition because the habit is almost always discontinued before the permanent incisors erupt. Thus there is no good reason for the dental practitioner to discourage parents from giving dummies to their children, provided of course that they are kept clean and are not dipped in honey or some other cariogenic substance.

Feeding

Suckling

Infant feeding takes place by the rhythmic pumping action known as 'suckling'. In the first few days after birth the lips are not readily poised, but a primitive rooting reflex exists and when the child is nursed it turns its head naturally to the breast. When a child is fed naturally, the nipple and areola are grasped between the upper gum pad and the dorsum of the tongue, which comes forwards over the lower gum pad. The lips form a seal and the mouth cavity is enlarged as the jaw is lowered. The central portion of the tongue is deeply grooved anteroposteriorly and its edges are everted. When the tongue is raised anteriorly this groove is obliterated from before backwards, followed by firm elevation of the jaws. The nipple is considerably extended and taken well back into the mouth, and the squeezing action is completed by contraction of the floor of the mouth. This action is called 'suckling' to differentiate it from 'sucking', which is the creation of an intraoral negative pressure (Ardran and Lind, 1958). In suckling, an intraoral negative pressure is created by the depression of the mandible at one stage of the cycle, but there is also a pumping and squeezing action, which is typical of 'milking'. There is no evidence that the jaws and dental arches of the bottle-fed child will be smaller or less well related than those of the breast-fed child. Postnormal occlusion is equally common among breast- and bottle-fed children and the adverse mechanical effects of artificial feeding have been greatly exaggerated.

Spoon feeding and weaning

Mixed feeding begins at between 4 and 6 months of age. At this time the lips are becoming more active. Lip activity manifests itself in a spluttering kind of lip play, which delights the parents. Between 4 and 6 months of age, coordination of lip movements brings about a change in feeding pattern. The child soon begins to pout and smack the lips, and the upper lip is drawn over the spoon. The child learns to suck in semi-solid food and to sip from a cup. The lower lip also becomes more active and is drawn in to prevent escape of food. This makes the mother's task in feeding the child considerably easier. Swallowing takes place with the gum pads widely separated.

Mastication

This complex pattern of activity is used to move food about the mouth, to break it up and insalivate it preparatory to swallowing. Premasticatory movements of the mandible can be seen before the eruption of teeth. These are at first mainly vertical but protrusive movements occur with the eruption of deciduous canines and lateral movements follow, becoming more purposeful with the eruption of the deciduous molars. The infant pattern of chewing becomes well defined by the end of the first year. By 18 months the child is able to enjoy meat and tougher foods, and lateral excursions of the jaw are more marked. Chewing is a complicated process that requires effortful attention. The 2-year-old child chews more automatically, and by 3 years the pattern is comparatively mature.

There is considerable variation in mastication from one individual to another. It is modified according to: the particular occlusion of the teeth; the relationship of the jaws; and the form of the articular surfaces of the temporomandibular joint. Mastication requires practice, but is probably built up on an underlying innate coordinating pattern, which once established does not require concentrated attention (Ahlgren, 1976).

Swallowing

In the infant the peristaltic type of action during suckling produces a stream of milk which passes down lateral channels on either side of the larynx and is prevented from entering it by a flap valve mechanism operating between the soft palate and dorsum of the tongue. The high position of the epiglottis behind the soft palate may enable suckling to occur without cessation of breathing. However, some authorities have described a discrete swallow with nasopharyngeal closure after two or three suckling movements.

Swallowing in the weaned infant does not follow the same pattern as in the older child or adult. Teeth are not yet present or are just erupting and the gum pads are widely separated. Food is scooped directly on to the dorsum of the tongue. The tip has developed and this facilitates the movement of food about the mouth. As food is passed back into the oropharynx, the gum pads do not come together and the lips and cheeks contract to meet the spread tongue.

As deciduous teeth erupt and the alveolar processes develop, the mouth becomes divided into the vestibule and the oral cavity proper. Alveolar bone and teeth now form the anterior and lateral rigid boundaries to the oral cavity when the teeth are occluded. Occlusion of the teeth during swallowing becomes more frequent and the lips usually play a progressively less important part in the swallowing of masticated food and saliva.

Swallowing action can be divided into three phases (Whillis, 1946; Ardran and Kemp, 1954). First, the intraoral mechanism by which the food is transferred from the anterior to the posterior part of the mouth; secondly, the passage of food through the isthmus of the fauces into the oropharynx; and thirdly, the movement of food down the oesophagus. The intraoral phase of swallowing is of particular interest to the orthodontist and differs in detail according to the type of food and the state in which it is swallowed. The term 'basic swallow' refers to the swallowing of saliva, an activity that occurs at frequent intervals through the day and night (Rix, 1946; Lear, Flanagan and Moorrees, 1963).

The intraoral phase of swallowing may be divided into two stages: the first is the action that moves the substance to be swallowed posteriorly and the second or 'mylohyoid phase' transfers the food into the oropharynx. Fluids taken into the mouth are swept on to the dorsum of the tongue and held in a groove formed by the eversion of the lateral margins and depression of the centre. This trough is obliterated from before backwards by progressive contraction of the transverse muscle fibres and the fluid is thus moved into the swallow-preparatory position on the posterior aspect of the dorsum of the tongue. For the 'mylohyoid phase' or second stage of the swallowing the teeth are normally occluded to fix the mandible, allowing a firm base for the contraction of the mylohyoid muscles elevating the floor of the mouth. The tongue is compressed against the palate and the lateral and anterior rigid walls of the cavity formed by the teeth and alveolar processes.

Semisolid food is usually insalivated to a paste and so rarely is there a true bolus. This paste is collected on the dorsum of the tongue and massaged against the palate.

During sipping from a cup, the teeth are not occluded and the tongue acts as a simple conveyor belt in the floor of the mouth; fluid is sucked on to the tongue by the creation of an intraoral negative pressure.

The teeth are not firmly occluded when swallowing soft and succulent foods. The pattern of swallowing here is similar to that used by the infant: the lips and cheeks contract to resist the spread of the tongue and the swallow is more in the nature of a gulp. Although swallowing is usually accompanied by firm occlusion of the teeth, there are wide variations.

Atypical swallowing patterns

Various atypical swallowing actions have been described and related to different forms of malocclusion (Rix, 1948; Rogers, 1961; Cleall, 1964). It was thought that the 'tooth-apart swallow', where lip activity is increased, was a factor restricting the development of the dental arches during growth. This view is no longer tenable because it is the interplay of the lingual, labial and buccal tissues, both in form and in resting posture, that dictates the arch perimeter.

Two principal atypical swallowing patterns are of clinical importance – adaptive and endogenous. Adaptive patterns of swallowing are particularly common where the lips are incompetent and there is a Class II, division 1 incisor relationship. The anterior oral seal is formed by contact between the lower lip or the tongue and the palatal mucosa. Swallowing takes place with the teeth parted and if the tongue habitually lies over the lower incisor edges, the overbite will be incomplete, but only to a small extent. In some cases with a Class II, division 1 incisor relationship the mandible is postured forwards to enable a lip seal to be obtained, and again swallowing will take place with the teeth parted.

Other adaptations of swallowing behaviour are found when there is an incomplete overbite or anterior open bite due, for example, to a digit-sucking habit or to skeletal factors. The tongue will generally ooze forwards to fill the gap and may contribute to the anterior oral seal. These many variations of swallowing behaviour are interesting and should be noted during orthodontic case assessment, but in general they do not impose limitations on the treatment of the malocclusion.

Endogenous atypical swallowing behaviour is an unusual condition associated with a rather forcible primary tongue thrust. This is not a habit activity and cannot be modified effectively. The thrusting of the tongue results in upper incisor proclination and a substantially incomplete overbite. Recognition of a true primary tongue thrust is important because overjet reduction will relapse under its influence. There are a few definite guidelines but the tongue seems to be particularly active in speech; circumoral contraction during swallowing is greater than would be expected from the degree of lip incompetence; and the overbite is incomplete to a substantial extent, usually without any other obvious explanation such as digit-sucking or a large lower facial height.

Speech

The first sounds made at birth are those of a 'baby cry'. At 1 month, throaty noises are produced and by 2–3 months, vowel sounds start to be used in conversations that have many of the rhythms and pacing of normal speech. Between 6 and 7 months of age, babies of different language groups start to show distinguishable differences in sound usage. Syllables with plosive consonants preceding vowels are made, coincident with increased lip play in feeding. These are soon put together to give the typical 'dada', 'baba', etc. Although these sounds bring delight to fond parents, they have no meaning. By repetition and by copying parents and older children, sounds begin to take on a meaning. By 1 year the infant may use several simple words and understand many more. Similarly, articulation may precede understanding by 'parroting' of words or phrases. At between 15 months and 2 years a child has his or her own jargon, and by 2 years most children can put several words together. They talk incessantly and are quick to imitate.

Speech may be an acquired skill, but is none the less built up on underlying coordinating patterns of motor activity. It is a complicated process involving the production of basic notes in the larynx, known as 'phonation', and modification of these by changing the shape of the cavities in the mouth, nose and throat, which is known as 'articulation'. Although there are classic descriptions of the position of the tongue and other articulating elements in various speech sounds, there is considerable individual variation, particularly when taking into consideration the variations in the shape and size of the oral cavity. The different ways in which sounds are put together in connected speech determine the articulatory movements.

Speech, being an acquired behaviour, is susceptible to the influence of bad habits. For normal speech it is important to have normal receptor mechanisms (good hearing), normal central connections and normal effector mechanisms. The special case of cleft palate is one problem that comes within the sphere of influence of the orthondontist (see Chapter 20).

Some children have a degree of tongue-tie that is not a problem in the development of speech. Most paediatricians recommend that this should be ignored, except when the ability to cleanse the mouth naturally is markedly impaired. It has been shown that a malocclusion is rarely the primary cause of a speech defect and conversely that speech defects are rarely the cause of a malocclusion. From the practical viewpoint an interdental lisp will disappear if it is merely an immature behaviour associated with a transient sucking habit (Hopkin and McEwen, 1955; Subtelny and Subtelny, 1962; Fawcus, 1966; Vig, 1973).

Some children appear to have a tongue that is less agile in performing the delicate movements required for certain speech sounds, of which the 'S' sound is one of the more precise. Children with difficulties in coordinating speech may also have difficulties in coordinating other body movements.

An extensive investigation has been carried out into the association between occlusal variation and anomalies of speech in Finnish children (Laine, Jaroma and Linnasalo, 1985; Laine, 1986; 1987). Although a number of relationships of this sort exist, the correlations are weak and orthodontic tooth movement is not likely to have any noticeable effect on speech, for better or for worse.

Facial expression

It has already been pointed out that in the newborn infant the facial musculature, particularly that of the middle third of the face, is rather flaccid; the lips may be just resting together or slightly parted and the upper lip is everted. Lip posture at this time does not relate closely to the future situation as the child grows and develops. Quite early on, expressive movements become meaningful and the face becomes more animated. Facial expression depends to some extent on the shape and configuration of the soft tissues.

The muscles of facial expression, varying as they do in anatomical configuration, also relate to the underlying bony structure. For example, where there is a retrusive mandible there may be a rather taut lower lip musculature, so that in expressive behaviour this may be drawn up in the form of a tight sling under the upper incisors (Fig. 2.6). Such activity may make for considerable difficulty in correcting the overjet.

Mandibular positions and paths of closure

When the mandible is habitually postured forwards there may be an upwards and backwards path of closure into centric occlusion, rather than simple hinge closure. This is a mandibular deviation. It is important to distinguish mandibular deviations from displacements, because the former are not associated with muscle or joint pain, whereas the latter may be.

Mandibular displacements are caused by premature contacts of the teeth that enforce a shift of the mandible to obtain a position of maximum occlusion. With a lateral displacement such as is produced by a unilateral crossbite (see Fig. 10.15), the position of maximal

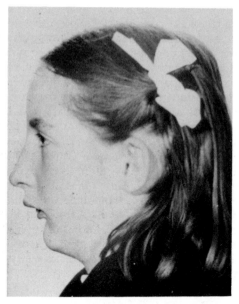

Figure 2.6 The very tight lower lip with a sling-like action under the upper incisors makes orthodontic correction of the associated Class II, division 1 incisor relationship problematic.

intercuspation is not one of centric relation. An anterior displacement may be caused by one or more instanding upper incisors. When all the incisors are instanding, the displacement is often associated with overclosure of the mandible, because the control of muscular contraction is disturbed and the occlusion is established with an overclosed position of the mandible. Posterior mandibular displacements are quite rare in an unmutilated dentition but can be found in Class II, division 2 cases where posterior teeth have been lost.

Mandibular displacements are associated with quite severe disruption of the pattern of activity of the muscles of mastication, which will often lead to pain and dysfunction in the long term. Treatment to eliminate the displacement is important.

Occlusal function

The occlusion of the teeth, the temporomandibular joints and the muscles of mastication should function harmoniously during mandibular movements. At rest, the mandible should be in a position of centric relation with the condyles in maximally retruded, unstrained positions within the glenoid fossae. Closure from rest to occlusion should be a hinge movement. There is often a slight anterior shift of up to 1 mm between the terminal hinge position and centric occlusion, and this is perfectly acceptable. A larger anterior shift or a lateral movement due to cuspal guidance is a displacement that may lead to muscular disharmony and tenderness.

When the mandible is protruded, with the teeth held lightly in occlusion, it moves downwards anteriorly as a result of incisal guidance and posteriorly as a result of condylar guidance, and this should result in disclusion of the cheek teeth. An incisor malrelationship may mean that this does not happen smoothly. For example, with a Class III incisor relationship or an anterior open bite, incisal guidance is lacking; and with a Class II incisor relationship, incisal guidance may be abrupt. In lateral excursions of the mandible, the condyle on the working side rotates and moves laterally by up to 1 mm – the Bennett movement. The non-working side condyle moves forwards and downwards on the articular eminence. On the working side, there should be either canine guidance or group function (see Fig. 1.3) of the occlusion. In an occlusion with canine guidance, all teeth except the canines are out of occlusion in lateral excursion. In an occlusion with group function, all or most of the teeth on the working side are in contact during lateral excursions (the buccal cusps of the lower teeth slide down the palatal surfaces of the buccal cusps of the upper teeth until a cusp-to-cusp relationship is obtained; the lingual cusps do not usually contact). Both canine guidance and group function are perfectly satisfactory. In some occlusions, for example with a Class II, division 2 incisor relationship, where the overbite is very deep, lateral excursions are very limited, owing to incisor locking. These patients chew with a chopping movement of the mandible and with little lateral excursion, but this does not seem to be a problem for the patient. The teeth on the non-working side should not contact in lateral excursion. Non-working side contacts create appreciable occlusal disturbances and may be associated with muscle and joint problems.

For the orthodontist, these simple guidelines will generally suffice for the evaluation of occlusal function before and after treatment. Wear facets or the use of articulating paper can reveal premature or non-working side contacts. Where orthodontic treatment is undertaken in conjunction with occlusal rehabilitation in an adult, a more detailed analysis of occlusal function may be necessary, with the help of models mounted on an adjustable articulator.

It should be remembered that some rebound often follows orthodontic treatment and that long-term minor occlusal changes occur for as long as facial growth continues, even when this is very slight as in middle age (Little, Reidel and Årtun, 1988). Orthodontic treatment must be planned to produce an occlusion that will settle well and will be stable. Occlusal objectives may vary with different treatment approaches. With edgewise appliances, for example, rather precise tooth positioning with little need for settling is the objective.

Many practitioners using the Begg technique deliberately overtreat arch malrelationships and deep overbites to allow for rebound and settling (Fletcher, 1981). Provided that this has been well judged, the tooth contacts will guide the settling so that an excellent occlusion results, just as happens in a developing normal occlusion where tooth contacts guide the erupting teeth.

References

Ahlgren, J. (1976) Masticatory movements in man. In *Mastication*, Wright, Bristol, pp. 119–130

Ardran, G. M. and Kemp, F. H. (1954) A radiographic study of movement of the tongue in swallowing. *Dental Practitioner*, **5**, 252–261

Ardran, G. M. and Lind, J. (1958) A cine-radiographic study of breast-feeding. *British Journal of Radiology*, **31**, 156–162

Ballard, C. F. (1955) Consideration of the physiological background of mandibular posture and movement. *Dental Practitioner*, **6**, 80–83

Ballard, C. F. (1962) The clinical significance of innate and adaptive postures and motor behaviour. *Dental Practitioner*, **12**, 219–228

Cleall, J. F. (1964) Deglutition – a study of form and function. DDS Thesis, University of New Zealand

Fawcus, R. (1966) An investigation into lingual sensory motor skills in children and adults with normal speech. *Dental Practitioner*, **17**, 70

Fletcher, G. G. T. (1981) *The Begg Appliance and Technique*, Wright, Bristol, p. 156

Gwynne-Evans, E. (1951) Organisation of the orofacial muscles in relation to breathing and feeding. *British Dental Journal*, **91**, 135–142

Harvold, E., Chierici, G. and Vargervik, K. (1972) Experiments on the development of dental malocclusions. *American Journal of Orthodontics*, **63**, 38–44

Hopkin, G. B. and McEwen, J. (1955) Speech defects and malocclusion: a palatographic investigation. *Dental Practitioner*, **6**, 123–131

Laine, T. (1986) Articulatory disorders in speech as related to size of the alveolar arches. *European Journal of Orthodontics*, **8**, 192–197

Laine, T. (1987) Associations between articulatory disorders in speech and occlusal anomalies. *European Journal of Orthodontics*, **9**, 144–150

Laine, T., Jaroma, M. and Linnasalo, A-L. (1985) Articulatory disorders in speech as related to the position of the incisors. *European Journal of Orthodontics*, **7**, 260–266

Larsson, E. (1985) The prevalence and aetiology of prolonged dummy and finger sucking habits. *European Journal of Orthodontics*, **7**, 172–176

Larsson, E. (1986) The effect of dummy sucking on the occlusion – a review. *European Journal of Orthodontics*, **8**, 127–130

Larsson, E. (1987) The effect of finger sucking on the occlusion – a review. *European Journal of Orthodontics*, **9**, 279–282

Lear, C. S. C., Flanagan, J. B. and Moorrees, C. F. A. (1963) The frequency of deglutition in man. *Archives of Oral Biology*, **10**, 83–99

Linder-Aronson, S. (1970) Effects of adenoidectomy on the dentition and facial skeleton over a five year period. In *Transactions of the Third International Orthodontic Congress* (ed. J. T. Cook) C. V. Mosby, St. Louis

Little, R. M., Reidel, R. A. and Årtun, J. (1988) An evaluation of changes in mandibular anterior alignment from 10 to 20 years post retention. *American Journal of Orthodontics and Dentofacial Orthopedics*, **93**, 423–428

Rix, R. E. (1946) Deglutition and the teeth. *Dental Record*. **66**, 105–108

Rix, R. E. (1948) Deglutition. *Transactions of the European Orthodontic Society*, 191–202

Rogers, J. H. (1961) Swallowing patterns of a normal population sample compared to those of patients from an orthodontic practice. *Journal of Orthodontics*, **47**, 674–689

Subtelny, J. G. and Subtelny, J. (1962) Malocclusion, speech and deglutition. *American Journal of Orthodontics*, **48**, 685–697

Thompson, J. R. and Brodie, A. G. (1946) The rest position of the mandible and its significance to dental science. *Journal of the American Dental Association*, **33**, 151–180

Vig, P. S. (1973) Evolutionary concepts relating to language and the morphology of the oral complex. *Transactions of the European Orthodontic Society*, 527–533

Vig, P. S., Showfety, K. J. and Phillips, C. (1980) Experimental manipulation of head posture. *American Journal of Orthodontics*, **77**, 258–268

Whillis, J. W. (1946) Movements of the tongue in deglutition *Transactions of the British Society for the Study of Orthodontics*, 121–129

Additional reading

Dubner, R., Sessle, B. J. and Storey, A. T. (1978) *The Neural Basis of Oral and Facial Function*, Plenum Press, New York

Lowe, A. A. and Sessle, B. J. (1973) Tongue activity during respiration, jaw opening and swallowing in the cat. *Canadian Journal of Physiology and Pharmacology*, **51**, 1009–1011

Luffingham, J. K. (1966) Intraoral pressures. PhD Thesis, University of London

Moss, J. P. (1980) The soft tissue environment of teeth and jaws. An experimental and clinical study: Parts 2 and 3. *British Journal of Orthodontics*, **7**, 205–216

Peat, J. H. (1968) A cephalometric study of tongue position. *American Journal of Orthodontics*, **54**, 339–351

Sims, F. W. (1958) The pressure exerted on the maxillary and mandibular central incisors by the perioral and lingual musculature in acceptable occlusion. *American Journal of Orthodontics*, **44**, 64–65

Tulley, W. J. (1964) The tongue, that unruly member. *Dental Practitioner*, **15**, 27–38

Chapter 3

Development of the occlusion

Since the beginning of this century, many studies have been made of the developing occlusion by the painstaking collection of serial models (Chapman, 1935; Friel, 1954). Some have concentrated on describing the ideal development of the occlusion, while others have also described what were perceived as acceptable variations (Sillman, 1951; Clinch, 1954; Moorrees, 1959; Leighton, 1968; 1969; 1971; Foster and Hamilton, 1969; Foster, Hamilton and Lavelle, 1969). Few adults achieve a dentition that approaches the ideal, with 32 teeth in good alignment. One study (Tulley, 1962) revealed that less than 10 per cent of a group of adults had a full complement of teeth without third molar impactions or late incisor crowding and only 5 per cent had anything approaching an ideal occlusion. Another, which defined ideal occlusion more strictly, found that only 2.3 per cent of 12-year-old Cardiff schoolgirls had 'anatomically correct occlusions' (Harkness, 1969).

The dental practitioner must have an understanding of the normal milestones in the development of the occlusion and the wide range of variation that is still functionally and aesthetically acceptable. This understanding must include an appreciation of the wide variation in the sequence and timing of eruption in the deciduous and permanent dentitions. Such knowledge will enable an appreciation of where there is a deviation from the normal that is likely to require treatment.

Postnatal development of the jaws

The neonate is without teeth for approximately the first 6 months of life (Fig. 3.1) and the gum pads in which teeth are developing are covered with dense fibrous periosteum and are divided into segmented elevations (Fig. 3.2). The segments relating to the second deciduous molars are not well defined until 5 months of age. The upper gum pad is horseshoe-shaped and the lower is U-shaped and somewhat flattened anteriorly. There is a well-defined groove distal to the crypts of the deciduous canines in both arches, which is known as the 'lateral sulcus' (Fig. 3.2). The arch of the upper gum pad is both wider and longer than that of the lower and the palatal vault is almost flat. The alveolar process is separated on the palatal side by a horizontal groove known as the

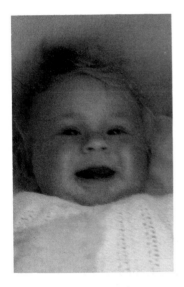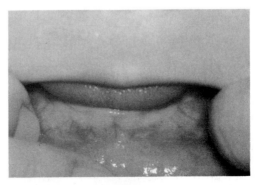

Figure 3.1 An infant of 3 months showing the gum pads.

'dental' or 'gingival groove', and the labial crest of the lower gum pad is slightly everted.

The gum pads are not brought together in function as the mouth at this stage is designed for suckle feeding. Although attempts have been made to define a true relationship between the upper and lower gum pads, any position of contact is artificial and difficult to record with accuracy. It has been shown that, despite considerable variation in the anteroposterior relationship of the gum pads, a normal occlusion may still develop. At birth the lower gum pad lies distal to the upper to a variable degree. This position is judged by the relationship of the lateral sulci (Fig. 3.2).

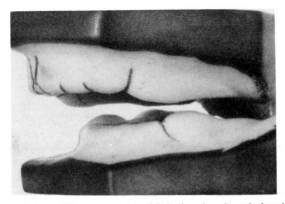

Figure 3.2 Lateral view of the gum pads at birth showing the relationship of the lateral sulci.

At this stage the tongue is blunt and quite large relative to the size of the jaws and it rests between the gum pads in contact with the lower lip, which forms the principal boundary to the anterior part of the oral cavity. The fraenum of the upper lip is attached to the crest of the gum pad and there is fibrous continuity with the incisive papilla in the palate.

Development of the deciduous dentition

An occlusal radiograph of the gum pads at birth shows there to be some crowding of the upper and lower deciduous teeth in their crypts (Fig. 3.3). This does not necessarily indicate that they will be crowded when they erupt.

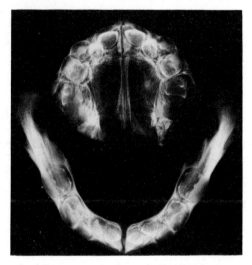

Figure 3.3 Radiograph of the gum pads shown in Fig. 3.2 demonstrating positions of the unerupted teeth in their crypts.

During the first year, the gum pads enlarge and the arches widen slightly to accommodate all the teeth. There is some adjustment in jaw relationship. The lower gum pad is only slightly distal to the upper by the time the deciduous incisors erupt.

The timing of tooth eruption is very variable but there appear to be no significant differences between the sexes in the primary dentition. Incisor eruption (Table 3.1) may begin at any time within the first year and parents often need to be reassured about this variation as they may have been told that teeth should start to appear by 6 months. Usually the lower central incisors erupt first, followed shortly by the upper central incisors. All the deciduous incisors are smaller, whiter and more upright than their successors and at first the overbite tends to be rather deep. This is not an indicator of the eventual overbite as it will reduce

Table 3.1 Typical ages of eruption and mesiodistal widths of the deciduous teeth

	Time of eruption (month)	Mesiodistal width (mm)
Maxillary teeth		
Central incisor	8	6.5
Lateral incisor	9	5.0
Canine	18	6.5
First molar	14	7.0
Second molar	24	8.5
Mandibular teeth		
Central incisor	6	4.0
Lateral incisor	7	4.5
Canine	16	5.5
First molar	12	8.0
Second molar	20	9.5

Eruption times vary considerably. Up to 6 months earlier or later than the times given is not unusual.
Mesiodistal widths vary by up to 20 per cent on either side of the figures given.
Calcification of the deciduous teeth begins between 4 and 6 months *in utero*.
Root formation is complete between 12 and 18 months after eruption.

over the next 3–4 years. In some instances the incisors erupt with spaces and these tend to close.

The first deciduous molars are the next teeth to erupt, at between 1 year and 18 months, followed by the deciduous canines and finally the second deciduous molars (Fig. 3.4). There is often space distal to the lower canine and mesial to the upper canine. This may be referred to as the 'primate space', after an equivalent space found in the primate dentition.

Completion of the deciduous dentition

In the past great emphasis was placed on describing the features of the 'ideal deciduous dentition' in terms of its good incisor occlusion, the presence of spacing between the incisor teeth and the 'end-to-end' relationship of the deciduous second molars. In the late 1960s, however, research by Foster and Hamilton (1969) revealed that there was little point in such assessments. Out of 100 2½ to 3-year-olds they examined, not one showed all these features. To take just one aspect as an example, increased overjet was present in 72 per cent of the children.

The deciduous dentition is rarely complete before the age of 3 years. At this time the incisors will usually show a greater or lesser degree of spacing. The overbite will virtually never be traumatic but almost all other vertical relationships are seen, many reflecting the presence of a more or less persistent digit habit. About half the 3-year-olds will have an anteroposterior relationship of the arches as shown in Fig. 3.4, with the distal edges of the upper and lower second deciduous molars flush;

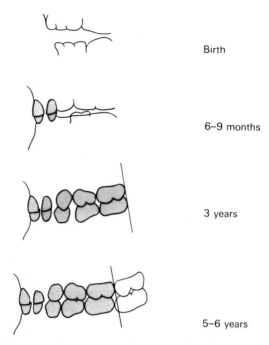

Birth

6–9 months

3 years

5–6 years

Figure 3.4 Development of the detention from birth to 6 years.

but about a quarter will show a more postnormal relationship. These common variations do not necessarily give any indication as to the occlusion that will be seen in the permanent dentition, for which reason intervention is never indicated at this stage in development.

There is some doubt as to whether there is any appreciable lateral or anteroposterior increase in arch size during the next 3 years but there is a definite change in the anteroposterior arch relationship. It is not clear whether this is due to the lower teeth moving forwards in relation to the upper teeth, or an actual change in jaw relationship. It is said that attrition of the deciduous teeth is necessary to allow this occlusal change. By the time the first permanent molars are due to erupt the distal edges of the second deciduous molars may no longer be flush in the vertical plane (Fig. 3.4) because of the change in arch relationships or because the lower primate space has closed.

By 5 years of age, the deciduous teeth have usually suffered some attrition and the incisors often have an edge-to-edge relationship and show varying degrees of spacing. (Fig. 3.5)

It has been found that if the primary teeth are significantly spaced by this time, there is a good chance of avoiding crowding in the permanent dentition, but this is by no means always true (Baume, 1950). In the lower arch, absence of later crowding can be assured only if the deciduous spacing is more than 6 mm (Leighton, 1971) (see Fig. 3.5).

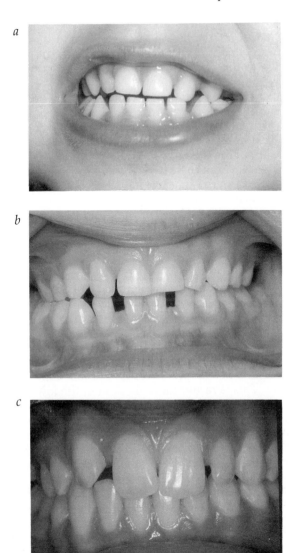

Figure 3.5 The considerable degree of spacing that is seen at the end of the mixed dentition where there is sufficient space for the lower permanent incisors to erupt without crowding: (a) at age 2 years 8 months; (b) the same child at 7 years; (c) at 16 years.

The change in the mixed dentition

Classically, the mixed dentition phase begins with the eruption of the first permanent molars at approximately 6 years of age, although in some cases it is the lower central incisors that are the first permanent teeth to erupt. The first permanent molars may be guided into a cusp-to-cusp relationship by the distal surfaces of the deciduous second molars if they are flush at this stage. If the lower arch has moved forwards relative to the upper, the permanent molars may erupt more nearly into full intercuspation (Bonnar, 1956).

The upper first permanent molars develop in the maxillary tuberosity with their occlusal surfaces facing distally and buccally as well as occlusally. Growth in maxillary length is necessary to allow them to erupt into the line of the arch. The mandibular molars develop under the anterior border of the ascending ramus of the mandible and growth in mandibular length is necessary if these teeth are to have room to erupt. Occasionally a maxillary first molar becomes impacted beneath the bulbous crowns of the second deciduous molar. Generally this will induce resorption of the distal root of the deciduous molar, which may then be lost prematurely (see Chapter 9).

The permanent incisors

The permanent incisors develop parallel to each other behind the roots of their predecessors with the lateral incisors rather more lingually positioned. They are larger than their predecessors and are accommodated by contributions from several factors. First, their predecessors will usually have been spaced to some extent. Secondly, the permanent incisors erupt into a more proclined and labial position than their precursors. Finally, there is an increase in intercanine width taking place at this time. This is rather more marked in the lower arch, and on average amounts to 2.5–3 mm. Teeth in the lower labial segment erupt before their upper counterparts. They are frequently quite rotated when they emerge but will align rapidly if space is available. Lower incisors, particularly the lateral incisors, may appear lingually and then, due to pressure from the tongue, move forwards into their correct positions as their predecessors are shed. Teeth in the upper labial segment develop on the palatal aspects of the roots of their predecessors and erupt downwards, outwards and forwards (Fig. 3.6). Here too the lateral

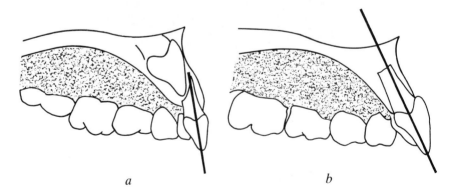

a   *b*

Figure 3.6 (a) Position of the upper permanent central incisor before eruption. (b) After eruption, the inclination of the upper central incisors may change under the influence of the lips and tongue.

incisor is more palatally placed than the central. It is important to recognize this pre-eruptive position because it explains why these teeth may be deflected from the normal path of eruption (see Chapter 9).

Except in the most crowded cases, when the upper central incisors first erupt, a midline diastema is normally present. The upper lateral incisors develop in a more palatal position than the central incisors and are overlapped by them, but become free to move labially as the central incisors erupt. Their apices always remain slightly more palatal than those of the central incisors. In particularly crowded cases, the lateral incisors may become trapped in anterior crossbite as they erupt.

It is at this time that parents may become concerned at the dental appearance of their child because, in addition to the midline diastema, the crowns of the upper lateral incisors have a slight distal inclination (Fig. 3.7). This arrangement was described by Broadbent as the 'ugly duckling' stage of dental development and should not be mistaken for a malocclusion. Treatment is not indicated for the diastema, which will gradually close as the upper lateral incisors and canines erupt (Fig. 3.8). The distal inclination of the lateral incisors reflects the fact that the developing permanent canines are high and closely associated with the roots of the lateral incisors at this time. As development proceeds, the canines move buccally and should be palpable high in the buccal sulcus, and the lateral incisors become more upright. The upper labial fraenum should no longer be attached to the crest of the alveolar process but to

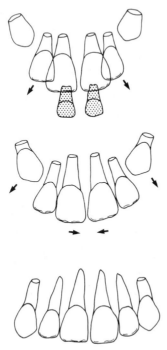

Figure 3.7 The pattern of eruption on the upper incisors in an uncrowded arch showing the change in inclination of the teeth and the closure of the midline ('physiological') diastema.

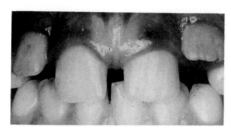 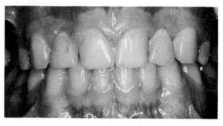

a   *b*

Figure 3.8 (a) A marked example of the 'ugly duckling' stage at 7½ years of age. (b) By 12 years of age the upper permanent canines have erupted and the incisor spacing has closed naturally.

its labial surface, quite clear of the incisors. If a low attachment persists it may cause interference with space closure (see Chapter 9).

In the absence of any digit-sucking habit, the overbite is little more than one-third the length of the crowns of the lower central incisors, but over the next few years it tends to reduce.

At this stage there are a number of common variations. The size of the diastema and the degree of distal tilt of the lateral incisors both vary considerably. The overbite may be reduced or incomplete, particularly if there is a residual digit-sucking habit. If a diastema is not present and the lateral incisors are slightly palatally displaced, this is a strong indication that crowding may remain and may even get worse with the eruption of the permanent canines.

The buccal teeth

The replacement of deciduous teeth by their successors in the buccal segments may begin as early as 7 years of age and is not always complete by the age of 12 (Table 3.2). There is a discrepancy in the total space occupied by the deciduous cheek teeth compared with that required for their successors. Although the permanent canines are wider than their predecessors, particularly in the upper arch, premolars are narrower than deciduous molars. Thus the combined mesiodistal width of the permanent canines and premolars is usually less than that of the deciduous canines and molars. The surplus space, or 'leeway space' as it is called, is greater in the lower jaw than in the upper (Fig. 3.9). This means that when all deciduous teeth have been replaced the upper first permanent molar will have drifted forwards to a lesser extent than the lower first molar. The normal cuspal relationship may not be established until this time (Angle, 1898). Surprisingly the direction of growth rotation does not appear to affect molar occlusion in a predictable way during this period (Brin *et al.*, 1982).

The sequence of eruption is variable. In the lower buccal segment the first tooth to erupt is either the lower first premolar or the lower canine. The lower second premolar sometimes erupts after the second permanent molar.

In the upper buccal segment the first premolar usually erupts first,

Table 3.2 Typical ages of eruption and mesiodistal widths of the permanent teeth

	Time of eruption (yr)	Mesiodistal width (mm)
Maxillary teeth		
Central incisor	7.5	8.5
Lateral incisor	8.5	6.5
Canine	11.5	8.0
First premolar	10.0	7.0
Second premolar	11.0	6.5
First molar	6.0	10.0
Second molar	12.0	9.5
Mandibular teeth		
Central incisor	6.5	5.5
Lateral incisor	7.5	6.0
Canine	10.5	7.0
First premolar	10.5	7.0
Second premolar	11.0	7.0
First molar	6.0	11.0
Second molar	12.0	10.5

The figures given both for eruption times and for mesiodistal widths commonly vary by up to 20 per cent on either side of the figures given. Calcification dates are variable but the permanent teeth have usually started to calcify as follows:

At birth $\frac{6}{6}$ by 6 months $\frac{1\ 3}{1\ 2\ 3}$ Between 8 and 14 years $\frac{8}{8}$

by 2 year $\frac{2\ 4}{4}$ by 4 years $\frac{5\ 7}{5\ 7}$

Root formation is normally completed 2–3 years after eruption.

followed by the canine. This tooth has a long path of eruption from its developmental position and this is one of the factors contributing to its frequently aberrant position. This is particularly likely to occur when the lateral incisor is unusually small or absent and this should always be checked for (see Chapter 9).

The canine erupts into a wider arc in the same way as the upper incisors and any remaining space between the upper central incisors should close at this time. The usual sequence of eruption of permanent teeth in the buccal segment is particularly significant if extractions for the relief of crowding are contemplated. The emergence of the upper first premolar well before the canine usually allows the premolar tooth to be extracted in good time to permit spontaneous alignment of the canine. The upper second premolar erupts a little before its lower counterpart.

In the lower arch, similar plans for the extraction of the first premolar may be frustrated if the canine erupts first. In such a case, spontaneous alignment of the canine following the later loss of the first premolar will usually be less favourable.

Planned extraction of the second premolar is usually accompanied by the use of a fixed appliance to align the teeth. This is because loss of this tooth is accompanied by unfavourable tipping of the first molar and first premolar unless this is avoided by the use of an appliance. The fact

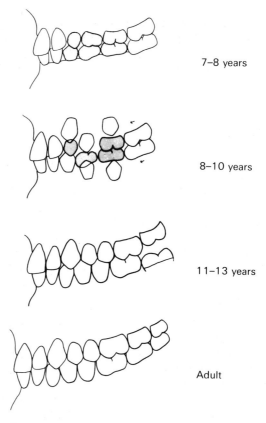

7–8 years

8–10 years

11–13 years

Adult

Figure 3.9 Changes from the mixed to the permanent dentition between 7 and 18 years of age.

that it is the last tooth of the series to erupt dictates a later start to active treatment.

To complete the full adult dentition the second molars erupt between 12 and 14 years, followed by the third molars whose eruption dates are usually quoted as being between 16 and 20 years. However, many are impacted and fail to erupt. These molars follow a similar path of eruption to that described for the first permanent molars. In the full dentition the upper buccal segments are tilted slightly outwards and the lower buccal segments tilted slightly lingually. The occlusal plane has a distinct upward curve (curve of Spee). The mandibular teeth are set one inclined plane in advance of the maxillary teeth because the mandibular incisors are smaller mesiodistally than the maxillary incisors (Fig. 3.9).

The maxillary teeth are half a cusp to the buccal of the mandibular teeth (i.e. they are not cusp-to-cusp) and the mesiobuccal cusp of the upper first permanent molar occludes with the anterior buccal groove of the lower first permanent molar (see Fig. 1.4).

A more reliable indicator of a normal arch relationship is that the upper permanent canine occludes in the embrasure between the lower permanent canine and first premolar. The lower incisors should occlude with the cingulum plateau of the upper incisors so that the overbite is about a third of the height of the lower incisor crowns and the overjet is approximately 2 mm.

Late changes in the permanent dentition

Three aspects of this later stage of development should be noted. First, there may be an increase in incisor crowding, particularly in the lower arch; secondly, there is usually an increase in the interincisal angle; and thirdly, there may be a slight increase in mandibular prognathism (Björk, 1951; Lande, 1952). The increase in incisor crowding is not found in every case, but a dentition that shows a slight slipping of the contact points of upper and lower incisors, at the time of eruption of the second molars, is likely to show an increase in crowding by 18–20 years of age.

Many factors may contribute to late incisor crowding. These include the tendency for prognathism to increase at this time as well as the effects of mandibular growth rotation described in Chapter 4, and soft tissue influences, all of which conspire to reduce the perimeter of the lower arch (Brodie, 1940; Tulley, 1957).

Another major factor contributing to incisor crowding could be continuing mesial drift of buccal teeth (Richardson, 1979). The cause of mesial drift is not fully understood, but the process appears to continue throughout life. Mesial migration of posterior teeth was much greater in primitive man where there was marked attritional wear (Begg, 1954) but is also seen in relatively modern populations where there is marked occlusal wear (Lysell, 1958). The process of mesial migration is almost certainly multifactorial and it seems likely that the same mechanisms which produce crowding in the intact unworn dentition of modern man are also responsible for the reappearance of lower incisor crowding after orthodontic treatment once any extraction space has closed.

The following have all been shown to be capable of making a contribution to mesial migration:

1 *Occlusal forces*. Due to the mesial inclination of upper and lower teeth the vertical forces of occlusion produce an anterior component of force (Osborn, 1961; Picton, 1962).

2 *Eruption of posterior teeth*. Posterior teeth have a mesial component of force as they erupt in monkeys (van Beek, 1979). The first and second molars move mesially as the shedding of the second deciduous molar allows this to occur. Whether the third molar makes a contribution to mesial migration by attempting to erupt against an intact arch is doubtful (Southard et al., 1991). In any case, late incisor crowding can still occur where third molars are missing (Bishara and Andreasen, 1983).

3 *Transseptal fibre contraction* (Picton and Moss, 1973). This mechanism may have been responsible for maintaining the integrity of contact points in the dentition of primitive man where there was marked

approximal wear but it is probably of little significance in the completed dentition of modern man.

4 *Continued vertical development of teeth.* Lower posterior teeth have a mesial inclination and therefore tend to shorten the arch as they erupt unless the anterior teeth are similarly inclined. Where these converge with the axes of the lower incisors, greater degrees of arch shortening are found, at least during the developing dentition (Sannin and Savara, 1972). As the lower face height continues to increase slowly throughout life (Tallgren, 1957; Forsberg, 1979), it is possible that this mechanism continues to make a contribution.

References

Angle, E. H. (1898) *Malocclusion of the Teeth*, S. S. White Dental Manufacturing Co., Philadelphia

Baume, L. J. (1950) Physiological tooth migration and its significance for the development of occlusion. *Journal of Dental Research*, **29**, 123

Begg, P. R. (1954) Stone-age man's dentition. *American Journal of Orthodontics*, **40**, 298–312

Bishara, S. E. and Andreasen, G. (1983) Third molars: a review. *American Journal of Orthodontics*, **83**, 131–137

Björk, A. (1951) Discussion on the significance of growth changes in facial pattern and their relationship to changes in occlusion. *Dental Record*, **71**, 197

Bonnar, M. E. (1956) Aspects of the transition from deciduous to permanent dentition. *Dental Practitioner*, **7**, 42

Brin, I., Kelley, M. B., Ackerman, J. and Green, P. A. (1982) Molar occlusion and mandibular rotation. *American Journal of Orthodontics*, **81**, 397–403

Brodie, A. G. (1940) Some recent observations on the growth of the face and their implications to the orthodontist. *American Journal of Orthodontics*, **26**, 471

Chapman, H. (1935) The normal dental arch and its changes from birth to adult. *British Dental Journal*, **58**, 201

Clinch, L. M. (1954) Analysis of serial models between three and eight years of age. *Dental Practitioner*, **71**, 61–72

Forsberg, C. M. (1979) Facial morphology and ageing: a longitudinal cephalometric investigation of young adults. *European Journal of Orthodontics*, **1**, 15–23

Foster, T. D. and Hamilton, M. C. (1969) Occlusion in the primary dentition. *British Dental Journal*, **126**, 76–79

Foster, T. D., Hamilton, M. C. and Lavelle, C. L. B. (1969) Dentition and dental arch dimensions in British children at the age of 2 to 3 years. *Archives of Oral Biology*, **14**, 1031–1040

Friel, S. (1954) The development of ideal occlusions of the gum pads and the teeth. *American Journal of Orthodontics*, **40**, 196

Harkness, E. M. (1969) A survey of 12 year old Cardiff schoolgirls. *Dental Practitioner*, **20**, 77–83

Lande, M. J. (1952) Growth behaviour of the human bony facial profile as revealed by serial cephalometric roentgenology. *Angle Orthodontist*, **22**, 78

Leighton, B. C. (1968) Some observations on vertical development and the dentition. *Proceedings of the Royal Society of Medicine*, **61**, 1273–1277

Leighton, B. C. (1969) The early signs of malocclusion. *Transactions of the European Orthodontic Society*, 353–368

Leighton, B. C. (1971) The value of prophecy in orthodontics. *Dental Practitioner*, **21**, 359–372

Lysell, L. (1958) Qualitative and quantitative determination of attrition and the ensuing tooth migration. *Acta Odontologica Scandinavica*, **16**, 267–292

Moorrees, C. F. A. (1959) *The Dentition of the Growing Child*, Harvard University Press, Cambridge, MA

Osborn, J. W. (1961) an investigation into the inderdental forces occurring between the teeth of the same arch during clenching the jaws. *Archives of Oral Biology*, **5**, 202–211

Picton, D. C. A. (1962) Tilting movements of teeth during biting. *Archives of Oral Biology*, **7**, 151–159

Picton, D. C. A. and Moss, J. P. (1973) The part played by the transseptal fibre system in experimental approximal drift of the cheek teeth of monkeys. *Archives of Oral Biology*, **18**, 669–680

Richardson, M. E. (1979) Late lower arch crowding: facial growth or forward drift? *European Journal of Orthodontics*, **1**, 219–255

Sannin, C. and Savara, B. S. (1972) Factors that affect the alignment of the mandibular incisors: a longitudinal study. *American Journal of Orthodontics*, **64**, 247–257

Sillman, J. H. (1951) Serial study of good occlusion from birth to twelve years. *American Journal of Orthodontics*, **37**, 481–507

Southard, T. E., Southard, K. A. and Weeda, L. W. (1991) Mesial force from unerupted third molars. *American Journal of Orthodontics and Dentofacial Orthopedics*, **99**, 220–225

Tallgren, A. (1957) Changes in adult face height due to ageing, wear and loss of teeth. *Acta Odontologica Scandinavica*, 15 (Supplement 24)

Tulley, W. J. (1957) Observations on the path of eruption of the incisors. *Transactions of the European Orthodontic Society*, 279–289

Tulley, W. J. (1962) Electromyographic study of the orofacial muscles in relation to the occlusion of the teeth and the form of the jaws. PhD Thesis, University of London

van Beek, H. (1979) The transfer of mesial drift potential along the dental arch in *Macaca irus*: an experimental study of tooth migration related to horizontal vectors of occlusal force. *European Journal of Orthodontics*, **1**, 125–129

Chapter 4

The classification of occlusion and malocclusion

Occlusal and facial patterns vary widely and in many circumstances it is convenient to categorize them into a small number of groups. The objective of any system of classification is to gather together cases with similar features or with a common aetiology. Individuals within a class should ideally resemble one another more closely in the relevant features than individuals in other classes. However, as with many biological attributes, there is a spectrum of continuous variation and the division between classes is arbitrary. This makes the designation of borderline cases difficult. Methods of classifying malocclusions and facial patterns have been developed intuitively and when modern statistical techniques are used to investigate the most efficient systems, these generally do not correspond with the time-honoured patterns, which nevertheless persist. However, the importance of classification in everyday clinical practice should not be exaggerated: the classification of a malocclusion cannot constitute an adequate description of it, nor is it the basis for the prescription of treatment.

Different methods of classification may be needed for different purposes, and an appropriate method must be adopted for the task in hand. The requirements for clinical categorization differ from those of epidemiology. Other methods of indexing are required for investigation into the relationships between dental irregularity and problems such as periodontal disease. In orthodontics, indices have described for:

1 occlusal classification (Angle, 1899; Simon, 1924; Ballard and Wayman 1964);
2 treatment need/priority –
   a aesthetic need (Banack, Cleall and Yip, 1972; Linder-Aronson, 1974; Cons 1986; Evans and Shaw 1987),
   b dental health need (Draker, 1960; Salzmann, 1968; Grainger, 1967; Summers 1971; Linder-Aronson, 1974; Brook and Shaw, 1989);
3 treatment complexity (Stephens and Harradine, 1988);
4 treatment change (Pickering and Vig, 1975; Elderton and Clark, 1983; Shaw et al., 1991);
5 for epidemiological purposes (Björk, Krebs and Solow, 1964; Baume et al., 1973).

Occlusal classifications

Angle's classification

The only internationally recognized classification of malocclusion is that of Angle, who was one of the founders of modern orthodontics. Angle divided the whole range of malocclusions into three main groups according to the anteroposterior relationship of the arches. Vertical and transverse malrelationships were not taken into account. In brief, a normal anteroposterior arch relationship is Class I (which Angle called 'neutroclusion'); a more distal than normal relationship of the lower arch to the upper is Class II ('distoclusion'); and a more mesial than normal relationship is Class III ('mesioclusion'). A more detailed description of these classes of malocclusion is given in the captions to Fig. 4.1.

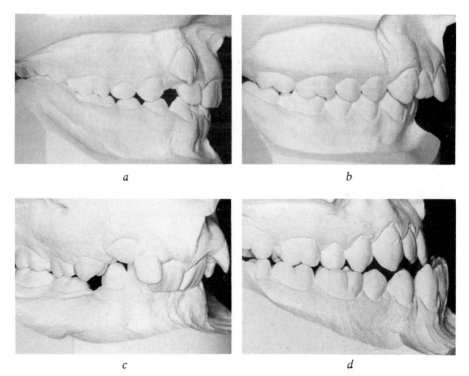

a   b

c   d

Figure 4.1 Angle's classes of malocclusion. (a) Class I: normal anteroposterior arch relationship. Angle stated that the mesiobuccal cusp of the upper first permanent molar should occlude with the anterior buccal groove of the lower first permanent molar. In Class II, Angle required the mesiobuccal cusp of the upper first molar to be at least one cusp width distal to the correct relationship, i.e. in what would today be called a 'full unit' Class II. However, nowadays this is not usually strictly adhered to and 'half a unit postnormality' is usually used. (b) In division 1 the upper incisors are of average inclination or are proclined so that the overjet is increased. (c) In division 2 the upper incisors are retroclined and the overjet is usually minimal but may be increased. (d) Class III: the lower arch lies prenormal to its correct relationship. Here again half a unit is usually taken as the determining factor rather than the full unit required by Angle.

Angle believed that the permanent molars developed in a constant relationship to the jaws and that their occlusion could be used to classify the jaw relationship. It is now recognized that this is not so and that skeletal and occlusal relationships must be assessed independently of one another.

There are difficulties in applying Angle's classification that arise because the original premise on which it is based (that the first permanent molar bears a fixed relationship to the dental arch) is untrue. To work at all, allowance is made when there has been drift of these teeth following early loss of deciduous molars, a judgement that may not be easy or reliable. In some cases where the upper first permanent molar is small, the correct relationship may be further back than described by Angle (see Fig. 1.4): the distobuccal cusp of the upper molar must occlude in the embrasure distal to the lower molar, otherwise it may not be possible to establish a correct premolar and canine relationship. Because of these problems, and obviously where first permanent molars are missing, it is important to take account of the general buccal segment occlusion, and in particular the canine relationships, before deciding on the classification.

Strictly interpreted, Angle's Class I includes anteroposterior buccal segment malrelationships of up to half a cusp width, and thus only quite severe discrepancies would be included in Class II and Class III categories. This requirement is generally relaxed, and milder arch malrelationships are included in Classes II and III (see Chapter 5 and Fig. 5.17).

Several studies have demonstrated low interexaminer agreement when using the original Angle classification (Salzmann, 1968; Jago, 1974; Gravely and Johnson, 1974). Modifications have been suggested to help to overcome this problem. For example, Gravely and Johnston proposed the inclusion of a 'Class II uncertain' category for those cases that did not fit easily into either of the two divisions proposed by Angle, but this has not been generally adopted.

Incisor classification

For general use, the incisor classification is simpler and more relevant than Angle's classification. Patients are generally more aware of incisor rather than buccal segment relationship; thus its correction is a central concern of much orthodontic treatment. Further, many of the problems associated with Angle's classification can be avoided if attention is focused on the incisor relationship.

In the incisor classification, first described by Ballard and Wayman (1964), Angle's terms are used and, in most cases, the classifications are concordant. This classification has now been widely adopted in the UK and forms the British Standards Institute's (1983) classification of malocclusion.

The incisor classification is based upon the relationship between the lower incisor edges and the cingulum plateau of the upper central incisors (Fig. 4.2). Problems can arise where the relationship differs between sides, but in these cases the classification should rest on the general features of the malocclusion.

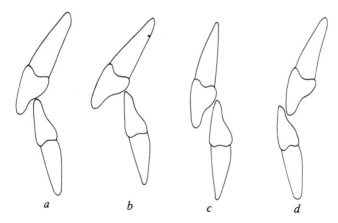

Figure 4.2 The incisor classification (see text): (a) Class I; (b) Class II, division 1; (c) Class II, division 2; (d) Class III.

Definitions

Class I. The lower incisor edges occlude with or lie immediately below the cingulum plateau of the upper central incisors (Fig. 4.2a).

Class II. The lower incisor edges lie posterior to the cingulum plateau of the upper central incisors. There are two divisions of Class II:
   division 1 – the overjet is increased and the upper central incisors are usually proclined (Fig. 4.2b);
   division 2 – the upper central incisors are retroclined; the overjet is usually minimal but may be increased (Fig. 4.2c).

Class III. The lower incisor edges lie anterior to the cingulum plateau of the upper central incisors. The overjet is reduced or reversed (Fig. 4.2d).

A recent study has shown that even with the incisor classification there could be low agreement between examiners (Williams and Stephens, 1992). Most of these disagreements arose from a failure on the part of some of the examining clinicians to appreciate that it was the cingulum plateau which formed the crucial feature of the incisor classification and that it was therefore not appropriate just to use the middle third of the visible palatal surface of the upper central incisor. Disagreement also arose where the upper incisors were upright but there was an increased overjet. Some observers classified these as Class II, division 1 whilst others identified these as Class II, division 2.
   It was found that the interexaminer reliability of incisor classification could be greatly increased by the following modifications:

a paying close attention to the palatal anatomy of the maxillary central incisor;
b introducing a Class II 'intermediate' subdivision to include those cases where the upper incisors were upright but the overjet was no more than 6 mm;

c using the Class III category only when three or more incisors were in
   Class III relationship.

Indices of malocclusion

Neither Angle's nor the incisor classification provide a measure of the
severity of a malocclusion. Thus different methods are required for
estimating the prevalence of malocclusion in a population, for deciding
on treatment priority where services are limited, and for investigating
the relationships between malocclusion and various aspects of dental
health, and health care provision.

Requirements of an index

The World Health Organization (1977) has proposed requirements for
an ideal index, and of these the most important are that it should:

a be reliable;
b be valid;
c be acceptable to the professionals and public;
d require a minimum of judgement to apply it successfully;
e be administratively simple.

Before any index is adopted, it must be thoroughly tested for its
validity (does it, in fact, measure what is required?); and reproducibility
(do observers consistently obtain the same values for a series of test
cases ?). Sadly few orthodontic indices have been exhaustively tested in
these respects.

Indices of treatment need

The aim of using such an index is to be able to rank occlusal disharmon-
ies according to their severity. The index can then be used for epidemiological purposes and to establish priorities of treatment. There are
many difficulties in devising a reliable index of malocclusion: for
example a localized irregularity such as an instanding upper incisor
may be a more serious problem than generalized mild crowding, which
will almost inevitably attract a higher score.

Two of the best established indices of malocclusion are the Handicapping Malocclusion Assessment Record (HMAR) (Salzmann, 1968), and
the Occlusal Index (OI) (Summers, 1971). Both perform reasonably well
for reproducibility and validity.

The HMAR allocates points for dental irregularities and arch malrelationships, which are multiplied by a weighting factor before the total
score is assigned. This can be done from orthodontic models. or at a
clinical assessment. In the latter case, further points can be allotted for
dentofacial deviations such as clefts of the lip and palate, facial asymmetry and functional disabilities. This assessment is quite rapid and
does not require special instruments.

The OI scores dental age, molar relations, overbite, overjet, posterior crossbite, posterior open bite, tooth displacement, midline relations and missing upper lateral incisors. A number of measurements are involved and the scoring is rather more complicated than for the HMAR, but it is a more reliable method of ranking malocclusion severity.

Table 4.1 The Index of Orthodontic Treatment Need – aesthetic components

Grade 1 (none)
1 Extremely minor malocclusions including displacements less than 1 mm.

Grade 2 (little)
a   Increased overjet greater than 3.5 mm but less than or equal to 6 mm with competent lips.
b   Reverse overjet greater than 0 mm but less than or equal to 1 mm.
c   Anterior or posterior crossbite with less than or equal to 1 mm discrepancy between retruded contact position and intercuspal position.
d   Displacement of teeth greater than 1 mm but less than or equal to 2 mm.
e   Anterior or posterior open bite greater than 1 mm but less than or equal to 2 mm.
f   Increased overbite greater than or equal to 3.5 mm without gingival contact.
g   Prenormal or postnormal occlusions with no other anomalies. Includes up to half a unit discrepancy.

Grade 3 (moderate)
a   Increased overjet greater than 3.5 mm but less than or equal to 6 mm with incompetent lips.
b   Reverse overjet greater than 1 mm but less than or equal to 3.5 mm.
c   Anterior or posterior crossbites with greater than 1 mm but less than or equal to 2 mm discrepancy between retruded contact position and intercuspal position.
d   Displacement of teeth greater than 2 mm but less than or equal to 4 mm.
e   Lateral or anterior open bite greater than 2 mm but less than or equal to 4 mm.
f   Increased and complete overbite without gingival or palatal trauma.

Grade 4 (great)
a   Increased overjet greater than 6 mm but less than or equal to 9 mm.
b   Reverse overjet greater than 3.5 mm with no masticatory or speech difficulties.
c   Anterior or posterior crossbites with greater than 2 mm discrepancy between retruded contact position and intercuspal position.
d   Severe displacements of teeth greater than 4 mm.
e   Extreme lateral or anterior open bites greater than 4 mm.
f   Increased and complete overbite with gingival or palatal trauma.
h   Less extensive hypodontia requiring prerestorative orthodontics or orthodontic space closure to obviate the need for a prosthesis.
l   Posterior lingual crossbite with no functional occlusal contact in one or both buccal segments.
m   Reverse overjet greater than 1 mm but less than 3.5 mm with recorded masticatory and speech difficulties.
t   Partially erupted teeth, tipped and impacted against adjacent teeth.
x   Supplemental teeth.

Grade 5 (very great)
a   Increased overjet greater than 9 mm.
h   Extensive hypodontia with restorative implications (more than one tooth missing in any quadrant) requiring prerestorative orthodontics.
i   Impeded eruption of teeth (with the exception of third molars) due to crowding, displacement, the presence of supernumerary teeth, retained deciduous teeth and any pathological cause.
m   Reverse overjet greater than 3.5 mm with reported masticatory and speech difficulties.
p   Defects of cleft lip and palate.
s   Submerged deciduous teeth

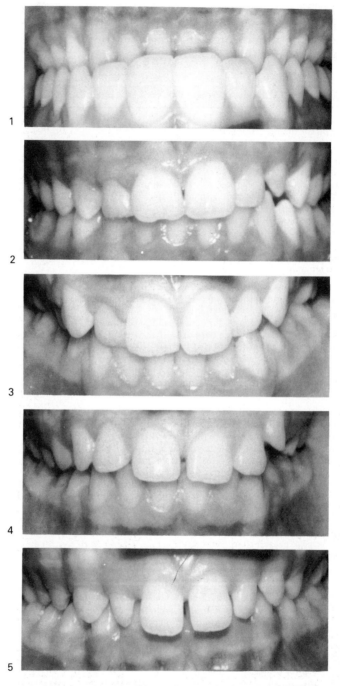

Figure 4.3 The SCAN index of aesthetic need (Evans and Shaw, 1987) by kind permission of the authors and the Editor of the *European Journal of Orthodontics*. More recently this has become known as the aesthetic component of the Index of Orthodontic Treatment Need.

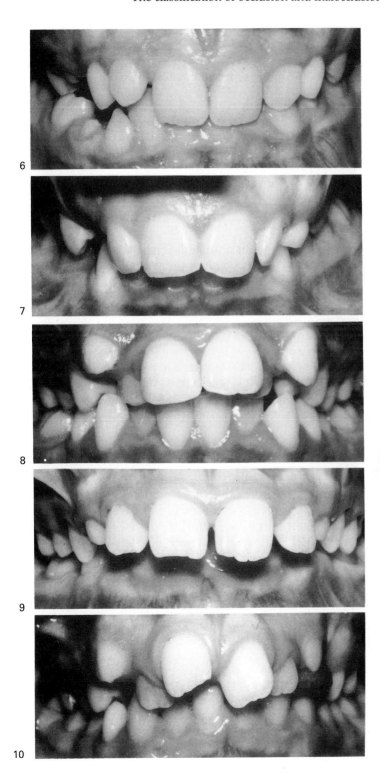

6

7

8

9

10

Treatment need – the dental health component

In Sweden the Dental Board have used an index for many years to categorize malocclusions into five grades of treatment need ranging from 'very great' to 'little'. Recently this index has been refined by Brook and Shaw (1989) into the dental health component of the Index of Treatment Need (Table 4.1). Using this a case may be rated from 5, 'urgent need' (Cleft lip and palate, overjets equal to or greater than 9 mm, impacted teeth, etc.) to 1, 'no need' (contact point displacements of less than 1 mm).

Treatment need – the aesthetic component

Most indices used in assessing treatment need contain a weighting for aesthetic impairment. However, it is more convenient to consider the aesthetic needs as entirely separate as most authorities now agree that orthodontic treatment can be justified on either aesthetic or functional grounds. The SCAN Index (Standardized Continuum of Aesthetic Need) developed by Evans and Shaw (1987) is based on a series of standardized photographs of the labial views of teeth with various degrees of irregularity (Fig. 4.3). Using these, a measure of aesthetic impairment may be made by choosing the photograph judged to show the same degree of aesthetic impairment. Surprisingly there is a good agreement between the decisions made by patients, parents and orthodontists.

Indices of treatment change

In order to evaluate the quality of treatment provided, indices have been developed that quantify treatment change in occlusal terms. The OI of Summers (1971), although not developed for this purpose, has been used to quantify treatment changes achieved with fixed and removable appliances and appears to give valid and reliable results.

More recently the PAR (Peer Assessment Rating) Index has been specifically developed to measure treatment change provided within the British National Health Service (Richmond et al., 1992). The originators of this index undertook an exhaustive study to validate the index by weighting the scores of various components from which it is made up so that it precisely reflects contemporary British orthodontic opinion. This means that regardless of who applies the Index the difference between the weighted scores derived from the pre- and post-treatment models can be directly and reliably interpreted as the verdict which a panel of British dentists would make about the degree of occlusal change achieved by the treatment. By applying the pre- and post-treatment scores to a nomogram, three categories of judgement ('great improvement', 'moderate improvement', 'no change') can be obtained for all severities and types of malocclusion.

Skeletal classification

As has already been pointed out, Angle believed that the first permanent molars had a definite devlopmental relationship to the jaws and so
he made no distinction between the skeletal and occlusal pattern, as he
believed that both were defined by the molar occlusion. This is incorrect
because (a) the dental lamina, which gives rise to the tooth germs, does
not develop in a constant relationship to the jaw, and (b) premature
loss of deciduous teeth in either arch usually leads to migration of the
first permanent molar.

Although jaw relationship influences the arch relationship (and hence
the molar relationship) and the two will often correspond, they must be
assessed separately. Indeed, because deciduous tooth loss is still
common it has become customary to assess skeletal, incisor and molar
relationship separately.

A detailed investigation of skeletal relationships can be undertaken
only with the aid of a lateral skull radiograph (see Chapter 7) but a
general evaluation sufficient for many clinical purposes can be obtained
by clinical assessment.

The appearance of nose and chin have a very important effect on the
facial characteristics, but of more immediate concern to the orthodontist
is the relationship of the dental bases, which are the parts of the jaws
that can be occupied by the apices of the teeth. Little periosteal
remodelling occurs at this level in response to tooth movement and so
the anteroposterior dental base relationship (the skeletal pattern)
imposes limitations on the possible tooth positions. Ideally the skeletal
pattern would be assessed at the apical level but there are no suitable
landmarks and so the depths of the concavities of the profiles of maxilla
and mandible, named points A and B respectively, are used instead
(see Fig. 6.7). The soft tissue, or integumental, profile does not follow
the skeletal profile exactly but variations in the thickness of the lips are
rarely sufficient to give a misleading impression of the skeletal pattern.
Some clinicians prefer to retract the lips and examine the skeletal
relationship at about the level of the mucogingival junction. When
assessing the skeletal pattern, the patient should sit or stand unsupported with the head in the free postural position. It helps if the patient
looks at an object at eye level, ideally at the reflection of their own eyes
in a wall-mounted mirror. The Frankfort plane should be more or less
horizontal when the head is positioned correctly. The clinical assessment of the skeletal pattern is subjective and so the definitions are
qualitative. With experience, the clinical assessment of the skeletal
pattern should closely match its measurement from a lateral skull
radiograph (see Chapter 6).

Definitions

Class I. The lower dental base is normally related to the upper. Point B
lies a few millimetres behind point A (see Fig. 6.7).

Class II. The lower dental base is retruded relative to the upper (Fig.
6.12).

Class III. The lower dental base is protruded relative to the upper (Fig. 6.21).

The use of classifications

It should be clearly understood from what has been said that the various classifications used in orthodontics are largely independent. A Class I incisor occlusion may be found in association with an Angle Class III molar occlusion in a patient who has a skeletal 2 dental base relationship. In the same way a patient with a Class II division 1 incisor malocclusion may have a very low rating for the index of aesthetic need but a high dental health need. Each classification helps to focus attention on a particular aspect of treatment planning.

At the present time, skeletal and occlusal classifications are used routinely. It is our belief that to these should be added the two indices of treatment need (aesthetic need and dental health need) because they force the clinician to pose the more fundamental question of whether the malocclusion should be treated and if so on what grounds.

References

Angle, E. H. (1899) Classification of malocclusion. *Dental Cosmos*, **41**, 248–264

Ballard, C. F. and Wayman, J. B. (1964) A report on a survey of the orthodontic requirements of 310 army apprentices. *Transactions of the British Society for the Study of Orthodontics*, 81–86

Banack, A. R., Cleall, J. F. and Yip, A. S. G. (1972) Epidemiology of malocclusion in 12 year old Winnipeg schoolchildren. *Journal of the Canadian Dental Association*, **12**, 437–455

Baume, L. J., Horowitz, H. S., Summers, C. J., Bacher Dirks, O., Britishown, W. A. B., Carlos, J. P., Freer, T. J., Harvold, E. P., Moorees, C. F. A., Salzmann, J. A., Schmuth, G., Solow, B. and Taatz, H. (1973) A method for examining occlusal traits developed by the FDI Commission on Classification and Statistics for Oral Conditions. *International Dental Journal*, **23**, 530–537

Björk, A., Krebs, A. A. and Solow, B. (1964) A method for epidemiological registration of malocclusion. *Acta Odontologica Scandinavica*, **20**, 606

British Standards Institute (1983) *Glossary of Dental Terms* (BS 4492), BSI, London

Brook, P. H. and Shaw, W. C. (1989) The development of an index of orthodontic treatment priority: *European Journal of Orthodontics*, **11**, 309–320

Cons, N. C. (1986) *The Dental Aesthetic Index*, Monograph on Health Questions, 1517, Derwen, Iowa City

Draker, H. L. (1960) Handicapping labiolingual conditions: a proposed index for public health purposes. *American Journal of Orthodontics*, **46**, 295–305

Elderton, R. J. and Clark, J. D. (1983) Orthodontic treatment in the general dental service assessed by the occlusal index. *British Journal of Orthodontics*, **10**, 178–186

Evans, R. and Shaw, W. (1987) Preliminary evaluation of an illustrated scale for rating dental attractiveness. *European Journal of Orthodontics*, **9**, 314–318

Grainger, R. M. (1967) *Orthodontic Treatment Priority Index*, Public Health Service Publication No. 1000, Series 2, No. 25, United States Government, Washington DC

Gravely, J. F. and Johnson, D. B. (1974) Angle's classification of malocclusion: an assessment of reliability. *British Journal of Orthodontics*, **61**, 286–294

Jago, J. D. (1974) The epidemiology of dental occlusion, a critical appraisal. *Journal of Public Dental Health*, **34**, 80–93

Linder-Aronson, S. (1974) Orthodontics in the Swedish Public Dental Service. *Transactions of the European Orthodontic Society*, 233–240

Pickering, E. A. and Vig, P. (1975) The occlusal index used to assess orthodontic treatment. *British Journal of Orthodontics*, **2**, 47–51

Richmond S, Shaw W. C., O'Brien K. D., Buchanan I. B., Jones R., Stephens C.D., Roberts C.T., Andrews M. (1992) The development of the PAR index (Peer Assessment Rating): reliability and validity. *EJO*, **14**, 125–139.

Salzmann, J. D. (1968) Handicapping malocclusion assessment to establish treatment priority. *American Journal of Orthodontics*, **54**, 749–765

Shaw, W. C., Richmond, S., O'Brien, K. D., Brook, P. and Stephens, C. D. (1991) Quality control in orthodontics: indices of treatment need and treatment standards. *British Dental Journal*, **170**, 107–112

Simon, P. A. (1924) On gnathostatic diagnosis in orthodontics. *International Journal of Orthodontics*, **10**, 755–762

Stephens, C. D. and Harradine, N. W. T. (1988) Changes in the complexity of orthodontic treatment for patients referred to a teaching hospital. *British Journal of Orthodontics*, **15**, 27–32

Summers, C. (1971) The occlusal index: a system for identifying and scoring occlusal disorders. *American Journal of Orthodontics*, **59**, 552–566

Williams, A. and Stephens, C. D. (1992) Modifications to the incisor classification of malocclusion to improve inter-examiner reliability. *British Journal of Orthodontics*, **19**, 127–130

World Health Organization (1977) *Oral Health Surveys: Basic Methods*, 2nd edn., World Health Organization, Geneva, p. 19

Chapter 5

Examination of the patient

The purpose of the examination is to record information that describes the nature of the malocclusion and from this to determine the underlying causes. From these data, general dentists should be able to decide whether treatment is necessary, whether they should undertake this themselves or whether the patient requires specialist advice.

The occlusion of every child who is receiving regular dental care should be examined briefly in the early mixed dentition to determine that all the teeth are present, correctly positioned, and of good form and prognosis. This examination should include extraoral radiography, and is best carried out at the stage at which the upper lateral incisors are erupting – about 7 or 8 years of age. It is at this time that interceptive measures may sometimes be indicated (see Chapter 9). However, for most children, the development of the dentition will be such that orthodontic treatment is best delayed until the first premolars and canines have erupted. At this stage, a full orthodontic assessment should be undertaken for all, even those few children who appear to have acceptable occlusions.

The format of the examination

A thorough and logical assessment of every case is essential: failure to follow a consistent procedure can result in important features being overlooked. Table 5.1 shows the structure of the examination.

The history

Medical history

Before orthodontic treatment is undertaken both a full medical history and a dental history are required. Fortunately very few medical conditions preclude the wearing of appliances. It is wise to delay orthodontic treatment in those suffering from epilepsy until this is well controlled, and patients with blood dyscrasias may need special management if extractions are required. Children with severe mental or physical handicap require very careful assessment. Every attempt

Table 5.1 The examination

A *History*

Reason for attendance
Medical history
Dental history
Social history

B *Examination*

1 Extraoral
Skeletal pattern
   a anterior/posterior (skeletal class).
   b vertical (face height/FMPA)
   c lateral (? facial asymmetry)
Soft tissue
   a lip competence
   b habitually apart/together?
   c resting (lower) lip line

2 Intraoral
General condition of the mouth
   a oral hygiene/caries rate
   b teeth present
Lower arch
   a labial segment (angulation, rotation, crowding/spacing)
   b canines (angulation, rotation, crowding/spacing)
   c buccal segments (crowding, local tooth displacement)
Upper arch
   a labial segment (angulation, rotation, crowding/spacing)
   b canines (angulation, rotation, crowding/spacing)
   c buccal segments (crowding, local tooth displacement)
In occlusion
   Incisors:
      class
      overbite
      overjet
      centre lines
      crossbite (? +displacement)
   Canines:
      relationship
   Buccal segments:
      molar occlusion
      crossbites (? +displacements)

3. Radiographic
Teeth present
Condition of:
   crowns
   roots
   surrounding bone

---

should be made to regard them as having equal access to orthodontic treatment and each case must be judged on its merits. Often parents will be most insistent that treatment be provided, but where the risks of causing harm outweigh the chances of conferring benefit, treatment should be sympathetically withheld. Often a great deal of time will need to be spent explaining just why treatment is not a reasonable course to follow. Sometimes this will be all that is required and the time spent will be greatly appreciated. For other parents it will be kind to arrange to recall the patient for review rather than to deny any prospect of future treatment.

A number of common, minor ailments can interfere with treatment. For example, recurrent aphthous ulceration can cause appliances to be worn intermittently and hay fever may prevent a patient from wearing a functional appliance during the summer months. It is important for both the dentist and patient to be aware of such problems before a treatment plan is drawn up. It is perhaps worthwhile mentioning that occasionally children are seen whose stature or general development is unusual for their age. Usually this will be a reflection of familial trends but very occasionally it may represent undiagnosed systemic disease such as coeliac disease or growth hormone deficiency.

Dental history

Previous dental history is of relevance in that irregular dental attendance and general lack of interest in dental treatment may prejudice cooperation with subsequent orthodontic treatment. Other aspects of particular relevance are any history of persistently poor oral hygiene, a high caries rate and any history of past injury to upper anterior teeth.

Social history

Because the enthusiastic support of both parent and patient are required if orthodontic treatment is to be successfully carried out, it is essential to obtain the views of both the child and parent before any treatment is planned. What are they concerned about? Do they understand what orthodontic treatment involves? Have other children in the family successfully completed treatment? How far away do they live? Do they have a car? If not, how reliable is public transport? How easy is it to get time off school? Do they holiday abroad? Clearly, if you are seeing the patient for routine treatment most of these answers will have been obtained at earlier visits.

The clinical examination

Provided that all relevant aspects are covered, the exact sequence of examination is a matter of individual preference. The approach outlined here is structured so that by the time the occlusion is examined in detail, the background information about the skeletal relationships, soft tissue pattern and dental status has been acquired and this can be important in interpreting the occlusal findings. It is also desirable to assess lip pattern and activity before dental status is checked comprehensively because after the intraoral examination the patient is less likely to behave in a relaxed and normal fashion. Indeed, much useful information about lip form and activity can be gained by observing the patient before the clinical investigation.

The extraoral examination

The extraoral examination is divided into two parts. First it is necessary to assess the skeletal framework upon which the dentoalveolar processes have developed and then to observe and record the muscular environment that envelopes them.

Skeletal pattern

The bony framework of the face which supports the dental arches should be assessed in all three dimensions, anteroposteriorly, vertically and transversely.

Anteroposterior

This part of the examination is best carried out with the patient seated upright in the dental chair with the head in the free postural position: that is, looking straight ahead with the eyes directed at the horizon. The face is examined in profile to determine the anteroposterior relationship of the basal parts of the jaws to each other. Although variations in lip thickness may disguise the skeletal relationship it is usually possible to gain an impression of the underlying anteroposterior jaw relationship in this way.

Ideally the maxillary base should lie about 2 or 3 mm anterior to the mandibular base when the teeth are in occlusion – skeletal Class 1 (Fig. 5.1). Note that the skeletal class relates upper and lower apical bases to each other and not to the face. In other words the classification

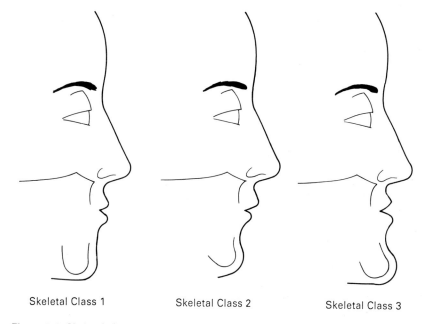

Skeletal Class 1   Skeletal Class 2   Skeletal Class 3

Figure 5.1 Skeletal class.

'skeletal 2' does not define whether the lower jaw is 'too far back' or the upper 'too far forward'. Some authorities have advocated palpation of the labial plates of alveolar bone in the regions of the incisor apices as a means of improving the clinical assessment of anteroposterior jaw relationship. However, if there is any degree of discrepancy, a cephalometric lateral skull radiograph is desirable.

Vertical

The space between the maxillary and mandibular dental bases is occupied by the teeth and their supporting alveolar processes. Excessively reduced lower face heights are associated with deep overbites, whilst greatly increased lower face heights may be the cause of anterior open bites. The latter are called 'skeletal' open bites to distinguish them from those caused by soft tissue influences. Because faces vary in size it is convenient to look at the lower face height in relation to the overall facial dimension.

   With the face still in profile, and the teeth in occlusion, an estimate should be made of the lower face height as a proportion of the total face height. Usually the distance from a point between the eyebrows to the junction of the nose with the upper lip will be roughly equal to the distance from the latter point to the underside of the chin (Fig. 5.2).

   The angle between the Frankfort and mandibular planes can also be used to make this estimate (Fig. 5.3). The face height is generally increased where this angle is raised and vice versa. However, because of the difficulty of judging angles, a more reliable clinical estimate may be made using the location of the point of intersection of these two

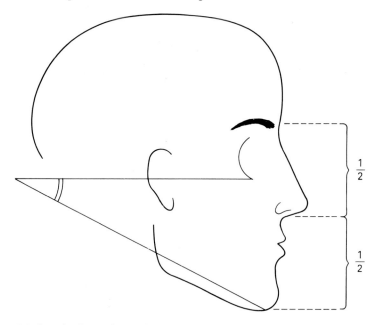

Figure 5.2 Anterior lower face height.

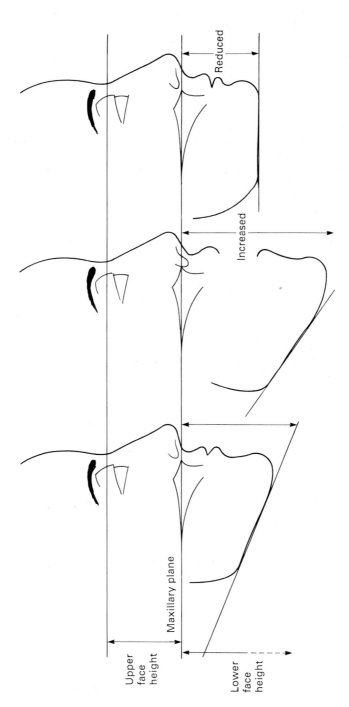

Figure 5.3 The relationship between anterior lower face height and the angle between the maxillary (of Frankfort) and mandibular planes.

planes rather than the angle between them. Where the planes meet at the back of the head (the region of the occiput), the angle will be within normal limits. If the angle is raised the point of intersection will lie within the contour of the skull; and where it is low the planes will intersect outside the skull (Fig. 5.2).

Once again the cephalometric radiograph provides the only really reliable way of obtaining an accurate determination of the face height, facial proportions and Frankfort/mandibular planes angle. Fortunately, the general practitioner is concerned only with identifying extremes and not with determining precise values.

Lateral

Two aspects of the lateral relationships of the jaws should be considered, as follows.

1 *Facial asymmetry*. Most patients have a roughly symmetrical lower face. To check this, it is best to view the patient's face either from in front or from above. It is then easy to detect an asymmetry of the jaws with respect to the face as a whole and, where asymmetry is present, it will be obvious which jaw is at fault.

Facial asymmetry may be the result of biological variation, pathology or a congenital abnormality. Fortunately, because the alveolar processes are moulded by the enveloping soft tissues, even quite marked asymmetry of the lower part of the face frequently fails to produce a disturbance in the occlusion of the teeth. Nevertheless, asymmetry should be checked for and, even if it appears to be of no significance, it should be regularly reviewed as such conditions may get progressively worse in the growing child (Fig. 5.4).

Where the occlusion is affected by asymmetry of the jaws this will

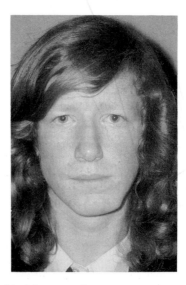

Figure 5.4 An example of facial asymmetry.

usually be in the form of a displacement of one incisor centre line so that the two centre lines do not coincide. More serious facial asymmetry may cause a buccal crossbite – that is, a disturbance in the relationship of the buccal teeth in the coronal plane such that the palatal cusps of the upper teeth no longer occlude in the fossae of their antagonists.

An apparent asymmetry of the lower part of the face when the teeth are in occlusion can also arise because the patient has adopted a displaced path of mandibular closure to avoid a premature contact as the teeth are brought into occlusion. This aspect will be covered under 'Intraoral examination' below.

2 *Arch widths.* Because the dental base is U-shaped the orthodontist is also concerned with the relative widths of the dental bases that support the cheek teeth. Usually the width of the upper jaw will be similar to that of the lower. Occasionally one jaw is very much wider than the other to such an extent that the occlusal relationships of the buccal teeth are affected and a buccal crossbite is seen. A crossbite is defined as a disturbance in the radial relationships of teeth. Crossbites are considered more fully under 'Intraoral examination' below.

Soft tissues

While the dental base determines the position of the apices of the teeth, the form and action of the lips and tongue are largely responsible for the positions that the crowns of the teeth occupy (Fröhlich, Thüer and Ingervall, 1991). Even the most talkative patient will have their lips and tongue active for only a fraction of the time. Hence it is the form of the lips and tongue that is of most importance, with functional activity playing a secondary role.

Lips

The examination of the lips covers three aspects – lip contour, lip line and lip seal. The patient should be sitting upright and relaxed. The first feature to examine is the contour of the lip musculature. Viewed in profile, are the lips everted (in which case the underlying teeth might be expected to be proclined), or are they rather vertical with no obvious outward curve at the red margin? The average lies between these two extremes (Fig. 5.5).

Next, still in this resting posture, where is the crest of the lower lip with respect to the upper incisor tips. Although this is referred to as the 'lip line' it is applied only to the relationship of the lower lip to the upper (central) incisors. In ideal incisor occlusion the resting lower lip covers between a third and a half of the labial surface of the upper central incisors. In Class II, division 1 malocclusion the lip line will be lower and often fail to 'control' the upper incisors whilst in a Class II, division 2 incisor relationship it will be much higher, sometimes covering the entire labial surface of the crown (Fig. 5.6).

Finally, do the lips form a seal at rest or are they too short to do this when the mandible is also in its resting position (lip incompetence)? Many patients with mild lip incompetence unconsciously hold their lips

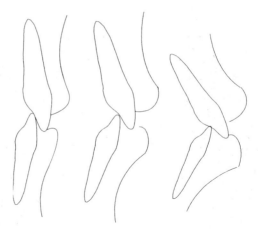

Figure 5.5 How variation in lip shape influences incisor position.

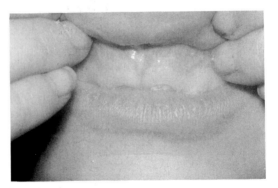

Figure 5.6 The Class II, division 2 incisor occlusion usually has a very high resting lip line.

together by slight circumoral contraction for a significant portion of the time and this can be difficult to detect at first (Fig. 5.7a). The tell-tale signs are a flattening out of the submental fold of the lower lip and a slight dimpling over the anterior surface of the chin where the fibres of the mentalis muscle (responsible for lower lip elevation) are inserted (Fig. 5.7b).

Lip incompetence is of greatest significance in Class II, division 1 malocclusion because the ultimate stability of the corrected incisor overjet depends on a lip seal being achieved. Fortunately, the desire to maintain a lip seal appears to increase until the late teens (Vig and Cohen, 1979) and so some quite unfavourable lip forms manage to retain corrected Class II, division 1 incisor occlusions. Nevertheless, cases with marked lip incompetence should be given a rather guarded prognosis.

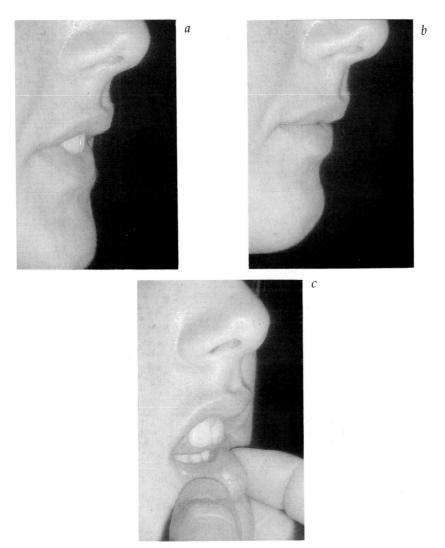

Figure 5.7 Incompetent lips: (a) at rest; (b) in their habitual posture; (c) in addition to circumoral contraction there is tongue/lip contact.

The tongue

Tongue position cannot be observed directly and any attempts to do so could interfere with what is being investigated. Even tongue size cannot be measured reliably and it is only gross variations from the normal that are worthy of record. Some positions of tongue activity can be inferred from the occlusion of the teeth. For example, it is to be expected that where the lips are incompetent the tongue will be used to produce a seal at the front of the mouth during swallowing. This can sometimes be demonstrated by pulling the lower lip downward and forward at the moment of swallowing and revealing the tip of the tongue interposed between the incisors. This 'adaptive' lip–tongue–alveolar process seal is probably used because it requires less effort than a seal produced by drawing the lips together (Ballard, 1961). Not surprisingly it is more commonly seen in Class II, division 1 malocclusions where the upper incisors make a lip seal more difficult. At other times in such cases the tongue may lie resting on the lower incisors, in which case it may prevent the full vertical development of the anterior dentoalveolar processes, leading to an incomplete overbite.

The adaptive tongue-to-lower lip seal tends to disappear as dental development proceeds, particularly if a Class II, division 1 incisor occlusion is corrected. Not too much importance should be attached to adaptive tongue thrusts. Unfortunately a very small number of individuals (not more than 1 per cent) have a swallowing activity accompanied by a thrusting behaviour that appears to be caused by an in-built neuromuscular defect (Fig. 5.8). It is highly desirable to distinguish between these two types of behaviour, although unfortunately this is not always possible.

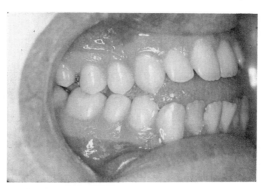

Figure 5.8 A tongue thrust.

Signs to beware of are:

a proclination of both upper and lower incisors;
b a tongue thrust associated with lip competence or only very mild incompetence;
c presence of a large part of the tongue between the anterior teeth at all times;
d a reversed curve of Spee in both arches;
e a marked lisp.

Habits

Although a great deal of emphasis was at one time placed on habits such as lip sucking, tongue sucking and pencil biting, the effects of these are now regarded as being of little significance to the developing occlusion. However, digit sucking nearly always has some effect on the dentition, the exact degree being dependent partly on the persistence of the habit and partly on the favourability of the soft tissues. Hence in a Class I case with ideal lip form, a thumb habit may cause no more than a slight reduction in the incisor overbite, whilst in a case with lip incompetence there may be a marked increase in overjet. Although a marked Class II, division 1 malocclusion may greatly improve if the owner can be persuaded to discontinue their habit early in the mixed dentition, it will rarely resolve completely.

Intraoral examination

Before the clinical examination can be completed, orthodontic records in the form of study models and radiographs are required. It is best to have reference (study) models and radiographs available at the time of the intraoral examination. This enables features such as tooth angulation, dental crowding and the presence of unerupted teeth to be confirmed at the time and is to be preferred to the alternative of attempting to fill in gaps in the intraoral assessment later when models and radiographs are available.

Reference models

Study models are helpful in assessing details of the occlusion and, of course, they provide an essential basis for measuring treatment progress. Orthodontic study models should reproduce all the erupted teeth, the palate and the full depth of the buccal sulcus (Fig. 5.9). Good

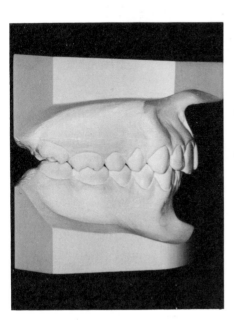
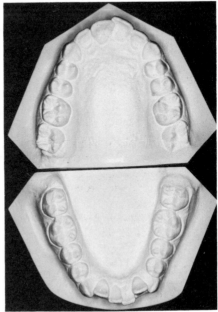

a   *b*

Figure 5.9 Orthodontic models correctly trimmed.

impressions are most readily obtained in trays with deep flanges. It may be helpful to build up the tray margins with soft wax. Careful trimming of the models is important because visual judgement of symmetry and arch form is influenced by the framing provided by the sides of models. The bases are trimmed parallel to the occlusal plane, leaving enough thickness to give a balanced form to the models. The heels must be perpendicular to the median palatal raphé of the upper and flush with one another so that when they are placed on a flat surface, the correct arch relationship is registered. The sides are trimmed symmetrically and equidistant from the median palatal raphé. Although the correct occlusal relationship of the arches should have been recorded with a wax wafer, it is necessary to check at the patient's next visit that the models are correctly related to one another.

Radiographs

In order to confirm the presence and condition of all teeth, radiographs must be available at the clinical examination. A minimum requirement is a panoral or equivalent view and an intraoral view of the upper labial segment. The intraoral view of the upper labial segment is required because supernumerary teeth, which are not rare in this region, may not be visible on a panoramic view if they lie out of the plane of the arch. For the practitioner who does not possess the apparatus for obtaining a panoral type of film, rotated oblique lateral views of the jaws should be obtained (Fig. 5.10). These can be taken with a standard dental radiographic unit provided that a suitable cassette with intensifying screens is employed. Cephalometric radiographs may be helpful in evaluating the more complex case, and their use is discussed in Chapter 6.

All possible precautions to minimize irradiation of the patient must

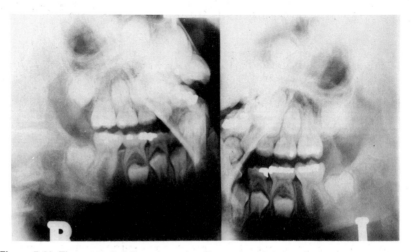

Figure 5.10 The rotated oblique lateral radiograph – bimolar views – can be taken with a conventional dental X-ray unit and should give an adequate view as far forward as the premolars.

be adopted. Filtration and collimation of the beam, the use of fast films and screening of the patient with a lead–rubber apron are all important. Where alternative views are possible, those involving less radiation to the patient should always be selected, and the number of films taken must be kept to the minimum required for adequate clinical evaluation.

Where there is any suspicion about the condition of any of the teeth, intraoral films may be required. In practice this usually means bitewings for the first molars, and periapical views of unerupted premolars where these appear to be hypoplastic on the extraoral film. Fractured incisors are adequately displayed on the naso-occlusal (standard occlusal) film.

If it is suspected that the maxillary canines are ectopic, localizing views will be needed. It is impossible to do this from the naso-occlusal film alone. The easiest combination for the general practitioner is a conventional periapical view of the canine region to supplement the naso-occlusal film. This gives just the right amount of tube displacement to enable the principle of parallax to be used (Fig. 5.11). Using the naso-

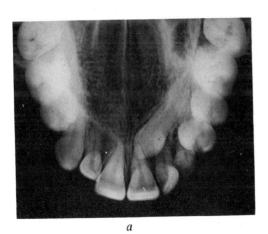 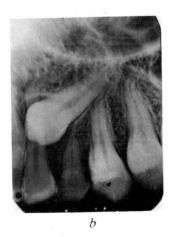

a   *b*

Figure 5.11 Standard occlusal and intraoral periapical films showing how an unerupted canine has apparently moved with the shift of the tube from overlapping the central incisor apex to overlap that of the lateral. The unerupted tooth has moved with the tube; by the principle of parallax it is therefore lying palatal to these teeth. Two periapical views can also be used. (See also Fig. 9.7.)

occlusal film, note the amount by which the crown of the unerupted canine overlaps the root of the lateral incisor. Now compare this with the intraoral film in which the tube has been moved distally around the arch. If the canine has apparently moved with the tube (i.e. there is less overlap in the intraoral film), the canine is palatally placed with respect to the lateral incisor root. If it moves in the opposite direction, it is buccal. If there is no apparent difference, the canine is lying within the ridge at the same depth as the lateral root. The same principle can be used to obtain vertical parallax between naso-occlusal and panoral films.

Although there are many ways in which the occlusion can be examined, there is almost unanimous agreement that the patient should be seated upright in the dental chair whilst this is being carried out. This is because it is extremely difficult to estimate the angulations of the incisor teeth to the face when the patient is semirecumbent. It is also essential to supplement your clinical examination with a close scrutiny of the study models. A ruler and a pair of dividers will be needed.

The recommended procedure is as follows:

1 Get a general idea of the condition of the mouth.
2 Examine each arch separately, looking in turn at incisors, canines and buccal teeth. Within each segment record in turn – crowding, angulations, rotations.
3 Examine the teeth in occlusion and record the anteroposterior and lateral relationships segment by segment.

Initially the findings should be recorded in rough. More will be said later on the most appropriate way to summarize findings in the case notes.

General condition of the mouth

If the patient is not being seen for routine dental care, this should be established at the beginning of the examination. Is the plaque control adequate for active treatment? Do the restorations appear to be of good quality? Are any teeth hypoplastic or of unusual form or size? Where a particular tooth has what appears to be a poor long-term prognosis it may be necessary to seek the view of the patient's general dental practitioner before a final decision about elective extractions can be made. Remember to check the gum margins of the teeth to ensure that they have an adequate zone of attached gingiva. If this is less than 1 mm, a more thorough examination of the fraenal and muscle attachments in this region will need to be made.

Examination of the arches

The use of models

While a visual assessment gives an impression of the space conditions in the arch, in some cases a more accurate estimate is required. Rather than arch size and tooth size *per se*, it is the amount of crowding and spacing that is of interest. Measurement can be helpful in marginal cases in deciding whether or not extractions will be required in the lower arch. A more reliable indication of upper arch space requirements is given by relating the upper canine teeth to the lowers and calculating how much space will be required to permit a Class I relationship. Allowance has to be made for any retraction of the lower canines that may be required to relieve lower labial segment crowding. Provided that the sizes of the upper and lower incisors match (see below), and the lower incisors are well aligned, a Class I canine relationship provides enough space to align the upper incisors with a normal overbite and overjet (Fig. 5.12a). (See also p. 145.)

Tooth size discrepancies. The upper incisor teeth are quite variable in size. If they are large in relation to the lowers and there is a Class I canine relationship with no lower arch spacing, then the upper incisors will be crowded or there will be an increase in overjet. The converse applies when the upper incisors are small relative to the lowers (Fig. 5.12b). It is important to recognize this problem before treatment is started and to plan accordingly. Often the discrepancy in size is due to upper laterals that are small. Collectively, the widths of the upper incisors should equal the total width of the lower incisors plus one lower canine.

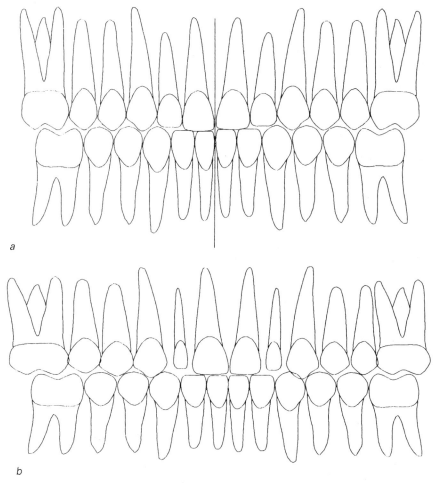

a

b

Figure 5.12 (a) Showing how a Class I canine relationship usually provides enough space to align the upper incisor where the lower arch is well aligned. (b) Where the upper incisor teeth are unusually small and there is a normal canine relationship there will be spacing in the upper labial segment unless there is crowding in the lower labial region.

Space discrepancy. Information obtained from the models gives an indication of space discrepancy. This information is most useful in the lower arch in mildly crowded cases where a decision has to be made whether or not to extract teeth. Sometimes it is possible to align the lower teeth provided that the leeway space is not lost by forward movement of the first permanent molars, and a space maintainer may be fitted on exfoliation of second deciduous molars. At the other extreme, where crowding is severe and extractions would provide just enough space, it is essential not to allow any forward movement of the permanent molars by the use of space-maintaining appliances (see Chapter 10).

Space analysis in the upper arch is less useful than in the lower. Extractions in the upper arch are determined by the need to obtain a buccal segment relationship with the lower arch that will allow alignment of the upper incisors in a normal relationship with the lowers. This will be influenced by whether or not extractions are required in the lower arch (see Chapter 8).

Examination of the lower arch

Labial segment. First count the teeth: three or five lower incisors are quite common and are easily missed. Tuberculate supernumerary teeth on the other hand, which are common in the upper labial region, are virtually unheard of in the lower incisor area.

Next, with the face in profile, estimate the angulation the lower labial teeth make with the lower border of the mandible. Usually the lower incisors are set at about 90° to the lower border. You will find it helpful to place your index finger along the lower border of the mandible and retract the lip with the thumb of the same hand to make this estimate.

Then, checking your clinical findings against the models, decide whether the lower incisors are crowded, acceptably aligned, or spaced. Some attempt should be made to grade the crowding (mild, moderate and severe are usually sufficient). Note local tooth irregularity: for example, are any teeth bodily displaced from the arch? This is fairly rare in the lower incisor region but quite commonly seen where maxillary lateral incisors are crowded. Any teeth that are significantly rotated should also be recorded. These are described with respect to the line of the arch. It is customary to identify the corner of the incisal edge that is most displaced from the arch and describe the direction in which it is displaced, hence: mesiolabial, distolingual rotation, etc. Are any teeth significantly tilted mesially or distally? Sometimes all the lower incisors appear to be splayed distally – aptly referred to as 'fanning'.

Canines. The examination of each canine area should be made in turn.

The angulation of the erupted canine has an important bearing on treatment planning. This angle should be estimated with respect to the occlusal plane, and the inclination of each canine classified as mesial, upright or distal. Any rotation is described in the same way as for incisors.

Is there enough space to accommodate each tooth? Where crowding exists the canine will usually be excluded buccally and if unerupted should be seen as a bulge. Part eruption and supra-eruption should be recorded.

Buccal segments. Sometimes the second deciduous molar will be retained at the time of the orthodontic examination. As a consequence it may be difficult to estimate the degree of crowding in the buccal segments until this tooth is shed. In general the excess space provided by a lower second deciduous molar is taken up by mesial migration of the first molar and should not be regarded as available for the relief of crowding anterior to this site.

Where a deciduous molar has been lost prematurely and the successional tooth is still unerupted, an estimate of the crowding can be made by using the dimension of a contralateral premolar as a guide. Remember that lower second premolars are quite frequently hypoplastic and, apart from the third molars, are also the most common teeth to be developmentally absent. If second premolars are crowded through early loss, they will usually be displaced lingually and delayed in their eruption. It is unusual to be able to palpate a lingually displaced premolar much before 13 or 14 years of age.

Despite the marked reduction in the prevalence of dental caries in children it is still extremely important to check the condition of the first permanent molar teeth thoroughly. Smooth surface caries, particularly lingually on the lower first molars, indicates a doubtful long-term prognosis. A check should also be made for recurrent caries around and beneath existing restorations in these teeth.

Examination of the upper arch

Labial segment. The angulation of upper incisor teeth is estimated with respect to the Frankfort plane. If a lateral skull radiograph is available the maxillary plane is used for this measurement.

Remember that supernumerary teeth, which are common in this area, can cause displacement as well as non-eruption of maxillary incisors. Deciduous and permanent central incisors are also frequently subjected to trauma. Fractured incisors are obvious, dilacerations less so. Discoloured anterior teeth or those with reduced translucency should always be viewed with suspicion, even where there is no other evidence of trauma.

Many of those cases with fractured teeth present problems that require expert advice. In such instances, it is extremely helpful for the orthodontist to have the practitioner's views about prognosis included in the referral letter.

Lateral incisors are quite often developmentally absent. They are also quite often small or 'peg-shaped'. Palatal invaginations are also common, so these should be specifically checked for, both clinically and radiographically (see below).

A naso-occlusal radiograph is always necessary, even where the region appears to be normal (Fig. 5.13). In addition to the conditions already mentioned, this radiograph will help to indentify other pathology affecting unerupted teeth such as hypoplastic enamel, short roots or the presence of a dens-in-dente.

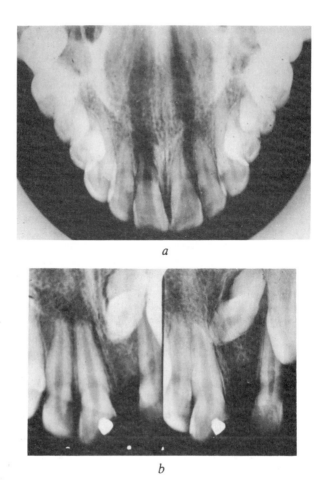

a

b

Figure 5.13 A standard occlusal film will also reveal other anomalies common in this part of the mouth.

Canines. Each canine area should be examined in turn. Canine angulation should be recorded in the same manner as in the lower arch and any rotation noted.

Is there enough space to accommodate each tooth? Where the canine is unerupted it will usually be palpable buccally, particularly if it is rather short of space. Palpation will also give some idea of the angulation of the unerupted tooth.

Unfortunately the maxillary canine is quite frequently misplaced and this possibility should be confirmed or excluded as early as possible. The prevalence of misplaced maxillary canines is very much greater where the lateral incisor is unusually small or is developmentally absent (Brin, Becker and Shalhav, 1986). If by 10½ years of age the canine cannot be palpated high up in the buccal sulcus it is almost certainly palatally misplaced and localizing radiographs must be taken to confirm this. The earlier this problem can be identified, the easier will be its treatment (see Chapter 9).

Buccal segments. Examination of the upper buccal segments is carried out precisely as in the lower arch. In the case of the upper first permanent molars the danger area for smooth surface caries is buccally rather than lingually.

The examination of the teeth in occlusion

Path of closure

As the teeth are brought into contact the mandible should make a simple hinge movement from its resting position with the condyles rotating in their glenoid fossae. Not infrequently, either as a result of dental crowding or skeletal discrepancy, two teeth meet prematurely. The mandible then makes a lateral or forward displacement from its path of closure by reflex lateral pterygoid activity. So well integrated does this pattern of muscle activity become that it is not possible to identify it just by observation. You should therefore get into the habit of ensuring that the patient's jaw is fully retruded when the incisor teeth are brought into occlusion. Place the knuckle of your curled index finger under the patient's chin and your thumb on the mental eminence. While applying gentle pressure ask the patient to relax until you are able to move the mandible freely up and down without resistance. Now bring the mandible up until the teeth occlude. If it is apparent that not all the teeth are fully in occlusion find the point of initial contact. If you cannot identify this, ask the patient to point it out to you. Then ask the patient to bring their teeth together 'in the way they usually do'. The displacement into centric occlusion will now be revealed. Note whether this is to the left, right or forwards or a combination. A few authorities use the term 'eccentric occlusion' to distinguish this type of occlusion from the undisplaced 'centric occlusion'. Whether or not you find a displacement, all the following assessments of incisor relationships are made with the teeth fully intercuspated.

Incisor occlusion

Overjet. This is recorded to the nearest millimetre by measuring from the labial surface of the lower incisor to the labial surface of the upper. It will usually be wise to record the distance for both central incisors. Get used to making the measurement in the middle of each incisal edge, keeping the ruler parallel with the occlusal plane. This will overcome the local effect of incisor rotation and reduce measurement error that may be caused by variation in head position.

Overbite. This is most easily assessed using the models. The overbite should be classified as either increased (more than 4 mm), average or reduced (less than 3 mm). Overbite should be further classified as either complete (i.e. the lower incisor tips touch opposing tooth or mucosa) or incomplete (Fig. 5.14).

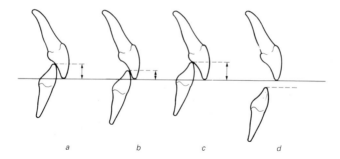

Figure 5.14 The classification of overbite: (a) average, (b) reduced, (c) increased, (d) an open bite. Where the lower incisors fail to contact opposing structures (tooth or palate) the overbite is said to be incomplete.

Incisor class (see Chapter 4). It will be recalled that this classification is based on the anatomy of the palatal surface of incisor crown (see Fig. 4.2). A common error is to forget that in the child only part of the full clinical crown is in the mouth. Many Class I incisor occlusions are identified incorrectly as Class II, division 1 relationships for this reason.

Incisor centre lines. Incisor centre lines can be affected by local dental irregularity, premature loss of deciduous teeth and by facial asymmetry. Although the incisor centre line has to be markedly displaced before patients and their parents become concerned about this feature of the occlusion, a mismatch between the upper and lower centre lines has an important bearing on the buccal occlusion.

The position of the incisor midline should be checked both with respect to the face and the opposing arch. This is best carried out standing behind the patient as described for the extraoral assessment of facial asymmetry. Then, using the study models, the cause of any discrepancy should be identified.

Canine occlusion

With the teeth in occlusion classify the anteroposterior relationship of the canines as Class I, half a unit Class II, etc. (see Chapter 4). Usually this will be closely correlated with the buccal occlusion but not invariably so (Fig. 5.15).

Buccal segment occlusion

Anteroposterior. The anteroposterior occlusion of the buccal teeth should be classified as described in Chapter 4. Generally the whole buccal segment will have the same type of occlusion and one can note that 'the left buccal segment is a full unit Class II'. If there has been premature loss of deciduous teeth, the canine, premolar and molar

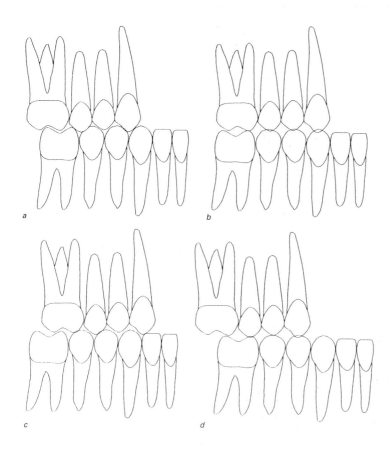

a   b

c   d

Figure 5.15 The classification of buccal occlusion based on Angle's classification: (a) Class I, (b) half a unit Class II, (c) a full unit Class II, (d) half a unit Class III.

occlusion will be different and it may be necessary to record them separately.

Buccolingual. Usually the buccal cusps of the upper teeth occlude buccal to those of the lower with the lingual cusps of the maxillary molars and premolars occluding in the fossae of their lower opponents. Where this is not occurring a crossbite is said to exist.

Posterior crossbites can be local or segmental and may be bilateral or unilateral. Where the upper teeth erupt with their buccal cusps lingual to those of the lower, a lingual crossbite is said to exist. If the lingual cusps of the upper teeth occlude buccally to the buccal cusps of the lower teeth there is said to be a buccal crossbite or scissors bite (Fig. 5.16). A typical example of a local crossbite would be a maxillary second premolar that erupts lingual to its correct occlusion where there is inadequare space following premature loss of its predecessor. A segmental crossbite, on the other hand, affects most of the buccal teeth and is often due to an underlying discrepancy in the widths of the arches. This may be dentoalveolar or skeletal in origin. For example, a digit-sucking habit is frequently the cause of a unilateral posterior

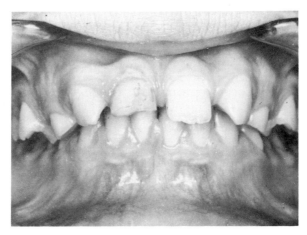

Figure 5.16 A scissors bite.

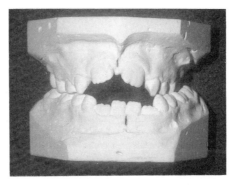

Figure 5.17 A common cause of a unilateral crossbite is a digit sucking habit. Often, as here, this is associated with a mandibular displacement; as a result the centrelines do not coincide.

crossbite through the action of tongue and cheek pressure on the maxillary teeth and alveolar process of the upper jaw (Fig. 5.17). On the other hand a gross Skeletal 3 anteroposterior dental base relationship will frequently be associated with a crossbite.

Unilateral (segmental) crossbites are usually associated with a mandibular displacement which should be checked for (see above, and also Fig. 10.15). Bilateral crossbites do not have associated displacements.

Crossbite and its treatment is considered more fully in Chapter 10.

The examination of radiographs

A cursory review of radiographs may not reveal important information and it is essential that each film is examined carefully and in an orderly manner, as follows.

1 *Identify and count the teeth*. Although this may seem self-evident it is easily overlooked. A systematic approach is required comparing the findings with the study models to ensure that teeth are correctly identified. By the age of 5 years, all permanent teeth except for third molars and possibly second premolars should be visible on radiographs. Occasionally, in boys, second premolars may develop as late as 8 years. Thus it can be difficult in a younger boy where there is not radiographic evidence of a second premolar to decide whether or not to extract the second deciduous molar in order to encourage space closure. Third molars are usually first visible on radiographs between 8 and 12 years of age but cases have been reported where they have not been evident until 14 years of age.

2 *Examine the tooth crowns*. Although the views obtained may not be ideal for demonstrating defects in tooth structure, there may be clues that need to be followed up with supplementary radiographs. Suspect areas below restorations, calcification of a pulp chamber, dens-in-dente involving the upper incisors and evidence of hypoplasia of the enamel of unerupted premolars are all features that may not be apparent clinically and yet need to be taken account of in planning treatment (Fig. 5.18).

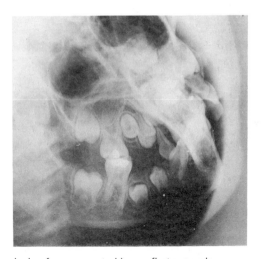

Figure 5.18 Hypoplasia of an unerupted lower first premolar.

3 *Examine the roots*. Dilaceration of roots may limit the possible correction of crown positions. Retarded root formation or failure of apical closure may indicate that the vitality of the tooth is in doubt and requires further investigation. Even in the absence of a history of trauma, fracture of upper incisor roots may be discovered and clearly influences the treatment plan: it may be best not to undertake orthodontic treatment or the decision may have to be made to extract the tooth, or to remove the apical fragment and root fill the tooth.

Root resorption is not uncommon, particularly in the upper incisor region. Sometimes there may be an obvious cause such as trauma or previous orthodontic treatment. More often there is no explanation and the resorption is termed idiopathic. Some individuals are susceptible to root resorption and several teeth may be affected. Teeth that have previously undergone root resorption seem to be particularly liable to suffer further resorption with orthodontic tooth movement, and even intact teeth in patients exhibiting idiopathic root resorption elsewhere may be at risk. It should also be remembered that teeth with short roots tip more than expected because the centre of rotation is closer to the crown. Clearly, in patients who have serious root resorption, appliance treatment should be undertaken with reluctance. If treatment is commenced, extensive movement of the root apex should be avoided and the patient should be made aware of the dangers of further root loss (see p. 271).

Apical or lateral root resorption may be caused by the crypt of an adjacent unerupted tooth. This is sometimes seen on an upper lateral incisor where the permanent canine is impacted against it (Fig. 5.19).

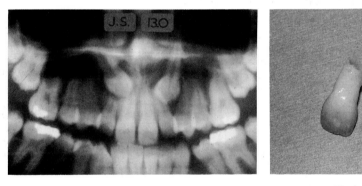

Figure 5.19 A canine that has resorbed the root of the upper lateral incisor.

4 *Supporting bone.* Areas of radiolucency or sclerosis may indicate some pathological process. Most common are periapical radiolucencies indicating that the tooth is not vital. The crypts around teeth whose eruption has been delayed should be examined for cyst formation.

As radiographs are taken at the first visit, before the intraoral examination, it is preferable where possible to examine them briefly at the first visit so that any additional views may be available as dry films at the time of the clinical examination.

Summarizing and recording your findings

The case assessment must follow a standardized procedure in order to ensure that no feature of the malocclusion is overlooked. The summary that appears in the notes serves a different purpose – to record all the essential features in such a way that a clear picture of the malocclusion is obtained. It is therefore important to be able to recognize the relevant features and their interrelationships and to summarize them in a coherent manner. In general a summary should include:

1 Details about the patient:
   name, sex, age;
   attitude to the malocclusion and to treatment;
   relevant medical history.
2 Classification (incisor class).
3 Skeletal base relationships.
4 Soft tissue environment.
5 Features of the malocclusion:
   teeth present;
   overjet and overbite where appropriate;
   degree of crowding or spacing (in terms of premolar units per arch);
   positions of individual teeth;
   molar occlusion.

Hence a summary might be as follows:

Christine B., 12 years 4 months. Concerned about prominent incisors. Willing to wear fixed or removable appliances but not keen on headgear. Slight asthma, uses inhaler.

On examination Class II, division 1 incisor relationship on mild Sk 2 base. Raised lower face height. Incompetent lips (slight). All teeth present (inc. 8s) and in good condition but Es retained.

Good lower arch. Upper incisors proclined and spaced. Overjet 8 mm, overbite increased and incomplete. Canines and molars Class II half unit both sides.

Note that in general only positive findings are recorded. The summary does not contain a statement confirming that features are 'normal'.

References

Ballard, C. F. (1961) The clinical significance of innate and adaptive postures and motor behaviour. *Transactions of the British Society for the Study of Orthodontics*, 63–72

Brin, I., Becker, A. and Shalhav, M. (1986) The position of the maxillary permanent canine in relation to anomalous or missing lateral incisors: a population study. *Journal of Orthodontics*, 8, 12–16

Fröhlich, K., Thüer, U. and Ingervall, B. (1991) Pressure from the tongue on the teeth in young adults. *Angle Orthodontist*, 61, 17–24

Vig, P. S. and Cohen, A. M. (1979) Vertical growth of the lips: a serial cephalometric study. *American Journal of Orthodontics*, 75, 405–415

Chapter 6

Cephalometric analysis

Skull radiographs have been used for a variety of purposes from the early days of radiography, but it was only in 1931 that Broadbent in the USA and Hofrath in Germany, independently of one another, developed a standardized system of cephalometric radiography that could be of use to the orthodontist. Subsequent research into facial growth and the results of orthodontic treatment had a major impact on orthodontic theory and practice. On the basis of early cross-sectional studies where average values for cephalometric measurements at different ages were compared with one another, it was concluded that the pattern of facial growth was rather stable and that orthodontic treatment had little or no effect upon it (Broadbent, 1937; Brodie, 1941). However, this method of analysis obscures individual variability and the work of Björk in particular has demonstrated the extent of this (Björk and Palling, 1955). The possible effects of orthodontic treatment upon facial growth are still a matter of controversy (see Chapter 7).

In clinical practice, cephalometric analysis is of value in assessing facial and dentoskeletal relationships as an aid to treatment planning. Evaluation of changes attributable to growth and treatment is important in monitoring treatment progress and standards. Broadbent (1937) had emphasized the three-dimensional nature of facial relationships and recommended that posteroanterior (PA) as well as lateral skull views should be obtained. Others have suggested that views of the skull base are of value for some measurements. However, cephalometric analysis has come to mean, almost exclusively, the measurement of lateral skull radiographs (Fig. 6.1). In part this is because the facial variations of greatest orthodontic importance are in the sagittal plane, and in part because other views are difficult to interpret and measure. In the PA view (Fig. 6.2), for example, few landmarks that are important in lateral skull radiographs can be identified and so the possibilities of three-dimensional analysis are very limited; and furthermore even minor variations in head position can result in distortion so that the apparent asymmetry of the skeletal structures can be exaggerated or even reversed.

Cephalometric radiographs are taken under standardized conditions so that measurements can be compared between patients and for the same patient on different occasions. The head is held in a cephalostat so that the mid-sagittal plane is at a fixed distance from, and parallel to, the film (Fig. 6.3). The target of the X-ray tube is also at a fixed distance

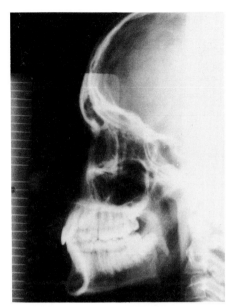

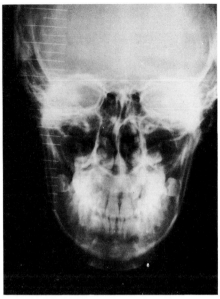

Figure 6.1 A lateral skull radiograph. Note the scale at the midsagittal plane which provides a permanent record of the enlargement of the radiograph.

Figure 6.2 Posteroanterior view of the patient shown in Fig. 6.1. Few landmarks common to both views can be identified reliably.

from the film, with the central ray directed through the ear rods of the cephalostat so that the enlargement at the mid-sagittal plane is constant (Fig. 6.4). Various recommendations have been made that the distances should be agreed internationally so that the enlargement would be standardized, but unfortunately these have not been adhered to. In most installations, the magnification is in the order of 10 per cent and provided that the magnification is known, linear enlargement can be compensated for. To this end it is good practice to suspend a metal scale of known length at the mid-sagittal plane of the head so that it appears in every film and provides a permanent record of the enlargement of that film (Fig. 6.1).

When the patient is positioned in the cephalostat, care should be taken to ensure that the ear rods are in fact in the ear canals and that the Frankfort plane is horizontal. The teeth should be in centric occlusion unless there is a mandibular displacement, in which case the mandible should be positioned in centric relation with the teeth in the initial contact relationship. If this is not done, a misleading impression of the skeletal relationships will be obtained. The patient should be posed with the lips in their habitual position.

Anatomy visualized on lateral skull and PA radiographs

The skull consists of three major components: the calvarium, the cranial

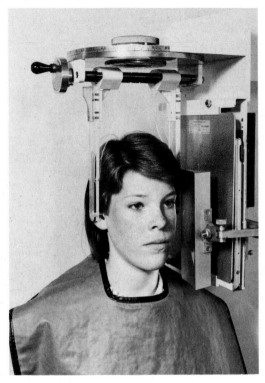

Figure 6.3 The cephalostat maintains the patient's head in a definite relationship to the film.

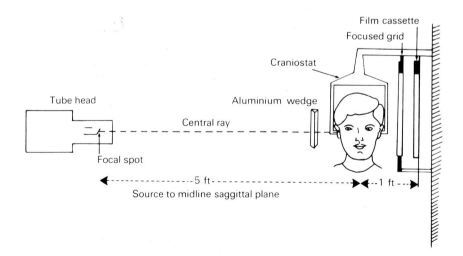

Figure 6.4 The relationship of film, patient's head and tube in a cephalometric installation.

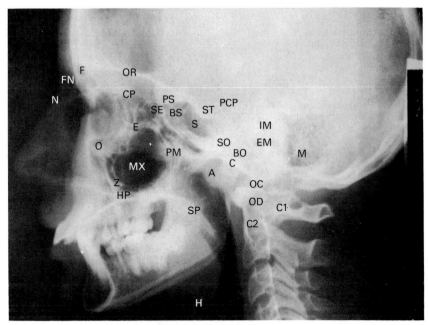

Figure 6.5 Anatomical features on a lateral skull radiograph. Key: A=adenoids; BO=basiocciput; BS=basisphenoid; C=condyle; CP=cribriform plate of ethmoid; C1=atlas; C2=axis; E=ethmoid air cells; EM=external acoustic meatus; F=frontal sinus; FN=frontonasal suture; H=hyoid bone; HP=hard palate; IM=internal acoustic meatus; M=mastoid air cells; MX=maxillary sinus; N=nasal bone; O=orbital margin; OC=occipital condyle; OD=odontoid process of axis; OR=orbital roof; PCP=posterior clinoid process; PM=pterygoid maxillary fissure; PS=planum sphenoidale; S=sphenoid air sinus; SE=site of sphenoethmoidal synchondrosis; SO=spheno-occipital synchondrosis; SP=soft palate; ST=sella turcica, the pituitary fossa; Z=zygomatic process of maxilla.

base and the facial skeleton. The calvarium is of little relevance to orthodontic assessment and in the interests of radiation protection, the radiographic beam should be collimated to exclude unnecessary radiation (Fig. 6.1). The radiographic anatomy of these views is shown in Fig. 6.5. Measurements are usually made on tracings (Fig. 6.6) and so the relevant aspects of the anatomy will be mentioned in the description of the tracing procedure.

Tracing a lateral skull radiograph

It is helpful when learning to identify the landmarks to obtain a radiograph of a dry skull. The absence of soft tissues improves the definition of the bony landmarks and it is instructive to compare the radiographic anatomy with the skull itself. Landmarks difficult to locate on the radiograph can be confirmed by fixing pieces of wire or lead shot to the skull before obtaining a further view. The tracing should be made under suitable conditions: a darkened room, a well-illuminated viewing

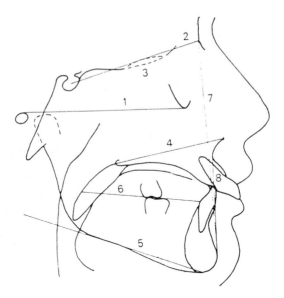

Figure 6.6 Lines of reference. 1 = Frankfort plane; 2 = sella-nasion line; 3 = de Coster's line; 4 = maxillary plane; 5 = mandibular plane; 6 = functional occlusal plane; 7 = facial plane; 8 = A–pogonion line.

screen blanked off with card to leave a window just large enough for the radiograph, a good quality tracing sheet fixed to the radiograph with clear adhesive tape, and a hard pencil (4H or 6H) are required. The **radiograph should be orientated with the Frankfort plane parallel to the bottom edge of the screen**, because a number of landmark definitions depend on head orientation.

The cranial base (Fig. 6.5)

Identify sella turcica and trace its outline, including the posterior clinoid processes. Proceed forward along the planum sphenoidale, across the sphenoethmoidal synchondrosis and along the cribriform plate of the ethmoid. The latter can be difficult to identify and must not be confused with the roofs of the orbits: the cribriform plate is flat or concave superiorly. The wedge-shaped contour of the posterior cranial base is traced easily, except at its posterior limit where the occipital condyles overshadow the basiocciput at the anterior margin of foramen magnum: the basiocciput in the midline does not curve inferiorly and terminates directly above the tip of the odontoid process of the second cervical vertebra.

The anterior surfaces of the frontal and nasal bones should now be traced. The nasal bone is thin and in an overexposed radiograph the anterior surface may be difficult to locate and care must be taken to trace it correctly. The frontonasal suture should also be indicated because the landmark nasion lies at its anterior limit. The frontal and nasal bones are, of course, not part of the cranial base but nasion is taken to represent its anterior limit because there is no alternative, reliably identifiable landmark.

The facial skeleton (Fig. 6.5)

The outline of hard palate is traced without difficulty. The posterior nasal spine may be obscured by unerupted upper molar teeth, but it lies directly below the inferior limit of the pterygomaxillary fissure and so the landmark can be constructed by dropping a perpendicular from the fissure to a line parallel to the nasal floor along the middle of the hard palate. The anterior nasal spine is difficult to locate, unless a wedge filter has been used (Fig. 6.4). It must not be confused with the alar cartilages of the nose, which are superimposed upon it and project further forward. The maxillary profile between anterior nasal spine and the alveolar crest can be very difficult to locate as the labial plate of bone is thin and the image of the soft tissues of the cheeks may be projected over it. The roots of the upper incisors give an approximate guide to its position.

The lateral and inferior borders of the orbit should be traced. Note their outline when viewed from the lateral aspect (Fig. 6.6). The inferior border can be particularly difficult to identify because of the complex pattern of bony trabeculae in this region but the roof of the maxillary antrum, which lies just below it, helps in its location. The root of the zygomatic process of the maxilla may also be identifiable below the orbit.

The external auditory meatus is difficult to locate: the head-holder of some cephalostats obscures it and if the central ray does not pass directly through both external auditory meati, the petrous parts of the temporal bones are superimposed upon them. The internal auditory meatus is often much clearer but should not be traced: it lies above and behind the external meatus. The glenoid fossa is level with the upper margin of the meatus and the mandibular condylar head, if it can be seen, gives a good indication of its height. Some authorities recommend that the ear rods of the cephalostat should be traced instead of the auditory meatus. This is not acceptable because at best they are positioned in the cartilaginous ear canals and may lie at some distance from the bony meati.

The posterior and inferior borders of the mandible are clearly visible. Where the sides are not superimposed, both should be traced and the 'average' position indicated by an interrupted line. The condylar heads can seldom reliably be identified on the lateral skull view, but if they are visible, their position can be indicated on the tracing. However, this should not encourage the use of landmarks on the condylar heads. If measurements are to be made to the condylar head, a second lateral skull view should be taken with the mouth open, so that it is forward on the articular eminence. This allows mandibular length to be measured but would seldom be of sufficient clinical importance to justify a second radiograph.

The exact outlines of the teeth can be difficult to identify with confidence, owing to their superimposition upon one another. The upper and lower central incisors and first permanent molars are traced. Because it is most clearly seen, the most prominent incisor is outlined, but in some cases this can give a misleading impression of the general position of the incisors and care should be taken in interpreting the results of a tracing where one incisor is particularly proclined or crowded labially. In these circumstances, the other central incisor should be traced as well. Many clinicians use a commercially produced stencil of tooth shapes to produce a clear outline of the tooth. Provided that the tooth to be traced is of average form and size, and provided that the stencil is located correctly so that the incisor edge and apex, and thus the long axis, are correctly shown, this is acceptable. However, there are considerable variations in incisor root length and crown-root angle, and a misleading impression of tooth form and position can be given when a stencil is used.

Soft tissues (Fig. 6.6)

The lips and facial integument, tongue, soft palate and nasopharynx may be traced to give an impression of their relation to the facial skeleton. However, unless the patient was carefully posed when the radiograph was taken, the positions of the lips in particular may be very misleading. If the lips are parted, no conclusions can be drawn about the mechanism of obtaining an anterior oral seal. A posterior oral seal is usually formed by contact between soft palate and tongue, but this

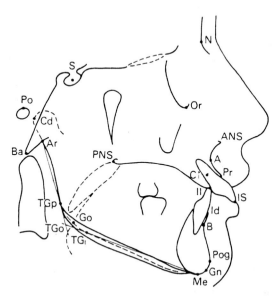

Figure 6.7 Cephalometric landmarks. A = point A; ANS = anterior nasal spine; Ar = articulare; B = point B; Ba = basion; C ↑ = centroid of upper incisor; Cd = condylion; Gn = gnathion; Go = gonion; II = incision inferius; IS = incision superius; Id = infradentale; Me = menton; N = nasion; Or = orbitale; Po = porion; Pog = pogonion; PNS = posterior nasal spine; Pr = prosthion; S = sella; TG₁ = inferior tangent point; TGₚ = posterior tangent point; TGₒ = constructed gonion.

may not appear patent on the radiograph if the patient was swallowing at the instant of exposure. The adenoids may be seen on the postero-superior wall of the nasopharynx but no firm conclusions should be drawn about the adequacy or otherwise of the airway from their appearance: even if they are large, the airway may be sufficient if the nasopharynx is wide, and if they seem to be small or absent, the airway may still be inadequate elsewhere (Montgomery *et al.*, 1979).

Cephalometric landmarks (Fig. 6.7)

The definitions assume that the radiograph is oriented with the Frank-fort plane horizontal. Many landmarks are bilateral but where the two sides are superimposed perfectly, only a single point is identifiable. Where the two sides are distinct, both should be traced and the midpoint taken as the landmark.

Anterior nasal spine (ANS)

The tip of the anterior nasal spine. This may be difficult to locate if a wedge filter has not been used to enhance profile detail. The spine must not be confused with the alar cartilages, which may be visible superimposed upon it.

Articulare (Ar)

The intersection of the posterior border of the neck of the mandibular condyle and the lower margin of the posterior cranial base. This constructed point does not exist and anatomically but is used to indicate the position of the mandibular joint relative to the cranial base. In some studies it has been used as an alternative to basion, which can be difficult to identify, in measurements of the cranial base; and others use it as an alternative to condylion in measuring mandibular length.

Basion (Ba)

The most posterior inferior point on the clivus (basiocciput). It lies on the anterior margin of foramen magnum and may be difficult to locate because it is overshadowed by the occipital condyles. It represents the posterior limit of the midline cranial base.

Centroid of the upper incisor root (C)

The midpoint on the root axis of the most prominent upper incisor.

Condylion (Cd)

The most superior posterior point on the head of the mandibular condyle. This point cannot be located reliably on a standard lateral skull radiograph because the shadow of petrous temporal obscures the condylar head. Articulare is often used as an alternative point.

Gnathion (Gn)

The most inferior point on the mandibular symphysis in the midline. It may be located by inspection or may be constructed as the intersection of the margin of the symphysis with the bisector of the angle between the facial line (N–Pog) and the mandibular line (TG–Me).

Gonion (Go)

The most posterior inferior point on the angle of the mandible. It may be located by inspection or may be constructed using the bisector of the angle between the ramal line (Ar–TG$_p$) and the mandibular line (TG$_i$–Me). The constructed point TG$_o$ may be used instead.

Incision inferius (II)

The tip of the crown of the most prominent lower incisor. In this text the point is also referred to as E – the lower incisor edge.

Incision superius (IS)

The tip of the crown of the most prominent upper incisor.

Infradentale (Id)

The intersection of the alveolar crest and the outline of the most prominent mandibular incisor.

Menton (Me)

The lowermost point of the mandibular symphysis in the midline. Where the chin is grooved, the most inferior points are bilateral but the midline contour can be seen slightly above them.

Nasion (N)

The most anterior point on the frontonasal suture. Where the frontonasal suture cannot be identified, the deepest point of the profile between the frontal and nasal bones should be taken. This is often slightly below true nasion and for consistency of identification might be a better point to use routinely. In dense radiographs, the anterior border of the nasal bone is difficult to see and care should be taken not to locate nasion too far back.

Orbitale (Or)

The most inferior anterior point on the margin of the orbit. Strictly speaking the left orbitale should be used for orienting the Frankfort plane but, unless there is a pointer to the lower border of the left orbit or a radiopaque mark is attached to the skin before the radiograph is taken, it is not possible to tell left from right and so the sides should be averaged. Orbitale is rather an unreliable landmark.

Pogonion (Pog)

The most anterior point on the bony chin.

Point A

This is also known as subspinale. It is *the most posterior point on the profile of the maxilla between the anterior nasal spine and the alveolar crest,* and is taken to represent the anterior limit of the maxillary apical base. It is difficult to locate reliably because the soft tissues of the cheeks may be superimposed upon it; and sometimes there is a ridge of bone passing inferiorly from the anterior nasal spine, which lies further forward than point A.

Point B

This is also known as supramentale. It is *the most posterior point on the profile of the mandible between the chin point and the alveolar crest.* It represents the anterior limit of the mandibular apical base.

Porion (Po)

The uppermost, outermost point on the bony external auditory meatus. This can be difficult to locate but it is on the same level as the upper border of the condylar heads, which may act as a guide if they can be seen.

Posterior nasal spine (PNS)

The tip of the posterior nasal spine. This may be obscured by unerupted molars in which case the landmark is constructed as the intersection of the line parallel to the nasal floor along the middle of the hard palate and the line perpendicular to it through the lower limit of the pterygo-maxillary fissure.

Prosthion (Pr)

The intersection of the alveolar crest and the outline of the most prominent maxillary incisor.

Sella (S)

The midpoint of the sella turcica.

TG_i

The inferior tangent point at the angle of the mandible. It is identified as the point of contact of the tangent to the angle of the mandible that passes through menton.

TG_p

The posterior tangent point at the angle of the mandible. It is identified as the point of contact of the tangent to the angle of the mandible that passes through articulare.

TG_o

The intersection of the lines Me–TG and Ar–TG. It is a constructed point that can be used as an alternative to gonion.

Cephalometric measurements

While cephalometric radiographs can be measured directly with computer-supported digitizers, most commonly the measurements are made on tracings. Both methods are subject to similar errors. Provided that due care is taken at each stage from positioning the patient to recording the measurements, errors should not be large. However, the validity and reliability of each measurement must be considered.

Validity is the extent to which the measurement represents the structure under consideration. If a measurement involves a landmark of questionable validity, it must be treated with caution. This problem has been discussed with the definition of landmarks. Measurements where the defining landmarks are not all in a plane parallel to the film are distorted according to the laws of perspective: linear measurements are foreshortened and angles are distorted (Fig. 6.8). If the lateral displacement of the landmarks is known, true values can be obtained but this is rarely done because most landmarks are difficult to identify on a PA film, and because it has become conventional cephalometric practice to use projections of measurements on to the film plane. Finally, where the relationship between pairs of points is measured as an angle subtended at a third point, or as the projected distance on to a line, variations in the position of the base point or line can give a misleading impression of the relationship of primary interest (Fig. 6.9).

Reproducibility is the closeness of repeated measurements of the same structure. This depends on a number of factors, including the quality of the radiograph, the clarity of the landmark and of its definition, and the skill and care of the observer. Some measurements, such as the angle SNB, should be highly reproducible because the landmarks are clear, while others such as SNA, where A may be difficult to locate, are less reliable. It is instructive for the clinician to trace the same group of radiographs on two separate occasions and to compare the reproducibility with results published by others (Gravely and Benzies, 1974; Houston, 1983) (Table 6.1).

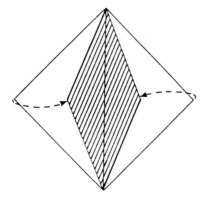

Figure 6.8 Effects of perspective. When a rectangle is viewed obliquely, the edges are foreshortened and the angles are affected according to the laws of perspective.

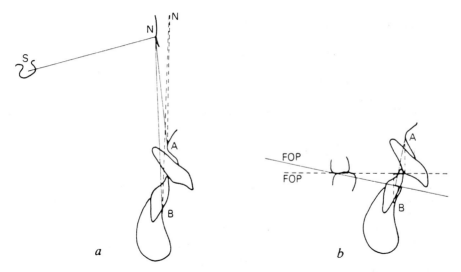

a *b*

Figure 6.9 Variations in a reference point or plane give misleading results.
(a) Anatomical variations in the position of nasion can affect the size of angle ANB
(b) Variation in the orientation of the functional occlusal plane affects the estimate of the skeletal pattern from projections to it.

Norms

If a measurement is to be intelligible, its average value and range of variation must be known. Most linear and some angular measurements vary according to age, sex and race and so for these, many different norm values are required. For this reason, most clinical cephalometric analyses use angular values that differ little with age or sex and so a single series of norms can be used for each racial group. The values used in this text are Caucasian and are derived from a number of groups of individuals with normal occlusions. Comparative values for some

Table 6.1 Cephalometric reproducibility – comparative figures

	σ	m
SNA	0.78	2.0
SNB	0.65	1.7
ANB	0.57	1.5
UI/Mx	2.23	5.8
Li/Md	1.68	4.4
MM angle	0.83	2.2

The sd of the measurement error for single readings (σ) in degrees determined by duplicated tracing (X_1, X_2), calculated from the formula $\sigma = \sqrt{\frac{\Sigma(X_1 - X_2)^2}{2n}}$, together with 1% confidence limits for single measurements (m). The values given are those for the best of three tracers reported by Gravely and Benzies (1974) and are based on a sample of cephalometric films selected at random ($n=100$).

Table 6.2 Some cephalometric norms for different racial groups

	Caucasian[1]		Negro[2]		Chinese[3]	
	Mean	SD	Mean	SD	Mean	SD
SNA	81.4	3.6	88.2	4.4	83.8	3.5
SNB	77.7	3.4	83.9	4.4	79.9	3.8
ANB	3.7	2.4	4.3	2.5	3.9	2.0
LI/Mn	94.7	6.5	101.2	7.0	98.4	7.6
UI/LI	125.5	10.0	112.8	9.5	121.7	7.8

[1]Data derived from: Riolo, M. L. *et al.* (1974) *An atlas of craniofacial growth,* Monograph No. 2, Center for Human Growth and Development, University of Michigan (sample: 12-year-old girls with no orthodontic treatment).
[2]Fonseca, R. J. and Klein, W. D. (1978) A cephalometric evaluation of American Negro women. *American Journal of Orthodontics,* **73**, 152–160 (sample: 40 adult women with Class I malocclusions.)
[3]Chan, G. K. (1972) a cephalometric appraisal of the Chinese. *American Journal of Orthodontics,* **61**, 279–285 (sample: 30 adult men with excellent occlusions.)

other racial groups are given in Table 6.2; 95 per cent of values lie within 2 sd of the mean (or average) and so measurements that fall beyond this range may be regarded as extreme.

Norms are of value in description, but they should not necessarily be taken as an indication of the need for treatment, nor as a treatment goal. Even in an individual with a good occlusion and a pleasing facial appearance, it is not uncommon to find several measurements at the limits of normal variation; and planning treatment to the average of a value, for example the inclination of the lower incisors, is no guarantee of stability.

Cephalometric measurements must not be evaluated singly and in isolation. It may well be the case that an extreme value for one measurement is compensated by variation in different structures. Thus true cephalometric analysis is the exploration of a pattern: how have the different dentofacial components fitted together to give the observed skeletal and occlusal relationships. Treatment is planned on the basis of

alterations of some of the components (generally dentoskeletal relationships) in a way that will harmonize with the overall facial pattern; and
that will give a result that is aesthetically and functionally acceptable
and will be stable.

Cephalometric analysis

Many different cephalometric analyses have been proposed. A number
of these are elaborate and the utility of some of the measurements is
obscure. Practical cephalometric analysis should concentrate upon features that have an immediate bearing on the orthodontic problem and
its treatment, and the clinical relevance of each measurement should be
clear. Cephalometric analysis may encompass: description of the dentofacial pattern; prediction of the changes that are expected to occur
with growth; prescription of treatment objectives; and retrospective
evaluation of growth and treatment changes.

It is desirable to avoid redundancy, but there is value in examining
some relationships in two different ways because, for structural reasons,
one measurement may be misleading. For example, the use of the angle
ANB to measure the skeletal pattern may be misleading because of
anatomical variation in the position of nasion (see Fig. 6.9); and an
independent measurement, such as the angulation of the line AB to the
occlusal plane, gives a useful check,

When two independent measurements reinforce one another, they
can be accepted with confidence; but when they do not, the reason for
any discrepancy must be sought. The cephalometric findings should be
integrated to give a coherent picture of the facial pattern of the
individual. An integrated approach to cephalometric analysis will be
illustrated by later examples, but first the individual measurements will
be discussed.

Descriptive analysis

Skeletal and dental relationships are generally measured by reference to
a point or plane. Variations in the position or orientation of the reference
structure can affect the measurement. It is important to recognize that
such structural effects can give erroneous results, which can usually be
discovered by looking at the general pattern of measurements, or by
making a separate assessment of the relationship in question, relative
to a different reference structure.

Lines of reference (see Fig. 6.6)

The true horizontal

If the patient can be posed with the head in the natural postural position
when the radiograph is taken, the true horizontal may be identified
(Solow and Tallgren, 1971). It is also possible to record this by attaching
radiopaque markers to the skin before taking the radiograph (Showfety,

Vig and Matteson, 1983). The problem lies in posing the patient reliably. The true horizontal would be particularly useful for the assessment of anteroposterior jaw relationships but, because positioning the patient correctly can be time consuming, this is seldom done. Attempts have been made to orientate cephalometric radiographs by reference to the semicircular canals of the vestibular apparatus, but these cannot be located reliably and so this approach has little application to clinical assessment.

Frankfort plane

This plane, which passes through porion and orbitale, was defined at a conference of craniometrists held in Frankfort (1884) as approximating to the true horizontal when the head is held in the normal postural position. It was designed to allow a comparison of the skulls of different species, and of races of man, and was subsequently adopted for use in cephalometric analysis. In fact, there is appreciable variation in the orientation of the Frankfort plane (up to 10° on either side of the true horizontal) and its identification on a lateral skull radiograph can be unreliable, owing to difficulty in locating its reference landmarks. However, it is one of the few planes that can be identified clinically as well as radiographically and so it can be useful in relating clinical impressions to radiographic findings, and in orientating profile photographs to match lateral skull radiographs.

Sella–nasion line

This line is taken to represent the anterior cranial base, which undergoes little change from growth or remodelling after about 6 years of age when the sphenoethmoidal synchondrosis fuses. This stable area is therefore valuable as a baseline in the measurement and comparison of jaw relationships between individuals and within the one case at different ages. A further advantage of this line is that the landmarks (S and N) are comparatively easy to locate reliably. Unfortunately nasion does not in fact lie on the anterior cranial base but at the outer limit of the frontonasal suture, which does remodel with growth. In most children, nasion drifts forwards along the original sella nasion line, but it can drift vertically and this will give an incorrect impression of the way the face has grown if serial radiographs are related to one another by means of this line (Fig. 6.10).

When jaw relationships are measured relative to the SN line, it is important to recognize that variations in its orientation and in the position of nasion in particular, can give a false impression of the true relationships (see Fig. 6.9).

De Coster's line (see Fig. 6.6)

This follows the floor of the anterior cranial base close to the midline from the anterior margin of the ethmoid bone to sella turcica. It passes along the cribriform plate of the ethmoid and the planum sphenoidale,

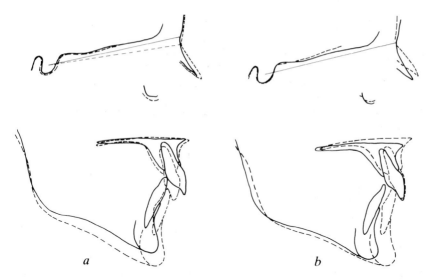

Figure 6.10 Superimposition of serial radiographs. (a) Superimposition on de Coster's line shows that nasion has drifted downwards with growth. (b) Superimposition of the same tracings on the sella-nasion line gives a different impression of facial growth in this case.

and includes the anterior wall and base of sella turcica. Little remodelling with growth takes place in the midline anterior cranial base after fusion of the sphenoethmoidal synchondrosis (Melsen, 1974) and so it is possible to use de Coster's line for the superimposition of serial radiographs taken after 7 years of age. Experience is required to do this reliably, and care has to be taken not to confuse the correct reference line with the roofs of the orbits or the crista galli, which may be more clearly visible on the radiograph. Minor remodelling changes do occur and so the comparison of serial radiographs taken more than 4 or 5 years apart must be undertaken with reservations.

Maxillary line (ANS–PNS)

The inclination of the upper incisors is commonly measured to this line. Where the anterior nasal spine curves upwards or downwards markedly, the maxillary line should be oriented parallel to the nasal floor (see Fig. 6.5) as is done when the posterior nasal spine cannot be seen.

Mandibular line

The inclination of the lower incisors is measured to the mandibular line; and its angulation to the maxillary line gives a measure of lower anterior face height. The mandibular line is defined in a number of different ways: the anterior landmark may be menton or gnathion and the posterior landmark may be TG_o or gonion. The measurements obtained will differ slightly according to the line used. The most convenient line, which is used in this book, passes through menton and TG_o.

Occlusal line

As with the mandibular line, several different definitions are found. Many authorities use the line passing midway between the tips of the mesiobucccal cusps of the upper and lower first permanent molars, and the lower incisor edges. This may give an unreliable assessment of the general line of the occlusion where there is a deep overbite.

The functional occlusal plane (FOP) is perhaps more useful for most purposes: it passes through the occlusion of the premolars or deciduous molars and the first permanent molars. The cuspal outlines of these teeth are often not clear and it may be difficult to locate the FOP accurately, particularly in the mixed dentition when only the first permanent molars may meet in occlusion.

It is important to recognize that whatever occlusal line or plane is used, its orientation may change with growth or treatment and so it is not an entirely satisfactory reference from which to evaluate other relationships.

The facial line (N–Pog)

This was used as a line of reference by Downs (1948) to help to assess the facial profile. The angle of the facial line to the Frankfort horizontal (the facial angle) indicates whether the profile is prognathic, retrognathic or orthognathic (the lower face is protrusive, retrusive or upright, respectively).

The line from point A to pogonion (A–Pog)

This line has been used in a number of cephalometric analyses to measure the anteroposterior position of the crowns of the incisor teeth. Williams (1969) stated that the best aesthetic results were obtained when the lower incisor edges lay on the A–Pog line; but it does not necessarily indicate a position of stability for these teeth. Many other cephalometric lines and planes of reference have been proposed, but in general they have little application to modern cephalometric analysis.

Measurement of skeletal relationships (Fig. 6.11)

Angle S–N–A (82±3°)

Prognathism of the maxillary apical base. The average value is 82° and a marked deviation from this usually indicates that either the position of nasion or the orientation of the S–N line is aberrant (see Fig. 6.9). Variation in the size of angle S–N–A is not usually important *per se* unless surgical change in the position of the maxilla is to be planned; but it should be taken into account when other measurements involving nasion, and in particular A–N–B are interpreted.

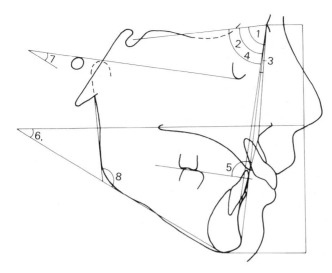

Figure 6.11 Cephalometric measurements of skeletal relationships. 1 = SNA; 2 = SNB; 3 = ANB; 4 = SNPog; 5 = A–B/FOP; 6 = MM angle 7 = FM angle; 8 = gonial angle.

Angle S–N–B (79±3°)

Prognathism of the mandibular dental base.

Angle S–N–Pog (80±3°)

Mandibular prognathism. It is interesting to compare the values of S–N–B and S–N–Pog. Where there is a well-developed chin but mandibular apical base retrusion, the facial appearance may be good although the apical base relationship is unfavourable, as is often the case in Class II, division 2 cases. Where S–N–Pog is smaller than S–N–B in Class II cases, the facial appearance is usually less good than the apical base relationship would suggest.

Angle A–N–B (3±1°)

The anteroposterior apical base relationship (skeletal pattern). Where the anteroposterior apical base relationship is favourable for a Class I occlusion, the A–N–B angle is usually in the range of 2–4°. However, apical base relationships beyond this range can be associated with a Class I occlusion if there is appropriate dentoalveolar compensation; and arch malrelationships occur even with favourable apical base relationships, where the inclinations of the teeth are unfavourable (Fig. 6.12). Following Angle's classification of arch malrelationships, the skeletal pattern is described as being Class I where the A–N–B angle is in the range 2–4°; and where the angle is greater than +4° or less than +2° as Class II or Class III, respectively (Fig. 6.13). As has been emphasized previously, the occlusal and skeletal relationships do not always match and they must be assessed independently of one another.

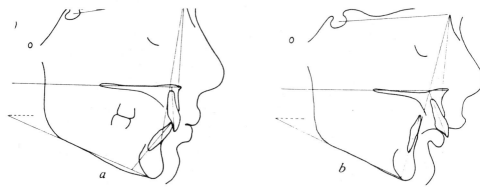

Figure 6.12 (a)Dentoalveolar composition. There is a Class II skeletal pattern (ANB = 6°) with the MM angle = 22°. The skeletal pattern is largely compensated by the proclined lower incisors (LI/Mn = 107°) and there is some compensation in the upper incisors (UI/Mx = 94°). The skeletal malrelationship is fully compensated and the incisor relationship is Class I. (b) Dentoalveolar exacerbation. The Class II skeletal pattern is moderately severe (ANB = 10°) and the MM angle is 25°. The overjet is even larger than would be expected from the skeletal pattern because the upper incisors are proclined (UI/Mx = 113°) and the lower incisors are retroclined (LI/Mn = 82°).

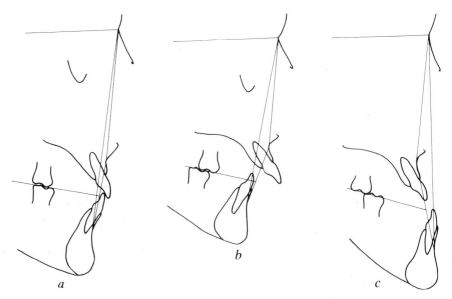

Figure 6.13 Different skeletal patterns. (a) Class I: ANB 2.5°, A–B/FOP 90°. (b) Class II: ANB 6°, A–B/FOP 100°. (c) Class III: ANB 7°, A–B/FOP 62°.

The value of A–N–B may be misleading where the position of nasion is unusual (see Fig. 6.9) and while a warning of this may be given by the value of S–N–A, this is not completely reliable.

Angle A–B/FOP (90±5°)

This measures the apical base by reference to the FOP. In a Class I skeletal pattern, the range is 85–95°. Clearly, variation in the orientation of the occlusal plane will affect this angle and changes in its size must not be taken as evidence of change in the skeletal pattern in treated cases where the orientation of the occlusal plane may have been altered.

If the FOP is to be used as a reference line, its angulation to the maxillary line should be checked: if this angle is within the range 6–14°, the orientation of the FOP is within 1 SD of the mean and it may be used with reasonable confidence to evaluate the skeletal pattern.

Harvold (1963) used the distance between the perpendicular projection of the points A and B on to the FOP to indicate the skeletal pattern, and this was subsequently adopted at the University of Witwatersrand and became known as the 'Wits analysis' (Jacobson, 1975). No figures for the range of normal variation were given and its construction is less convenient than the angle described above.

Maxillary–mandibular planes angle (Mx–Mn or MM angle) (27±5°)

This angle provides a measure of the divergence of the intermaxillary space anteriorly. Variations are usually attributable to the slope of the mandibular plane. The anterior intermaxillary height is of interest because if it is appreciably increased or reduced, there is often an anterior open bite or a deep overbite, respectively, and these being of skeletal origin can be difficult to correct. A high MM angle is often associated with a posterior pattern of mandibular growth rotation, and a low angle with an anterior growth rotation.

The size of the MM angle is, of course, largely determined by the ratio of anterior and posterior intermaxillary heights and so an independent estimate of the anterior intermaxillary height is desirable. This is provided by the ratio of lower and middle facial heights.

Face height ratio (Me–Mx/N–Me) (50–55 per cent)

This ratio is used to estimate the anterior intermaxillary height but it can, of course, be affected by variations in mid-facial height. When the MM angle and the face height ratio are inconsistent, they must be interpreted with caution and the reason for the discrepancy should be sought.

Frankfort–mandibular planes angle (FM angle) (27±5°)

This angle is highly correlated with the MM angle and there is little point in measuring both. The FM angle is less reliable, owing to problems in locating the landmarks that determine the Frankfort plane; but it does have the advantage that it can be measured clinically

Gonial angle (Ar–TG$_p$/TG$_i$–Me) (126±5°)

The slope of the posterior border of the mandibular ramus varies little and so this angle essentially measures the slope of the mandibular plane and is highly correlated with the MM angle. There is little value in measuring both.

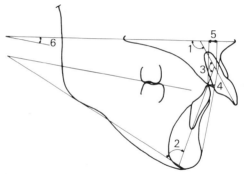

Figure 6.14 Dentoskeletal relationships. 1 = Upper incisor to maxillary planes angle (UI/Mx). 2 = Lower incisor to mandibular planes angular (LI/Mn). 3 = Interincisor angle (UI/LI). 4 = Lower incisor edge to A–Pog distance (E ↓ –A–Pog). 5 = Lower incisor edge to upper centroid projection (E ↓ C ↑). 6 = Functional occlusal plane to maxillary planes angle (FOP/Mx).

Dentoskeletal relationships (Fig. 6.14)

Upper incisor to maxillary plane angle (UI/Mx) (108±5°)

The orientation of the upper incisors is important functionally and aesthetically, and the existing inclination will determine the types of tooth movement that are required to correct any anomalies in the incisor relationships. For example, a case with a moderate Class II, division 1 incisor relationship is treated much more readily if the upper incisors are proclined than if they are retroclined. Further insight into the tooth movements required to correct incisor malrelationships is obtained from the edge–centroid relationships (see below).

Where there is an unusually large crown–root angle, this measurement may give an incorrect evaluation of the orientation of the incisor crowns, which is the important factor in appearance and occlusal relationships.

Lower incisor to mandibular plane angle (LI/Mn) (92±5°)

Although it is usually stated that this angle should ideally lie within the range indicated, it cannot be evaluated adequately without taking account of other variables. The average and range of variation given is appropriate only where the maxillary mandibular planes angle and skeletal pattern are within normal limits.

The labiolingual position of the crowns of the lower incisors and thus their inclination is influenced by the balance between the lips and tongue; when the lower border of the mandible is inclined steeply relative to the maxillary plane, there tends to be compensatory retroclination of the lower incisors, and vice versa when the mandibular plane is more horizontal than average (Fig. 6.15). Thus there is an inverse relationship between the size of the MM angle and the expected inclination of the lower incisors to the mandibular plane: for every

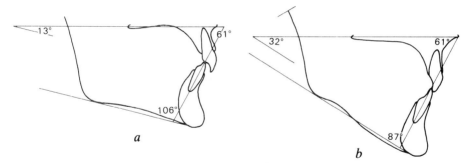

Figure 6.15 The inverse relationship between the lower incisor angulation and the MM angle. (a) The lower incisor angle is 106° (14° above the average) but the MM angle is 13° (14° below the average). The lower incisor angle is therefore considered to be 'normal' for this patient. (b) The MM angle is 5° above the average (27°) and so the lower incisor angle, which is 5° below the average, is considered normal for this patient. Note that the lower incisor to maxillary plane angle is 61° in both cases, which is average for this population group.

degree that the MM angle exceeds 27°, the expected value of the lower incisor inclination (92°) should be reduced by 1°; and vice versa where the MM angle is less than 27°. In order to avoid adjusting the lower incisor angle in this way, some authorities measure the inclination of the lower incisors to the maxillary or to the Frankfort plane, which does not vary with the slope of the mandibular plane.

Where there is a Class II or Class III skeletal pattern and the soft tissue pattern is favourable, dentoalveolar compensation is often found and so the lower incisors may be proclined or retroclined, respectively. This is, of course, a favourable feature and so the lower incisor angulation should not be interpreted without reference to the skeletal pattern. Formulae for the expected degree of dentoalveolar compensation according to the skeletal pattern have been suggested, but it is more instructive to assess this by taking account of the relationships of the lower incisor edge to the A–Pog line and to the upper incisor centroid, as described below.

Interincisor angle (UI/LI) (133±10°)

The interincisor angle is associated with the depth of overbite when there is incisor contact: if the interincisor angle is wide, then even if incisor contact is achieved during the eruption of the teeth or as a result of orthodontic treatment, they will tend to erupt past one another (Fig. 6.16) and the wider the interincisor angle, the deeper the overbite. However, the importance of a wide interincisor angle is greater in cases with a Class II rather than a Class III skeletal pattern (Fig. 6.16). In fact, it is the anteroposterior relationship of the incisor apices, rather than of the apical bases, that is important but this is not usually assessed in cephalometric analysis. A better and more direct assessment is given by the lower edge/upper centroid relationship, as described below.

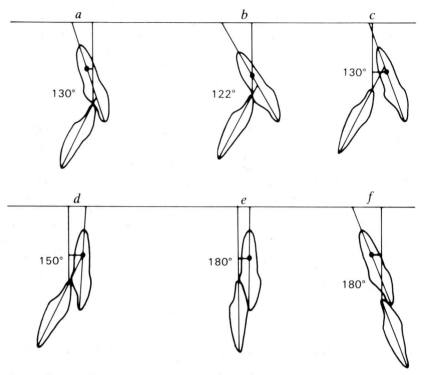

Figure 6.16 Interincisor relationships and overbite. The interincisor angle is given on the diagrams. (a) In a Class I incisor relationship with an average inclination of upper incisors, the lower incisor edge lies in advance of the upper incisor centroid and so the overbite is within normal limits. (b) In this Class II incisor relationship, the upper incisors are proclined and so the interincisor angle is reduced. E ↓ is directly below C ↑ and so provided that the tooth is tipped back around the centroid, the overbite reduction should be stable. For greater security of overbite reduction, C ↑ should be moved 1–2 mm palatally. (c) A Class II, division 1 incisor relationship where E ↓ lies well behind C ↑ . Simple tipping of the upper incisor will merely produce a Class II, division 2 incisor relationship, with a deep overbite. Stable overbite reduction depends upon a change in the E ↓ and C ↑ relationships. (d) A Class II, division 2 incisor relationship. Overbite reduction will be stable only if the E ↓ and C ↑ relationship can be changed. (e, f) In both these cases, the interincisor angle is very wide (180°). In (e), there is a Class II, division 2 incisor relationship with an adverse E ↓ C ↑ relationship. When the E ↓ lies in advance of C ↑ (f) then the overbite will not be deep, in spite of the wide interincisor angle.

Lower incisor edge to A–Pog distance (E ↓ A–Pog) (0–2 mm)

It is found that in well-balanced faces with good occlusions, the lower incisor edge lies on or close to the A–Pog line; and in treated cases with a skeletal malrelationship, the most satisfactory occlusal and aesthetic relationships are generally obtained when the lower incisors are in this position. In many cases with a favourable soft tissue pattern, this is also the position of lower incisor stability, which the teeth will have adopted naturally. However, this is not always the case and the A–Pog line should not be used to predict the position of lower incisor stability: it takes no account of soft tissue balance and its orientation is greatly influenced by the prominence of the chin. The A–Pog line does provide a measure of the extent of dentoalveolar compensation for skeletal malrelationships; and it can be useful to monitor the changes in the position of the lower incisor crowns that have occurred during treatment.

Lower incisor edge to upper incisor centroid distance (E ↓ C ↑ 0–2 mm)

This is measured as the distance between the perpendicular projections of the lower incisor edge and the centroid of the upper incisor root (Fig. 6.16) on to the maxillary plane (Houston, 1989). This relationship is closely associated with overbite depth in that the further behind the centroid the lower edge lies, the deeper the overbite is liable to be, except, of course, if the overbite is incomplete. The edge–centroid relationship allows for the influence on the incisor relationship of both the skeletal pattern and the lower dentoalveolar compensation. In planning treatment it focuses attention on the tooth movements that will be required to obtain a satisfactory incisor relationship, and in particular a stable overbite.

Functional occlusal plane to maxillary plane angle (FOP/Mx) (10±4°)

This measurement is correlated with the divergence of the intermaxillary space (MM angle). If it is beyond the normal range, the FOP must be used with caution as a plane of reference (e.g. in the A–B/FOP angle) because the result may give a misleading impression of the relationship that it is intended to measure.

Soft tissue analysis

Changes in tooth position have a small but variable effect on lip positions (Wisth, 1974) and one should be aware of this in planning treatment. For example, when upper incisors are retracted, the upper lip will drop back, more at the vermilion border than at the base, and the lip will tend to flatten. The form and position of the lower lip can alter markedly when a large overjet is corrected and it lies in front of the upper incisor rather than behind them. When a bimaxillary proclination is reduced, the lip protrusion is also affected, particularly in patients who previously had difficulties in obtaining a lip seal. Lip position always changes less than tooth position and the relationship varies appreciably in different individuals. The dentist should be aware of the relationship of the teeth to the rest of the face and to the soft tissues in particular.

However, people rarely see themselves in profile and are seldom viewed by others, except orthodontists, in this way; and so some of the features that are evaluated may have little impact on the patient in everyday life. There are a number of problems with soft tissue analysis. If cephalometric radiographs rather than profile photographs are used, the soft tissues may not be visualized readily unless a wedge filter has been used (see Fig. 6.4) and the patient may not have been posed correctly with the lips in their habitual posture. A major difficulty is that soft tissue assessment is purely aesthetic, and opinions differ as to what is acceptable: to one a slight fullness of the lower face may be pleasing, while to another this is considered unattractive.

The orthodontist's ability to produce changes in the soft tissue profile ' is strictly limited. Stability of treatment is imperative, and if it is acknowledged that facial growth cannot be controlled at will, the possible positions of the incisors are constrained by the skeletal relation-ships, by soft tissue balance, and by growth. Thus it is facile to base treatment planning on changes in soft tissue profile. Naturally the possible effects on lip form of any proposed changes in incisor position should be evaluated when treatment is planned; and if alternative approaches to treatment are feasible, this is a factor to consider in choosing between them. It should be remembered that published cases illustrating the importance of soft tissue planning are selected specially for that purpose and may not be typical results of the approach to treatment planning that is being advocated. In many cases, the major contribution to an improvement in integumental profile is growth and facial maturation. Soft tissue analysis has a more important role in planning surgical correction of skeletal malrelationships where there may be a wider choice of procedures and their effects on the integumen-tal profile are greater than with tooth movement by orthodontic appliances.

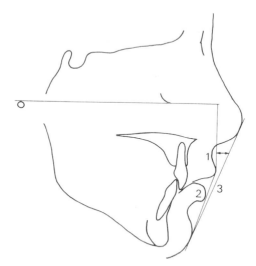

Figure 6.17 Soft tissue profile analysis. 1, the upper lip tangent is perpendicular to the Frankfort plane. The depth of the concavity of the upper lip should lie 1–4 mm behind this. In this case the upper lip curl is 3 mm. 2, The H (or harmony) line of Holdaway is drawn tangential to the upper lip and chin. The vermilion borders of the lower lip should lie within 1 mm of the H line. 3, The E (or aesthetic line) of Ricketts. The vermilion borders of both lips should lie close to this line. Note that during the later stages of facial growth, growth of the nose in particular carries the E line forwards so that the relation of the lips to it may well change after the completion of orthodontic treatment.

Many reference lines have been proposed for analysis of the integumental profile and some of these are shown in Fig. 6.17. They are an aid to description of facial appearance and of soft tissue change associated with growth and treatment. As explained above, they are of limited value in planning treatment, although manoeuvres that would cause deterioration in lip form should be avoided if possible.

Lines of reference (Fig. 6.17)

Upper lip tangent

This is a line perpendicular to the Frankfort plane and tangential to the vermilion border of the upper lip (Holdaway, 1983).

H line, the harmony line of Holdaway (1983)

This is tangential to the soft tissue chin and to the vermilion border of the upper lip.

E (aesthetic) line (Ricketts, 1957)

This is the line tangential to the tip of the nose and to the chin.

Measurements

Upper lip curl

The upper lip profile should be concave, the depth of the concavity lying 1–4 mm behind the upper lip tangent. This is a more useful measurement than the nasolabial angle, which can be misleading if the base of the nose slopes markedly.

Lower lip pout

The vermilion border of the lower lip should be close to the H line, and preferably within 1 mm of it.

Lips to aesthetic line

The vermilion borders of both lips should ideally lie close to the aesthetic line (Ricketts, 1957).

Practical cephalometric analysis

The evaluation of a single cephalometric film is concerned with description, prescription and prediction. Description involves comparison of the individual's values with cephalometric norms in order to build up a coherent picture of skeletal and dentoskeletal relationships. Inferences may then be made about the aetiology of the malocclusion: e.g. what is

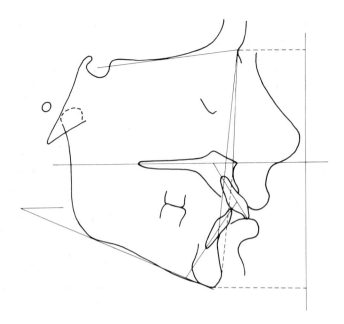

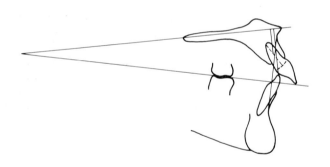

Measurement	Mean ± normal range	This case
SNA	82±3°	81°
SNB	79±3°	77°
ANB	3±1°	4°
A–B/FOP	90±5°	90°
MM<	27±5°	23°
Face-height ratio	50–55%	49%
FOP/Mx	10±4°	12°
UI/Mx	108±5°	121°
LI/Mn	92±5°	102°
UI/LI	133±10°	114°
EI–APog	0–2 mm	+1·5 mm
EICI	0–2 mm	+2 mm

the contribution of skeletal relationships and how much dentoalveolar compensation has taken place?

Prescription involves the planning of possible changes in incisor positions, together with an appraisal of their practicability and stability. This has to be done in conjunction with the clinical findings on such as the soft tissue pattern. Once the changes in incisor position and relationship have been decided, other tooth movements can be planned from the models and clinical findings. Prediction of the alterations that can be expected as a result of growth, and of the changes in tooth position that will be stable, is a necessary part of treatment planning.

All prediction involves a margin of uncertainty. As discussed in Chapter 8, the best guide to stability of the labial segments is the existing position of the lower incisors. Many attempts have been made to discover some reliable basis for individualized prediction, but without success. The best that can be done is to assume that the individual will experience average growth changes. Fortunately the facial pattern remains fairly stable with growth, and appreciable changes in jaw relationship are unusual, at least during a course of orthodontic treatment of average duration. However, it is important to be aware of the general trends of growth and to recognize whether these are liable to be helpful or otherwise (Chapter 4). For example, growth in facial height and forward growth of the mandible relative to the maxilla are helpful in Class II cases but adverse in Class III.

Practical cephalometric analysis is best described by applying it to a number of cases (Figs. 6.18–6.21). Many cephalometric analyses have been described but most have fallen into disuse. Downs' (1948) and Steiner's (1953) analyses are illustrated in Figs. 6.22 and 6.23. Simplistic analyses where one or two variables are considered to hold the key to the facial pattern are suspect; and analyses where measurements are used which have little obvious biological or clinical relevance are to be avoided.

Figure 6.18 A 12-year-old boy with a Class II, division 1 malocclusion. SNA and SNB are both within normal limits although slightly below average. The ANB angle is within the range of a Class I skeletal pattern. This is supported by the A–B/FOP angle at 90°. The orientation of the FOP to the maxillary plane is within normal limits.

The face height ratio and the MM angle are both a little reduced but again within normal limits. Thus the skeletal relationships do not impose limitations on the correction of the malocclusion.

The lower incisors are quite proclined at 102° to the mandibular plane: even allowing for the slightly low MM angle, the adjusted value is 98°. However, the lower incisor edge is only slightly in advance of the A–Pog line, indicating that they are quite well placed within the face and should allow a satisfactory position of the upper incisor edges following their retraction.

The upper incisors are proclined and, as is to be expected from the inclination of upper and lower incisors, the interincisor angle is reduced. The lower incisor edge lies 2 mm in advance of the upper root centroid which indicates that tipping the upper incisors about a fulcrum close to the centroid should produce a satisfactory incisor relationship. There is liable to be a slight residual overjet due to the proclination of the lower incisors, but this should not present problems of aesthetics or stability.

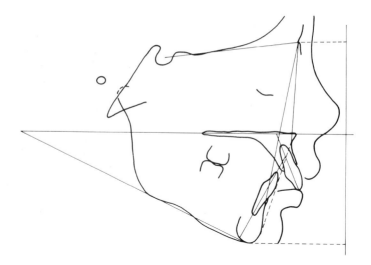

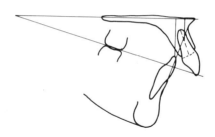

Measurement	Mean ± normal range	This case
SNA	82±3°	79°
SNB	79±3°	72°
ANB	3±1°	7°
A–B/FOP	90±5°	94°
MM<	27±5°	25°
Face-height ratio	50–55%	54%
FOP/Mx	10±4°	16°
UI/Mx	108±5°	113°
LI/Mn	92±5°	93°
UI/LI	133±10°	128°
EI–APog	0–2 mm	–2 mm
EⱮCↃ	0–2 mm	–5 mm

Evaluation of growth and treatment changes

When growth and treatment changes are to be examined, a comparison of the cephalometric measurements from the two radiographs gives a general impression of the changes that have occurred, but a detailed investigation requires direct superimposition of the tracings (Fig. 6.24). A valid superimposition can be undertaken only by using reference structures that have not changed during the interval in question, and these are few in number

In order to obtain a realistic impression of the changes of interest, an appropriate region of superimposition must be used. In order to examine the overall changes in facial pattern, superimposition on the anterior cranial base is appropriate (Fig. 6.24a). For a clear impressoin of changes in the intermaxillary space and in upper incisor position, superimposition on maxillary structures is required (Fig. 6.24b); while superimposition on mandibular structures will reveal details of the changes in position of the lower teeth (Fig. 6.25c).

Superimposition on cranial base structures

Superimposition on the S–N line with registration at sella usually gives quite a reliable picture of overall facial growth, but if nasion has drifted upwards or downwards with growth, a rotational artefact will be introduced (see Fig. 6.10), which will produce the greatest errors at the mandibular symphysis as this is furthest from the centre of rotation at sella (Baumrind, Miller and Molthen, 1976). Superimposition on de

---

Figure 6.19 An 11-year-old girl with a Class II, division 1 malocclusion. SNA and SNB are both reduced in value, SNB being particularly low; and the ANB angle is increased at 7°. As the angle SNA is reduced, the ANB angle may slightly underestimate the severity of the Class II skeletal pattern. The A–B/FOP angle is only slightly increased at 94° but this too underestimates the severity of the Class II skeletal pattern, because the FOP is rather steeply inclined. The skeletal pattern is definitely Class II and is more severe than the cephalometric measurements indicate, a conclusion reinforced by the clinical assessment. Lower face height appears to be close to average according to the MM angle and face height ratio.

The lower incisors are of average inclination but their edges lie a little behind the A–Pog line. Thus there is no lower incisor compensation for the Class II skeletal pattern. The upper incisors are a little proclined but the lower incisor edge upper root centroid relationship is very unfavourable at −5 mm. This will have to be corrected either by advancement of the lower incisor edges or palatal movement of the upper incisor roots, or a combination of both. Bodily retraction of the upper incisors to reduce the overjet completely would be technically difficult and would set the upper incisors rather far back in the face. There is probably not enough palatal bone at apical level to retract the incisors fully. The patient does not suck a digit and the overbite is incomplete so the lower incisors have not been restrained by either of these factors. It is possible that when a lip seal is obtained anterior to the upper incisors, the lower labial segment might be stable if advanced a little, but this is questionable. As this is an 11-year-old girl, the face is still growing and it is reasonable to hope that the skeletal pattern will improve. If facial growth were adverse, orthodontic treatment would be very difficult. If this were an adult patient, serious consideration would have to be given to surgery to correct the skeletal pattern, in conjunction with orthodontic treatment.

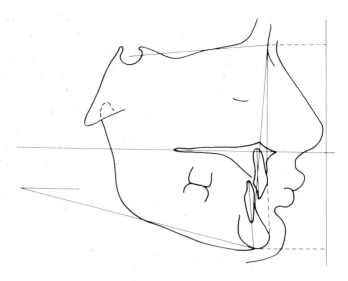

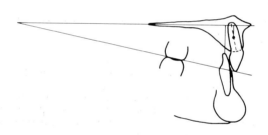

Measurement	Mean ± normal range	This case
SNA	82±3°	85°
SNB	79±3°	81°
ANB	3±1°	4°
A–B/FOP	90±5°	91°
MM<	27±5°	13°
Face-height ratio	50–55%	47%
FOP/Mx	10±4°	12°
UI/Mx	108±5°	93°
LI/Mn	92±5°	71°
UI/LI	133±10°	184°
EÌ–APog	0–2 mm	−10 mm
EÌCÌ	0–2 mm	−4·5 mm

Coster's line is more reliable, provided it is done with expertise. Various methods of relating the radiographic images by superimposition have been attempted, but tracing is simplest and is of sufficient accuracy for routine use. It is important that the tracing is done with great care, taking the precautions mentioned on pp. 83–84. The cortical plate of the basisphenoid in particular is quite thick, and so its periosteal surface should be traced. A good knowledge of skull anatomy is necessary and it is quite common to see tracings superimposed upon the roofs of the orbits, which do undergo periosteal remodelling. The most accurate superimposition is obtained by tracing the first radiograph and superimposing that tracing on the second film, registering the appropriate cranial base structures (Ekstrom, 1982). Although superimposition on cranial base structures is potentially very accurate, large errors can arise if it is not done expertly and this can give a very misleading impression of the changes that have in fact occurred.

Superimposition on maxillary structures

Unfortunately, the maxilla is subject to extensive periosteal remodelling and there are no really satisfactory stable sites for superimposition. The maxillary plane is often used but the hard palate descends by apposition

---

Figure 6.20 An 11-year-old girl with a Class II, division 2 malocclusion. SNA and SNB are above average and so the ANB angle may be biased towards Class II. However, it is still within the range of normal at 4°. This is supported by the A–B/FOP angle of 91° which is probably reliable because the inclination of the FOP to the maxillary plane is within normal limits. Thus the skeletal pattern is Class I. It is apparent from inspection that the chin is well developed and this could be confirmed by measuring the S–N–Pog angle.

The MM angle is very low and lower face height is slightly small relative to total face height, a common finding in Class II, division 2 cases. The lower incisors are very retroclined, particularly when the low MM angle is taken into account. Their expected inclination would be 106° (14° above average) but they are only at 71° to the mandibular plane. Thus the lower incisor edge lies far behind the A–Pog line. Given the well developed chin, it is not surprising that the lower incisors are behind the A–Pog line, but they are severely retruded. This is a very unfavourable position for the lower incisor edge, as is confirmed by the lower edge upper root centroid projection of −4.5 mm. This, together with the retroclination of the upper incisors and the large interincisor angle, explains the very deep overbite.

Treatment planning is difficult. It would not be possible to correct the incisor relationship by retraction and apical torque of the upper incisors: there is not sufficient bone palatal to the upper incisor apices. In addition, the incisors would be far too retruded within the face. It is possible that the lower incisor retroclination can be explained to some extent by unfavourable dentoalveolar adaptation during favourable mandibular growth: the lower incisors are trapped behind the upper incisors and even if the skeletal relationship had improved with growth after they had erupted, this would not be reflected by an improvement in the incisor relationship. If this had happened, some lower incisor advancement would be stable following a change in the upper incisor position, but this is difficult to quantitate. In addition, it is reasonable to expect favourable changes during further growth. Orthodontic correction of this incisor relationship is feasible only if the lower incisor edges can be advanced by several millimetres to a stable position.

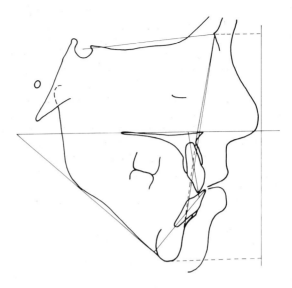

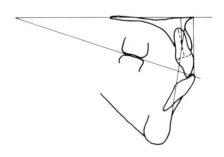

Measurement	Mean ± normal range	This case
SNA	82±3°	74°
SNB	79±3°	75°
ANB	3±1°	−1°
A–B⁄FOP	90±5°	81°
MM<	27±5°	41°
Face-height ratio	50–55%	57%
FOP/Mx	10±4°	18°
Ul/Mx	108±5°	99°
Ll/Mn	92±5°	90°
Ul/Ll	133±10°	131°
E↓–APog	0–2 mm	−8 mm
E↓C↑	0–2 mm	+6·5 mm

of bone on the oral surface and resorption on the nasal surface. This does not always take place uniformly along the length of the palate and so some rotational artefacts may be introduced by the use of the maxillary plane. However, at least where radiographs are taken within a few years of one another, these rotational effects are quite small and should not introduce serious errors. The other problem is the antero-posterior registration of the superimposition. Errors in this will give an erroneous impression of the tooth movements that have been achieved, and of the changes in the apical base relationship (Fig. 6.25). Commonly, the contour of the palate at the base of the alveolar process is used but, although this is not affected by tooth movements, it is a site of periosteal remodelling with growth and is not entirely satisfactory. Björk, on the basis of studies where metallic implants were inserted as markers in the jaws of children, found that the anterior surface of the zygomatic process of the maxilla is the one site in the maxilla that undergoes little periosteal remodelling with growth (Björk and Skieller, 1979). This structure is not always easily seen on a lateral skull radiograph, and it is much too short to provide a satisfactory base for superimposition. However, it can be used for anteroposterior registration of superimposition on the maxillary plane (see Fig. 6.24b). This is a registration requiring great care.

Superimposition on mandibular structures

Björk found that the mandible undergoes rather complex remodelling changes, which may be associated with anterior or posterior growth

---

Figure 6.21 A Class III malocclusion in a 9-year-old boy. There is no mandibular displacement on closure. There is a definite Class III skeletal pattern with an ANB angle of −1°. However, both SNA and SNB are below average and this probably means that the severity of the Class III skeletal pattern is underestimated by the ANB angle. The A–B/FOP angle is considerably reduced at 81° and, although to some extent this may reflect the steep cant of the FOP (18° to the maxillary plane), it still indicates a definite Class III skeletal pattern. The MM angle is very high and the lower face height is a larger than average proportion of total face height. This is not a favourable feature because it may mean that, with growth, the overbite will reduce and perhaps be lost altogether, which could prejudice the stability of any incisor correction.

The lower incisors are at 90° to Mn, but taking account of the MM angle, the expected value is 78° (92−14°) and so the lower incisors are very proclined. The upper incisors are a little retroclined and so there has been no dentoalveolar compensation for the Class III skeletal pattern. Retroclination of the lower incisors and proclination of the upper incisors could correct the reverse overjet without producing an unacceptable inclination of these teeth and, provided the overbite was maintained, this could be stable. However, the long-term stability depends on growth. A 9-year-old boy expects appreciable further growth. Vertical growth will tend to reduce the overbite and anterior growth will tend to exacerbate the Class III skeletal pattern, both factors that may lead to relapse in the incisor relationship. Even if the incisor correction were to remain stable, the aesthetic acceptability of the skeletal pattern would have to be assessed clinically. Treatment planning is difficult and this case lies at the limits of orthodontic treatability.

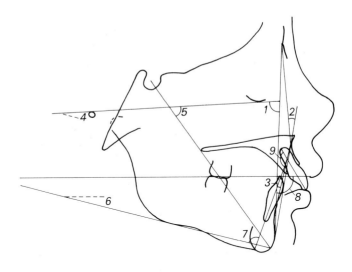

		Downs' norm		
		Mean	Range	This case
1.	Facial angle	88°	82–95	84
2.	Angle of convexity	0°	–8·5–10	15
3.	AB/facial plane	–5°	–9–0	11
4.	FM angle	22°	17–28	17
5.	Y axis	60°	53–66	57
6.	Cant of occlusal plane	9°	1–14	14
7.	1 to mandibular plane	91°	81–97	96
8.	1 to occlusal plane	105°	93·5–110	111
9.	Interincisor angle	135°	130–150	128
10.	1 to A-Pog	3 mm	1-5	10

Figure 6.22 Downs' analysis of case in Fig 6.19. The interpretation of the measurements is as follows. The facial angle towards the lower end of the normal range indicates a retrognathic lower face. The large angle of convexity (AB to facial plane angles) reflects the Class II skeletal pattern. The FM angle is low, indicating a reduced lower facial height but it is surprising that the cant of the occlusal plane is at the upper end of the norm range: with a low FM angle it could have been expected to be low as well. The lower incisors are proclined, as shown by their angulation to the mandibular and occlusal planes, reflecting mild dentoalveolar compensation for the Class II skeletal pattern. The upper incisor edge is far in advance of the A–Pog line but the interincisor angle is low, indicating that the overjet should not be reduced by tipping the upper incisor teeth palatally, because they would become too retroclined.

Note that this analysis leads to slightly different conclusions about this case than the recommended procedure (see Fig. 6.19), which gives a more useful insight into the cephalometric relationships.

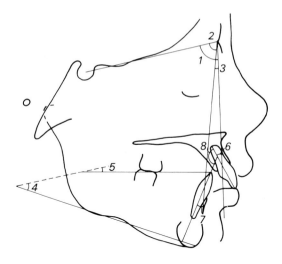

Measurement	Steiner norm	This case
1. SNA	82°	79
2. SNB	80°	72
3. ANB	2°	7
4. Go–Gn/S–N	32°	31
5. Occlusal plane/S–N	14°	12
6. 1̄ to NA	22°	27
	4 mm	6·5
7. 1̄ to NB	25°	18
	4 mm	3
8. Interincisor angle	131°	128

Figure 6.23 Steiner's analysis of case in Fig. 6.19. The low values of angles SNA and SNB reflect a retrognathic lower face and ANB shows that the skeletal pattern is Class II. The orientation of the mandibular plane (Go–Gn) and of the occlusal plane to SN are about normal. The upper incisors are slightly more proclined and a little more ahead of NA than the norm. The lower incisors are a little retroclined and fractionally retruded to NB. The interincisor angle is slightly low.

Steiner's analysis does not give as detailed a picture of dentoskeletal variables as is desirable. Measurement of the incisor position relative to the lines NA and NB is not sufficiently informative about their positions.

rotations (Björk and Skieller, 1972). However, he described a number of stable structures, the contour of the mandibular canal and the inner contour of the cortex of the mandibular symphysis being the most useful of these. This superimposition (Fig. 6.246) can be used to evaluate the remodelling in the mandible that has occurred with growth, and the changes in lower incisor position.

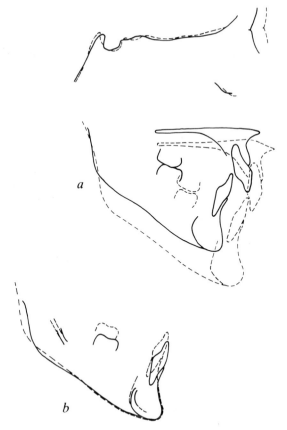

Figure 6.24 (a) Superimposition on stable structures gives a general impression of the overall changes in facial pattern that have occurred with growth. Here, nasion has grown forwards. The maxillary complex and palate have descended relative to the anterior cranial base, in part as a result of sutural growth, and in part as a result of periosteal drift. It is not possible to distinguish these contributions from this superimposition. The mandible has descended about twice as far as the maxillary complex and in this patient has grown forwards to a similar extent.
(b) Superimposition on stable structures in the mandible, in particular the inner cortex of the lingual and inferior border of the mandibular symphysis and the cortical outline of the mandibular canal. This reveals the periosteal remodelling that has occurred at the lower and posterior border of the mandible; and the amounts and directions of movement of the mandibular dentition.

Superimposition on maxillary structures is not very reliable and may be misleading (see Fig. 6.25). The palate has descended during growth as a result of periosteal remodelling and this superimposition does not reveal the full extent of eruption of the maxillary dentition.

Conclusion

Cephalometric radiography is valuable in dental and skeletal relationships in difficult cases. However, it should be used only to supplement the clinical examination, not as a substitute for a clinically based diagnosis and treatment plan.

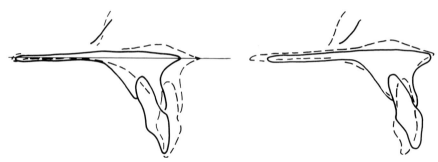

Figure 6.25 Incorrect anteroposterior registration of the maxillary superimposition gives a totally erroneous impression of the nature of any orthodontic tooth movement. Apposition of bone takes place both at ANS and at PNS. Registration at ANS gives a misleading impression of the amount of palatal movement of the upper incisors that has been achieved by treatment. Registration at PNS gives a misleading impression of labial movement of the upper incisor apices. These problems are compounded by the inferior drift of the palate which obscures the descent of the dentition that may have occurred during growth and treatment. Unless metallic implants have been placed in the maxilla prior to taking the first radiograph, it is not possible to be confident about the reliability of this superimposition where appreciable growth has taken place between registrations.

References

Baumrind, S., Miller, D. and Molthen, R. (1976) The reliability of head film measurements. *American Journal of Orthodontics*, **70**, 617–644

Björk, A. (1955) Cranial base development. *Americal Journal of Orthodontics*, **41**, 198–225

Björk, A. and Palling, M. (1955) Adolescent age changes in sagittal jaw relation, alveolar prognathy and incisal inclination. *Acta Odontologica Scandinavica*, **12**, 201–232

Björk, A. and Skieller, V. (1972) Facial development and tooth eruption. *American Journal of Orthodontics*, **62**, 339–383.

Björk, A. and Skieller, V. (1979) Growth of the maxilla in three dimensions as revealed radiographically by the implant method, *British Journal of Orthodontics*, **4**, 53–64

Broadbent, B. H. (1931) A new X-ray technique and its application to orthodontics. *Angle Orthodontist*, **1**, 45–66

Broadbent, B. H. (1937) The face of the normal child: Bolton standards and technique. *Angle Orthodontist*, **7**, 183–233

Brodie, A. G. (1941) Growth patterns of the human head from the third month to the eighth year of life. *American Journal of Anatomy*, **68**, 209–262

Downs, W. B. (1948) Variations in facial relationships; their significance in treatment and prognosis. *American Journal of Orthodontics*, **34**, 812–840

Ekstrom, C. (1982) Facial growth rate and its relation to somatic maturation in healthy children. *Swedish Dental Journal* (Supplement), **11**, 1–99.

Gravely, J. F. and Benzies, P. M. (1974) The clinical significance of tracing error in cephalometry. *British Journal of Orthodontics*, **1**, 95–101

Harvold, E. (1963) Some biologic aspects of orthodontic treatment in the transitional dentition. *Americal Journal of Orthodontics*, **49**, 1–14

Holdaway, R. A. (1983) A soft tissue cephalometric analysis and its use in orthodontic treatment planning, Part 1. *American Journal of Orthodontics*, **84**, 1–28

Houston, W. J. B. (1983) The analysis of errors in orthodontic measurements. *American Journal of Orthodontics*, **83**, 382–390

Houston, W. J. B. (1989) The incisor edge–centroid relationship and overbite depth. *European Journal of Orthodontics*, **11**, 139–143

Jacobson, A. (1975) The 'Wits' appraisal of jaw disharmony. *American Journal of Orthodontics*, **67**, 125–133

Melsen, B. (1974) The cranial base. *Acta Odontologica Scandinavica*, Supplement 62

Montgomery, W. M., Vig, P. S., Staab, E. V. and Matteson, S. R. (1979) Tomography: a three-dimensional study of the nasal airway. *American Journal of Orthodontics*, **76**, 363–375

Ricketts, R. M. (1957) Planning treatment on the basis of facial pattern and an estimate of its growth. *Angle Orthodontist*, **27**, 14–37

Showfety, K. J., Vig, P. S. and Matteson, S. R. (1983) A simple method for taking natural head position cephalograms. *American Journal of Orthodontics*, **83**, 495–500

Solow, B. and Tallgren, A. (1971) Natural head positioning in standing subjects. *Acta Odontologica Scandinavica*, **29**, 591–607

Steiner, C. C. (1953) Cephalometrics for you and me, *American Journal of Orthodontics*, **39**, 729–755

Williams, R. (1969) The diagnostic line. *American Journal of Orthodontics*, **55**, 458–476

Wisth, P. (1974) Soft tissue response to incisor retraction in boys. *British Journal of Orthodontics*, **1**, 199–204.

Chapter 7

Facial growth

The control of growth of an organism or tissue depends on the interaction between genetic (the genotype) and environmental factors. The result of this interaction is the phenotype. For cells, the environment includes all influences external to them, including tissue fluids and other cells. The genetic control of growth of one organ may influence growth of another and so some genetic factors act indirectly: they are known as epigenetic factors. The extent of environmental influences depends on the tissue under consideration and on the severity of these external effects; while the nature of response of the cells is genetically determined.

Any organ or tissue requires an adequate level of nutrition and an appropriate hormonal balance if growth is to be within normal limits: nutritional deprivation and hormonal deficiencies stunt growth. However, given favourable environmental conditions, many features of the individual are determined largely by genetic factors. For example, the ultimate stature of a child and its general physical constitution are affected little by normal variations in environmental conditions. However, other features (for example fat deposition and muscle growth) are very sensitive to environmental variation, although individual differences in response are under genetic control. Thus the observed charactristics of the individual depend on a complex interplay between genetic and environmental influences.

The elucidation of the relative importance of genetic and environmental factors is difficult and, in the field of craniofacial growth, many of the problems are still unresolved. Information has been derived from experiments on animals where the external conditions can be varied in a controlled manner and the response observed; from clinical investigations of the effects of different forms of treatment in children; and from studies of families and of twin pairs in an attempt to assess the hereditability of different features. A few of the obvious problems of interpreting such information are that findings in experimental animals may not be applicable directly to other species; human variability in growth makes the response to treatment difficult to discern; and in studies of the likeness of related individuals, environmental effects may be underestimated because the conditions within families tend to be rather similar.

The orthodontist is concerned with the interaction between genetic and environmental factors in determining facial growth for a number of reasons. If external factors have an effect on facial growth in general, and on jaw relationships in particular, they could be important in the aetiology of malocclusion, and interception and prevention would have to be considered. For example, in the past, the role of bottle feeding of infants and of oral respiration have been considered important in the aetiology of malocclusion. It is now generally recognized that factors such as these have little or no influence on jaw malrelationships. Of equal interest is whether orthodontic treatment, as an environmental factor, is capable of influencing jaw growth or relationships. Clearly if jaw growth could be controlled, the treatment of many malocclusions would be simplified. The question here is not whether jaw and occlusal relationships are normally under genetic control, but to what extent the normal controlling factors can permanently be overridden by orthodontic appliances. The fact that certain occlusal relationships have a high heritability does not mean that they cannot be changed by orthodontic means; and permanence of the induced changes depends on the degree to which the natural controlling factors can adapt to the new tooth positions.

The complexity of the interaction between genetically determined and environmental factors makes discussion of the control of growth confusing except for the simplest circumstances, and it is clearer to talk in terms of intrinsic and extrinsic influences upon growth. The level of interest may be the cell, the structured tissue, the functional region or the entire organism. When speaking of the organism, extrinsic factors include environmental factors such as nutritional availability and exercise. At cellular level, extrinsic factors comprise nutritional and hormonal variations and interaction with other cells, which may in turn be influenced by genetic and environmental factors.

Intrinsic control implies that given common extrinsic factors, variation between individuals or within the one individual are determined at that level. For example, the epiphyses of the short bones of the hand (see Fig. 7.3) grow by different amounts and fuse at different times, and these variations reflect differences in control intrinsic to the cartilages themselves.

In considering the extent to which a particular feature can be influenced by extrinsic factors, it is convenient to speak of the tightness of intrinsic control. Some features, for example blood groupings, are under tight intrinsic control at cellular level and are unaffected by even the severest environmental variations. At the other extreme are features that are more loosely controlled. Skin colour, at least in the white races, depends to a large extent on the amount of ultraviolet light to which it is exposed and a tan can be acquired or lost quite rapidly. However, different skin types respond in different manners to the same intensity and duration of exposure to light, and these differences are at least in part the result of intrinsic variation.

In considering craniofacial growth, the tissues of primary interest are bone and muscle.

Bone growth

Bone grows either by replacement of cartilage or by periosteal activity, and these two processes differ in the extent of their intrinsic control at tissue level. Experimental results suggest that the amount of cartilage growth is under rather tight intrinsic control. The most convincing support for this comes from experiments where bones have been transplanted into different sites (e.g. spleen or brain). Noel and Wright (1972) reported that when tail vertebrae from very young rats were transplanted, the amount of growth in length was at least as great as would normally have been expected; and Chalmers and Ray (1962) found that tibiae from young mice transplanted into immunologically compatible litter mates grew in length nearly to the normal extent. It might have been expected that transplantation would have impeded growth through interference with the blood supply and so these results indicate clearly that the amount of growth at epiphyseal plates is controlled primarily by factors within the cartilages themselves.

Epiphyseal bone growth is susceptible to some extrinsic influences: hormonal and nutritional deficiencies impair growth and it has been found that tension in the periosteum constrains epiphyseal growth to a small extent (Crilly, 1972). Presumably tensions in muscles, tendons and ligaments could have similar minor effects.

In contrast, periosteal activity is very susceptible to extrinsic influences. Pressure applied to the periosteum stimulates the appearance of osteoclasts and bone resorption occurs; whereas if the periosteum is pulled away from the bone surface, osteoblastic activity and bone formation follow. However, control of periosteal activity is not merely a simple matter of pressure and tension. Even under the one muscle attachment, adjacent areas of periosteum may be formative and resorptive. In order to maintain the form of a growing bone, complex patterns of periosteal bone formation and resorption occur and the mechanism of the control of these fields is obscure. Periosteum also responds to bone deformation. It has been known for centuries that a bone that had been fractured and healed in malalignment would gradually remodel towards its original form, and these observations were the basis of Wolff's 'Law of the transformation of bone', which stated in an abbreviated form that 'wherever in a bone pressure and tension stresses are caused, bone formation takes place; but wherever relief from pressure or tension occurs, bone substance disappears' (Enlow, 1968).

The link between the physical deformation of the bone and the biological response of the periosteum has been the subject of much speculation. Stress, strain and changes in surface curvature have all been suggested as crucial factors but none of these provides an adequate explanation (Wright and Yettram, 1979). It has also been suggested that changes in the surface electrical charge of the bone prompt the cellular response (Bassett and Becker, 1962). It is known that bone behaves as a piezoelectric material and that changes in surface charge do occur with deformation. A negative charge is associated with bone formation and a positive charge with bone resorption. It has also been found that the application of direct current to bone can promote remodelling and accelerate tooth movement (Davidovitch *et al.*, 1980), but whether this is a specific effect or merely the result of perturbation of cellular activity, as is also produced by magnetic fields, is not yet clear (Norton, Hanley and Turkewicz, 1984). A major problem with any theory that postulates that electrical phenomena are responsible for bone remodelling is that the electrical fields from normal muscle activity are much stronger than any that can arise from bone deformation (McDonald and Houston, 1990).

Sutures and periodontal ligaments can be regarded as periosteal modifications that respond to physical forces in a similar manner to periosteum: tension is associated with bone formation and compression with resorption, a phenomenon upon which orthodontic tooth movement depends.

Muscle growth

The diameter of muscle fibres is determined by the work they under-take, and muscular development can be achieved by the appropriate exercises. The length of muscle fibres is affected by the distance through which they habitually have to contract (Crawford, 1954). If the range of action of a muscle is increased experimentally in the growing animal, the number of sarcomeres in the fibres may be increased: sarcomere contraction is determined by their structure and thus the potential range of action of a muscle fibre is determined by their number. Fibres may be arranged in series and so the shortening of the muscle may be greater than that of the individual fibre. Growth in length of a muscle and the separation by growth of its bony attachments must be coordinated. In most muscles, the fibres at one or both ends have a tendinous attachment. This may be a well-defined tendon or aponeurosis, or it may be in the form of discrete connective tissue fibres attached to the periosteum. This tendinous attachment provides a means of adjustment during growth between the length of muscle fibre or muscle belly, and the distance between its bony attachments.

Growth characteristics of different tissue systems

Different tissues and organs exhibit different patterns of growth. The classic work on this topic was undertaken by Scammon (1930) who, on a cross-sectional basis, constructed growth curves for neural, lymphoid and general somatic tissues (Fig. 7.1). Most somatic tissues increase steadily throughout the period of growth, with a modest acceleration at the time of puberty and levelling off to a plateau soon after this. In contrast, tissues of neural origin such as brain and eyes are relatively advanced at the time of birth and reach a plateau soon after 6 years of age. This is relevant to growth of the calvarium and orbits because skeletal growth at these sites follows the pattern of growth of the neural tissues. Lymphoid tissues reach their maximum size in childhood and regress later. It is quite common, therefore, to find that partial nasal

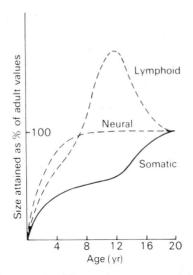

Figure 7.1 Growth curves for different tissue systems (after Scammon (1930)).

obstruction associated with adenoid enlargement improves during the adolescent period.

Growth in stature

Growth in stature has been investigated more thoroughly than has growth in facial dimensions, which follow a similar pattern. It is therefore useful to consider this first. Stature follows a general somatic curve of growth, with a steady diminution in velocity after birth except for a brief reversal during the pubertal growth spurt (Fig. 7.2). After the peak of the pubertal spurt, growth declines rapidly. This is relevant to orthodontic treatment in that some aspects, such as overbite reduction, are much simpler while there is still appreciable facial growth than after growth has ceased.

Pubertal growth spurt

On average, the peak of the growth spurt occurs at 12 years in girls and at 14 years in boys. There is, however, appreciable individual variation with a standard deviation of nearly 1 year (Tanner *et al.*, 1976). This means that in approximately 2 children out of 3, the growth spurt will occur within 1 year of the average time, and in 19 out of 20 it will occur within 2 years of the average. The growth spurt is a manifestation of physical maturity and attempts have been made to identify other aspects of physical maturity that would give a better guide to the timing of the growth spurt. Skeletal age, estimated from the developmental stages of the bones of the hand and wrist (Fig. 7.3), has proved to be useful in helping to predict adult stature but the correlation with the timing of

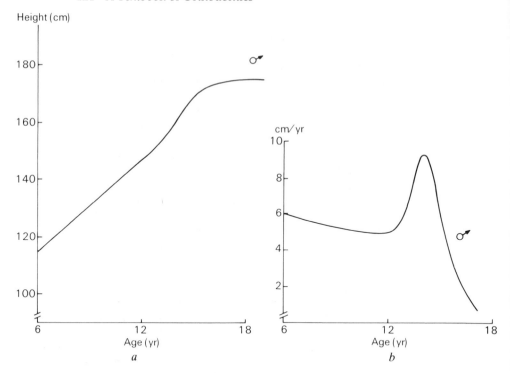

Figure 7.2 Growth curves for stature: (a) height gained; (b) velocity.

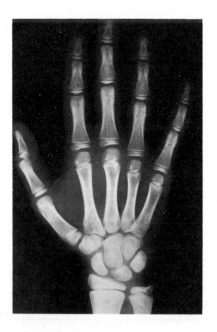

Figure 7.3 Hand–wrist radiograph.

the growth spurt appears to be rather low (Houston, 1980) and it is doubtful whether this offers a better basis for the timing of the growth spurt than does chronological age. Dental development is not correlated with the timing of the pubertal growth spurt and so it is not of predictive value. The secondary sex characteristics appear at the time of puberty but variations in their timing are not sufficiently well correlated with the timing of the growth spurt to be of practical predictive value. However, it has been found that menarche in girls and the change to adult voice characteristics in boys occur soon after the peak of the growth spurt and so these features can reasonably be used to indicate whether or not its peak has passed (Hägg and Tarranger, 1980).

It may be considered that there has been too much emphasis on the relationship of the timing of the growth spurt to orthodontic treatment. The relevant question in the treatment of patients where growth is important is whether or not an appreciable amount of growth can still be expected. Where growth would be helpful – such as in Class II cases where a deep overbite has to be reduced and where favourable growth changes might improve the skeletal pattern – it is probably best to proceed with treatment as soon as dental development justifies this. In most cases this will be when the upper permanent canines are just emerging. If dental development is retarded and the child has reached the average age of the peak of the growth spurt, treatment should be commenced in order at least to reduce the overbite while awaiting the eruption of more teeth. This is a problem only in severe Class II cases because milder occlusal problems can be managed without help from growth.

In some circumstances it is important to know that growth is virtually complete. Surgical correction of jaw malrelationships is usually delayed until after the pubertal spurt. In moderately severe Class III cases at the limits of orthodontic treatment, it may be best to delay orthodontic intervention in case unfavourable facial growth changes occur that would take the malocclusion beyond the bounds of orthodontic correction. In a patient showing signs of having passed the peak of the growth spurt (adult voice in boys/menarche in girls) and who is gaining height at less than 7 cm per year, it can be concluded that growth is almost complete. This can also be confirmed from hand–wrist radiographs showing fusion of the radial and ulnar epiphyses. Facial growth continues at a very slow rate well into adult life and may be responsible for minor changes in incisor crowding. However, this is not relevant to the timing of orthodontic treatment or of orthognathic surgery.

Skull growth

The calvarium

The calvarium comprises the bones and parts of bones that develop from the membranous coverings of the brain: the frontal, parietal and squamous parts of the temporals and occipital. In the fetus, ossification centres appear in the membranes covering the brain and the osseous

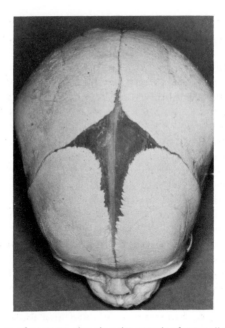

Figure 7.4 Calvarium of neonate showing the anterior fontanelle.

territories expand until they meet. Some of these forming bones fuse while others remain separated by sutures, which may usefully be regarded as periosteal modifications. At birth the bony covering of the brain is incomplete (Fig. 7.4) and the remaining membranous areas are known as fontanelles. The bone margins extend to cover the fontanelles during the first year. The factors determining the location and timing of fusion of the sutures are still obscure. The calvarial sutures lie over the different reflections in the dura mater and so tension in the membranous coverings of the brain during growth may determine suture location (Smith and Töndury, 1978). Premature sutural fusion occurs in certain developmental abnormalities (e.g. Crouzon's syndrome) and fusion can be precipitated experimentally by transplanting periosteum across the suture or by glueing the adjacent bones together (Persson *et al.*, 1979). However, the factors determining normal suture fusion are not clear.

Soon after birth, the bones of the calvarium are seen to consist of two plates the outer and inner tables, separated by cancellous bone – the diploäe. The inner table follows the contours of the brain while the outer table becomes elevated into ridges according to the functional demands made upon it: the temporal and nuchal crests provided extended sites for muscle attachment, although in man they are not very prominent; the mastoid process similarly provides a site of muscle attachment and the supraorbital ridges develop, possibly in response to the distribution of stresses in the calvarium generated by mastication and other muscular forces.

The calvarium is of little direct relevance to the orthodontist, but its structural and functional simplicity in comparison with other regions of the skull makes it a useful model in which to investigate sutural and periosteal growth; and findings from this region have been applied by analogy, though not always wisely, to growth of the facial skeleton.

It is helpful to consider skeletal growth in terms of functional areas rather than anatomically individual bones. The calvarium incorporates the squamous parts of complex bones that also contribute to entirely distinct functional areas, and the growth and control of these different parts of single bones is almost completely independent. Although the temporal bone has squamous and petrous parts, their functions and patterns of growth are quite distinct. The squamous part is more closely related to the other bones of the calvarium in its origin and control of growth than it is to the rest of the temporal bone.

There is good clinical and experimental evidence that the sutures of the calvarium have little if any independent growth potential: growth at the sutures does not force apart the adjacent bones but rather the suture responds to external forces separating the bones, which in the calvarium are provided largely by the increased volume of the brain and cerebrospinal fluid. Nature's experiments of hydrocephaly where the volume of cerebrospinal fluid is increased, and of microcephaly where brain growth is deficient, demonstrate how sutural growth is augmented or diminished, respectively. These conditions have been reproduced experimentally in animals, with similar effects on calvarial growth (Young, 1959); and it has been demonstrated that when sutures are transferred to non-functional sites, no growth occurs, while transplantation across an epiphysis results in growth in the suture to match that in the epiphyseal cartilaginous plate (Ryoppy, 1965). While growth of the sutural tissues may not be sufficient to generate the forces to separate the bones, the bone edges do have a certain independent growth potential: for example, when they are growing towards one another to form sutures, they do so at a rate greater than the separation of the bone edges due to brain growth, otherwise the suture would never be established!

The various ridges and surface modifications of the calvarium are the result of local periosteal activity. This is not a simple matter of muscular tension pulling out processes on the bone surface: the direction of growth is often opposite to that of muscle pull, and below a single area of muscular attachment, both apposition and resorption may be seen. Rather the expansion of the muscle seems to promote an expansion of the local periosteal area, with the production of crests and ridges accordingly. Where the outer and inner tables diverge appreciably from one another, the intervening area may be pneumatized as in the frontal sinus and mastoid air cells, which has the effect of maintaining strength without excessive weight.

The cranial base

The cranial base comprises the bones that originate from the chondrocranium of the embryo – the plate of cartilage that develops on the ventral surface of the brain. The bones that arise from this cartilage include the ethmoid, body of sphenoid, basiocciput and petrous temporals. The cartilages that remain between these bones – in particular between the body of the sphenoid and the ethmoid anteriorly, and the occipital posteriorly – form sites at which growth occurs by proliferation of cartilage cells. These cartilaginous joints, or synchondroses, are analogous to the epiphyses of long bones except that the growth plate is symmetrical, with cartilage proliferation and bone growth occurring on both sides.

The extent to which growth of the cranial base synchondroses is under tight control is still a matter of controversy, and the relative inaccessibility and complexity of the area makes conclusive experimental investigations difficult. However, the weight of evidence currently available suggests that they are comparable to epiphyses in that the control of the growth is under rather tight genetic control and they are not very susceptible to external influences.

The length and growth of the cranial base has an important effect on jaw relationships (Björk, 1955). The upper facial skeleton is related by its articulation to the anterior cranial fossa while the mandible, through the temporomandibular joint, is related to the middle cranial fossa. Growth at the synchondroses – in particular at the spheno-occipital synchondrosis – carries the maxilla upwards and forwards relative to the mandible and so contributes to the depth and height of the face (Fig. 7.5).

The spheno-occipital synchondrosis fuses at about the age of puberty (12–14 years), while the sphenoethmoidal synchondrosis fuses at 6–7 years of age (Melsen, 1974). This means that the floor of the anterior cranial fossa in the midline is rather stable from the age of 7 years and so provides an area within the craniofacial complex that can be used as a frame of reference for the superimposition of serial lateral skull radiographs of a child (Fig. 7.6). This gives a somewhat distorted view of the pattern of facial growth – for example the temporomandibular joint appears to be displaced downwards and backwards – and this should be remembered when comparing serial radiographs in this way.

The importance of cranial base growth is illustrated well in conditions where it is deficient. In the disorders known collectively as achondroplasia, the cranial base is short and so the maxilla is retruded. In most individuals with mandibular retrusion, it is found on average that the cranial base is longer than in groups with mandibular protrusion (Hopkin, Houston and James, 1968). In these cases, cranial base length is one of a number of factors that may contribute to the overall jaw malrelationship.

The facial skeleton

The facial skeleton serves a variety of functional requirements: vision, respiration, olfaction, mastication, deglutition and speech are only some of the functional demands on the facial region and it is not surprising that it is structurally complex. Growth has to be integrated so that none of the functional requirements is encroached upon.

In the neonate, the facial skeleton is a smaller proportion of the head

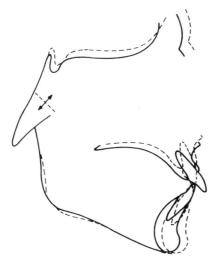

Figure 7.5 Growth at the spheno-occipital synchrondrosis carries the anterior cranial base upwards and forwards. The tracings are superimposed on the basiocciput. Solid line, age 12 years; broken line, age 15 years.

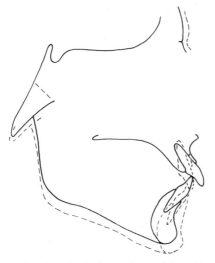

Figure 7.6 The conventional method of superimposition of lateral skull radiographs on the structures of the anterior cranial base gives the impression that the mandible is displaced downwards and backwards with growth. Compare this picture with the alternative superimposition of the same records given in Fig. 7.5. Solid line, age 12 years; broken line, age 15 years.

than in the adult (Fig. 7.7). This reflects the different pattern of growth of the calvarium, which follows a neural growth curve, and the facial skeleton, which follows a typically somatic pathway. Thus the face in the adult is considerably more prominent than in the young child. Within the face, the proportions change: the greatest amount of growth

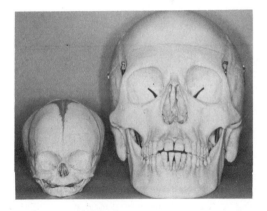

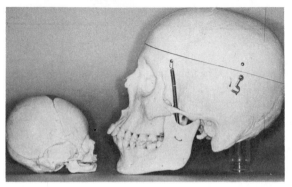

Figure 7.7 Neonate and adult skulls. Note the differences in the skeletal proportions.

is in facial depth and the least in width, so that on average the face becomes relatively longer and narrower.

In the neonate, the eyes are relatively large as they follow a neural growth curve and will grow less than will the rest of the face. Conversely the young child's nose is small and the adult form of nose is attained only after puberty. Jaw relationships also change with growth and this is discussed in the section on growth of the intermaxillary space.

Thus with growth, the character of the face changes in ways that are subtle and complex and which have a bearing on the appearance of the dentition. At the most obvious level, a child of 8 years of age with a good occlusion may appear to have teeth that are too large and prominent relative to the rest of the face. The face will continue to grow, however, and particularly with growth of the nose and chin, and maturation of the facial soft tissues, the teeth will become much less dominant.

Lip posture often changes at around the time of puberty. In many young children, the lips are parted habitually but most of them will maintain a lip seal after puberty. This may in part reflect differential growth in lip length and in lower face height, and in part a greater self-awareness with age. These changes can well affect the positions of balance of the teeth and this can be relevant when planning orthodontic treatment. For example, for the child with a Class II division 1 malocclusion, overjet reduction may not be stable at 9 or 10 years of age because the lower lip will not control the retracted upper incisors, but by 13 or 14 years of age the lip posture may have matured sufficiently to ensure stability.

The upper facial skeleton

The maxilla and other bones of the upper facial skeleton are related to one another and to the bones of the cranial base at sutures. The maxilla grows downwards and forwards from the anterior cranial base, in part by displacement with growth at the suture system, and in part by drift resulting from periosteal remodelling (Fig. 7.8).

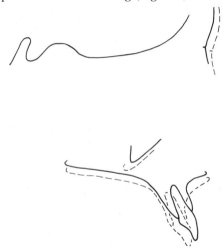

Figure 7.8 The maxilla grows downwards from the anterior cranial base, in part by displacement (growth at the sutures), and in part by drift (periosteal apposition and resorption of bone). Solid line, 12 years; broken line, 14 years.

The pattern of growth of the upper facial skeleton has been studied extensively by histological methods and by the use of serial radiographs of children where metallic markers have been inserted into the maxilla to act as fixed reference points (Björk and Skieller, 1977). Sutural separation continues until facial growth is nearly complete. In general, periosteal apposition of bone occurs on the outer and anterior surfaces of the maxilla, on the oral surface of the hard palate and at the alveolar processes, while resorption is seen on the nasal surface of the hard palate and on the walls of the maxillary antrum. This extensive remodelling means that there are no stable natural landmarks that can be used to relate serial radiographs of the one child in order to display the individual pattern of periosteal activity. Björk has reported that the anterior surface of the zygomatic process is relatively stable but this is too limited in extent to form a reliable area for superimposition (Björk and Skieller, 1977).

These studies with metallic implants have demonstrated that the pattern of maxillary growth may be more complex than had previously been thought. The downward displacement of the maxilla associated with growth at sutures may have a rotational component, which in turn is masked by periosteal remodelling and compensatory drift of the teeth. The determinants of sutural growth in the upper face have been a matter of much controversy. The classic view was that growth at the suture itself was responsible for the displacement of the maxilla and that, in this respect, sutures were akin to the epiphyseal plates of long bones. However, the appropriate comparison is with sutures of the calvarium, which, as already discussed, have virtually no independent growth potential: they are sites at which growth can occur, not centres of active growth (Koski, 1968). It is now generally accepted that the facial sutures are sites where growth can occur in response to separating forces generated elsewhere.

A major gap in our knowledge is the identification of the primary growth centres. The cartilaginous nasal septum has been implicated by several authorities (Scott, 1953). Early experiments where the nasal septum was removed surgically in animals showed major disturbance of upper facial growth, but there was also scar tissue formation and disruption in blood supply, which in themselves would affect skeletal growth. Subsequent, less traumatic experiments demonstrated that when the nasal septum is dislocated or partially removed, suture growth is reduced though not inhibited (Wexler and Sarnat, 1965). In children with clefts of the lip and palate, it is found that the lesser segment, which is isolated from the nasal septum, exhibits less sutural growth than would be expected normally, but growth is not inhibited. Growth of the eyeballs is important in growth of the orbit and if an eye is lost early, orbital growth is severely affected. there are probably also effects on the sutural growth of the surrounding bones, including the maxilla. Growth of the eyeball is nearly complete by 7 years of age, while sutural growth continues for a much longer period and so it could be a factor only in younger children. Suggestions have been made that nasal airflow has an important influence (for example, see Fränkel, 1980) but these have no scientific foundation. Indeed, in children with congenital nasal obstruction, upper facial growth is nearly normal and even in these children, any slight deficiency can not be attributed to the lack of nasal airflow (Freng, 1979).

It is probably a mistake to seek a single key factor as being responsible for upper facial growth: growth of the eyeball, of the nasal septum, of the sutural tissues and even tension within the muscles and fascia attached to the maxilla probably all play a part, the importance of which may vary from time to time and from case to case.

One of the reasons why the mechanisms controlling growth of the upper facial complex are of such interest is the possibility of growth being influenced by external factors or by treatment. It has been convincingly demonstrated in experimental animals that growth of the circummaxillary sutures can be reduced or inhibited by the application of distally directed traction to the maxilla (Elder and Tuenge, 1974): provided that the traction is of a sufficient magnitude to override the normal controlling mechanisms and is applied continually, it is hardly surprising that sutural growth should be prevented. Anterior traction can accelerate growth at the circummaxillary sutures and so increase the displacement of the maxilla relative to the cranial base (Nanda, 1978). Unless the growth of the basic controlling mechanisms is altered too, it must be anticipated that maxillary growth will rebound after removal of the appliances and this is indeed found.

Although there is much talk of the orthopaedic effects of extraoral traction to the maxilla in children, it is difficult to affect maxillary growth permanently to a clinically important extent. The extraoral appliances would have to be worn continually over an appreciable period of time, which is not generally acceptable socially. In children at the age when orthodontic treatment is usually undertaken, the amount of sutural growth is rather small and so, even if this were inhibited completely, the effects would be minimal. Significant sutural resorption is not likely to be obtained because of the complexity and large surface area of the sutures, and so appreciable retraction or advancement of the maxilla is not obtained, even with the most assiduous wear of the relevant appliances. As mentioned above, the small changes that are produced may well be lost by rebound unless treatment is continued until growth has ceased. A major practical problem is that the appliances have to be attached to the teeth, which move more readily than do the bones of the facial skeleton, and the amount and duration of extraoral traction that can be used may well be limited by the risk of unwanted tooth movements, particularly when anterior traction is applied to the maxilla. It has to be accepted that appreciable changes in maxillary position that might be desirable in a number of malocclusions, cannot be obtained in a child by orthodontic means. However, force systems that could result in unfavourable growth changes should be avoided.

The mandible

The mandible develops in membrane, in association with but not arising from Meckel's cartilage. Secondary cartilages do appear in the mandible, the most important of these being the condylar cartilage (Fig. 7.9). The classical view was that growth of the mandibular condyle was under tight genetic control and thrust the mandible downwards and forwards from its articulation within the skull. Many investigators disagree with this and argue this cartilage is more like a periosteal modification than a primary growth cartilage, and that growth at this site occurs secondarily to growth elsewhere carrying the mandible downwards and forwards (Moss, 1969). It has also been argued that control of growth does not lie within the condylar cartilage itself but that it is influenced by the actions of the adjacent musculature, and in particular by the lateral pterygoid muscle. At the present time, no conclusive evidence is available to settle this dispute. What is clear is that normal growth at the condylar cartilage

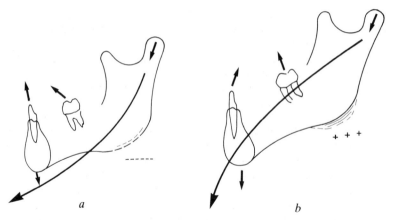

Figure 7.9 Growth rotations of the mandible occur when there is a discrepancy in the amounts of growth in anterior and posterior facial heights. The amount of rotation is masked by periosteal remodelling in the mandible and dentoalveolar adaption. (a) Anterior growth rotation; (b) posterior growth rotation.

is required if mandibular length and the relationship of the mandible to the upper facial skeleton are to be within normal limits.

The greater part of mandibular growth is the result of periosteal activity (Fig. 7.9) and much of this occurs in response to the functional demands of the muscles attached to the mandible. The coronoid and angle are muscular processes whose presence and development depend on the presence and development of the temporal muscle, and the medial pterygoid and masseter, respectively: in experiments in animals where the muscle is ablated or denervated, the corresponding muscular process fails to develop or is vestigial (Avis, 1961). The presence and growth of the alveolar process is dependent on the development and position of the teeth: in children with anodontia, there is no alveolar process; and following the extraction of teeth, the alveolar process is resorbed. The alveolar processes grow to keep pace with eruption of the teeth and when the teeth are moved by an orthodontic appliance, the alveolar process is remodelled accordingly.

The extent to which condylar growth can be modified in amount or direction by external influences is clearly a matter of clinical orthodontic interest. Destruction of the condylar cartilage as a result of infection or disease results in a very severe facial deformity because not only does the mandible fail to grow in overall length but it is attached to the temporal bone by the capsule, which may well be scarred. The facial deformity is much less severe if the mandible can be freed of such ankylosis because it is then carried into a more normal relationship with the upper facial skeleton by the musculature and other soft tissues (Rowe, 1983).

The cartilage of the mandibular condyle has been the subject of extensive study and widespread disagreement. Some have maintained that the condylar cartilage is comparable to epiphyseal cartilage of long bones in that the control of growth lies within the cells themselves. Others have pointed out that developmentally and histochemically the condylar fibrocartilage is very different from the hyaline cartilage of epiphyseal plates: it is a secondary cartilage and it is thus possible that the control of its growth is different.

It has been suggested by some authorities that the condylar cartilage is merely a local periosteal modification at the joint surface, and that its growth is controlled in the same way as is periosteum elsewhere. Experimental studies in animals have shown that cellular proliferation in the condylar cartilage can be influenced by appliances that displace the jaw forwards (McNamara, 1980); but it is in fact much more difficult to control its activity than in the case of periosteum, sutures or periodontal ligaments. The evidence suggests that while epiphyseal cartilages (and cartilages of the synchondroses) are under tight intrinsic control and periosteal activity is under rather loose intrinsic control, condylar cartilage lies somewhere between the two. Although claims have been made that condylar growth can be influenced in children by some types of appliance, the average changes reported are small and seem to be of questionable clinical importance. This may be because it is difficult to generate the stimuli that would be most effective in influencing condylar growth, and because orthodontic treatment is normally undertaken for older chilren where the major part of growth has already been completed and where the condylar cartilage is less responsive to environmental variation.

Growth rotations

The classical view of mandibular growth based upon the analysis of lateral skull radiographs is that it grows downwards and forwards relative to the anterior cranial base in a more or less linear fashion (see Fig. 7.5). However, Björk has shown that in many children, some degree of mandibular rotation occurs during its descent (Björk and Skieller, 1972). These findings were based upon examination of lateral skull radiographs of children who had metallic implants placed in the bone of the mandible to provide fixed reference points. The extent of rotation is masked by periosteal remodelling so that the mandibular plane appears to descend in a nearly parallel fashion (Fig. 7.9). Anterior rotations are more common than are posterior rotations but in most children they are small in amount. Rotations are important for their effects on normal occlusal development and because they may influence the ease with which overbite changes are achieved by orthodontic treatment.

Occlusal changes with mandibular growth rotations

Where there is an anterior growth rotation, and in the absence of compensating tooth movements, the lower incisors would become more retroclined within the face. However, dentoalveolar adaptation under

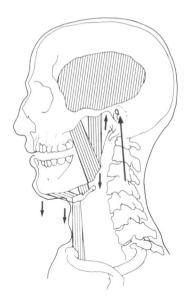

Figure 7.10 Growth of the cervical column means that the muscles and fascia between cranium and thorax stretch and this influences the level of hyoid bone and the mandibular symphysis.

the influence of tongue and lips results in a labial tipping of the incisors so that their inclination to reference lines within the upper facial skeleton is more or less maintained (Fig. 7.10). Full adaptation to the rotation may not occur because of contact with the upper incisors and because at the same time the mandible may be growing forward relative to the maxilla. When the mandible rotates anteriorly, the posterior teeth have an upward and forwards pattern of eruption, and particularly if there has been incomplete adaptation of the incisors, crowding will develop in the incisor region due to the shortening of the arch. With a posterior pattern of mandibular rotation, the incisors adapt by tipping back and, although the buccal teeth will have a posteriorly directed path of eruption, shortening of the arch again tends to occur, with crowding of the labial segment (Fig. 7.9). Thus mandibular growth rotations are one of the factors that contribute to the development of incisor crowding in the permanent dentition (Björk and Skieller, 1972).

Mechanisms of growth rotations

A mandibular growth rotation is merely a manifestation of a discrepancy in growth of anterior and posterior facial heights. Where posterior facial height increases more than does anterior facial height there will be an anterior growth rotation and vice versa (Houston, 1979). Growth in posterior facial height depends on the vertical components of growth at the condyle and at the spheno-occipital synchondrosis. Anterior facial height growth depends on the relative growth of the muscles of mastication, the suprahyoid muscles and the associated fascia. As the head is carried vertically by growth of the cervical column, the entire chain of muscles and fascia between the cranium and the thorax grows and stretches, and the bones forming links in that chain – the mandible and hyoid – descend relative to the cranial base (Fig. 7.10).

Growth of the intermaxillary space

The intermaxillary space lies between the maxillary and mandibular dental bases. Its dimensions depend on the relationship between maxilla and mandible. The teeth and alveolar processes grow vertically to establish an occlusion and this is maintained by continued dento-alveolar development as the intermaxillary space grows in height. Where the intermaxillary height is excessive, the teeth and alveolar processes may fail to maintain an occlusion (Fig. 7.11). Skeletal open bites of this

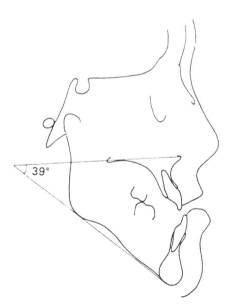

Figure 7.11 Skeletal anterior open bite. The anterior intermaxillary space is too great to be bridged by growth of the teeth and intermaxillary processes.

sort tend to worsen with facial growth and in the most severe cases, only the last standing molars will meet. Orthodontic correction is not usually feasible in these cases, because extrusion of the teeth may not be accompanied by alveolar bone growth, and so the periodontal support of the teeth would be reduced. In addition, these patients usually have incompetent lips and they would show too much tooth if they were extruded into occlusion. Surgical correction of the vertical jaw discrepancy is required in these cases, if they are to be treated at all.

As the teeth erupt into the intermaxillary space, they are guided towards one another by the tongue, lips and cheeks. Thus dentoalveolar compensation will often minimize any occlusal mismatch that would otherwise have arisen from variations in apical base relationships. The compensation may be inadequate to establish a normal occlusion where there are severe apical base discrepancies, and may break down altogether when the soft tissue pattern is unfavourable. for example in the child with a Class II skeletal pattern and incompetent lips, a Class II, division 1 relationship may be established, that is more severe than the dental base discrepancy because the lower lip fails to control the upper incisor position.

Prediction of facial growth

In certain cases, it would be useful to be able to predict the pattern of facial growth and the timing of the pubertal growth spurt. Jaw relationship can change appreciably during growth and, particularly for cases at the limits of appliance correction of their malocclusion, even minor changes in skeletal relationships may be important. The average tendency is for the mandible to become more prognathic than the maxilla, which is helpful in Class II cases but may make a Class III case untreatable, or may cause it to relapse. Currently available methods of growth prediction depend upon adding average increments of growth to the existing skeletal patterns. As the major part of facial growth has already been completed by the age that orthodontic treatment is usually started, and because most individuals do not differ greatly from the average in their growth pattern, this procedure gives a reasonably reliable estimate of future changes due to growth, in most cases. However, some cases differ appreciably from the average and it is in these individuals for whom growth prediction would be most important, that it is least reliable (Houston, 1979).

Growth changes during the average course of orthodontic treatment are not usually great enough to interfere with the outcome of treatment, and provided that good, stable occlusal relationships are established, dentoalveolar adaptation will maintain the occlusion in spite of minor changes in jaw relationship. It is normally prudent to plan treatment for Class II cases on the basis of the existing jaw relationship, and any growth changes that occur will usually be favourable and enhance stability. Orthodontic treatment is directed towards attaining specific occlusal goals, and the clinician will automatically allow for any growth changes during treatment, often being unaware of them and taking credit for favourable changes. Class III cases at the limits of orthodontic correction should be evaluated conservatively: growth changes in jaw relationships are often unfavourable and if this would prejudice the result, it may be more prudent to defer intervention until growth is nearly complete.

References

Avis, V. (1961) The significance of the angle of the mandible: an experimental and comparative study. *American Journal of Physical Anthropology*, **19**, 55–61

Bassett, C. A. L. and Becker, R. O. (1962) Generation of electric potentials by bone in response to mechanical stress. *Science (New York)*, **137**, 1063–1064

Björk, A. (1955) Cranial base development. A follow-up X-ray study of the individual varition in growth occurring between the ages of 12 and 20 years and its relation to brain case and face development. *American Journal of Orthodontics*, **41**, 198–225

Björk, A. and Skieller, V. (1972) Facial development and tooth eruption. *American Journal of Orthodontics*, **62**, 339–383

Björk, A. and Skieller, V. (1977) Growth at the maxilla in three dimensions as revealed radiographically by the implant method. *British Journal of Orthodontics*, **4**, 53–64

Chalmers, J. and Ray, R. D. (1962) The growth of transplanted foetal bones in different immunological environments. *Jornal of Bone and Joint Surgery*, **44B**, 149–164

Crawford, G. N. C. (1954) An experimental study of muscle growth in the rabbit. *Journal of Bone and Joint Surgery*, **36B**, 294–303

Crilly, R. G. (1972) Longitudinal overgrowth of children radius. *Journal of Anatomy (London)*, **112**, 11–18

Davidovitch, Z., Mathew, M. D., Finkelson, B. S., Steigman, S., Shanfeld, J. L., Montgomery, P. C. and Korostoff, E. (1980) Electric currents, bone remodelling and orthodontic tooth movement. *American Journal of Orthodontics*, **77**, 14–32; 33–47

Elder, J. R. and Tuenge, R. H. (1974) Cephalometric and histologic changes produced by extraoral high-pull traction to the maxilla in *Macaca mulatta*. *American Journal of Orthodontics*, **66**, 599–617

Enlow, D. H. (1968) Wolff's law and the factor of architectonic circumstance. *American Journal of Orthodontics*, **54**, 803–822

Fränkel, R. (1980) A functional approach to orofacial orthopaedics. *British Journal of Orthodontics*, **7**, 41–51

Freng, A. (1979) Dentofacial development in long lasting nasal stenosis. *Scandinavian Journal of Dental Research*, **87**, 260–267

Hägg, U. and Tarranger, J. (1980) Menarche and voice change as indicators of the pubertal growth spurt. *Acta Odontologica Scandinavica*, **38**, 179–186

Hopkin, G. B., Houston, W. J. B. and James, G. A. (1968) The cranial base as an aetiological factor in malocclusion. *Angle Orthodontist*, **38**, 250–255

Houston, W. J. B. (1979) The current status of facial growth prediction: a review. *British Journal of Orthodontics*, **6**, 11–17

Houston, W. J. B. (1980) Relationships between skeletal maturity estimated from hand–wrist radiographs and the timing of the adolescent growth spurt. *European Journal of Orthodontics*, **2**, 81–93

Koski, K. (1968) Cranial growth centres: facts or fallacies? *American Journal of Orthodontics*, **54**, 566–583

McDonald, F. and Houston, W. J. B. (1990) An *in vivo* assessment of muscular activity and the importance of electrical phenomena in bone remodelling. *Journal of Anatomy*, **172**, 165–175

McNamara, J. A. (1980) Functional determinants of craniofacial size and shape. *European Journal of Orthodontics*, **2**, 131–159

Melsen, B. (1974) The cranial base. *Acta Odontologica Scandinavica*, Supplement 62

Moss, M. L. (1969) The differential roles of periosteal and capsular functional matrices in oro-facial growth. *Transactions of the European Orthodontic Society*, 193–206

Nanda, R. (1978) Protraction of maxilla in rhesus monkeys by controlled extra-oral forces. *American Journal of Orthodontics*, **74**, 121–141

Noel, J. F. and Wright, E. A. (1972) The growth of transplanted mouse vertebrae. *Journal of Embryology and Experimental Morphology*, **28**, 633–645

Norton, L. A., Hanley, K. J. and Turkewicz, J. (1984) Biolectric perturbations of bone. *Angle Orthodontist*, **54**, 73–87

Persson, K. M., Roy, W. A., Persing, J. A., Rodeheaver, G. T. and Winn, H. R. (1979) Craniofacial growth following experimental craniosynostosis and cranioectomy in rabbits. *Journal of Neurosurgery*, **50**, 187–197

Rowe, N. L. (1983) Ankylosis of the temporomandibular joint. *Journal of the Royal College of Surgeons (Edinburgh)*, **27**, 167–209

Ryoppy, S. (1965) Transplantation of epiphyseal cartilage and cranial suture. *Acta Orthopaedica Scandinavica*, Supplement 82.

Scammon, R. E. (1930) The measurement of the body in childhood. In (ed. J. A. Harris, C. M. Jackson, D. G. Paterson and R. E. Scammon) *The Measurement of Man* University of Minnesota Press

Scott, J. H. (1953) The cartilage of the nasal septum. *British Dental Journal*, **95**, 37–43

Smith, D. W. and and Töndury, G. (1978) Origin of the calvaria and its sutures. *American Journal of Diseases of Childhood*, **132**, 662–666

Tanner, J. M., Whitehouse, R. H., Marubini, E. and Resele, L. F. (1976) The adolescent growth spurt of boys and girls of the Harpenden growth study. *Annals of Human Biology*, **3**, 109–126

Wexler, M. R. and Sarnat, B. G. (1965) Rabbit snout growth after dislocation of nasal septum. *Acta Otolaryngolica*, **81**, 305–313

Wright, K. W. and Yettram, A. L. (1979) Analytical investigation into possible mechanical causes of bone remodelling. *Journal of Biomechanical Engineering*, **1**, 41–49

Young, R. N. (1959) The influence of cranial contents on postnatal growth of the skull in the rat. *American Journal of Anatomy*,**105**, 383–409

Chapter 8

Treatment planning

Principles of treatment planning

Orthodontic treatment can be justified only when it is reasonable to expect that it will produce a worthwhile and lasting improvement in dental appearance and/or the health of the masticatory system. Thus the aims of treatment are to produce an occlusion that is stable, functionally adequate and aesthetically satisfactory.

Stability is a primary requirement and imposes limitations on the scope of acceptable changes in tooth positions. For example, proclination of lower incisors to correct a Class II incisor relationship, or expansion of the arches to relieve crowding might superficially seem to be attractive but in general will not be stable and so should not be undertaken except in special circumstances that are discussed in Chapters 10–13.

Whatever the reason for orthodontic treatment, it is important that the result is functionally acceptable. Premature contacts, non-working side contacts in lateral excursion and other potential causes of occlusal dysfunction should not remain after orthodontic treatment. Incompetent orthodontic treatment may create these occlusal anomalies and leave the patient worse off than before. With simple removable appliance treatment it may not be possible to correct all potentially traumatic tooth relationships, but provided that no new malfunctions are introduced and the expectation of future functional problems is remote, this may have to be accepted. However, where fixed appliance treatment is undertaken, care should be taken to correct functional malrelationships even if these were not the primary justification for the orthodontic treatment. It is not acceptable to deal with the post-treatment occlusal functional irregularities in the mixed and early permanent dentition by grinding the permanent teeth. Subsequent minor occlusal changes associated with continuing facial growth may well mean that the occlusal reshaping which has been undertaken prejudices the future functional status of the occlusion and of later occlusal adjustment that might be required.

Aesthetic considerations apply principally to the alignment and relationship of the labial segments. Particularly where there are severe incisor rotations or the overbite and overjet are greatly increased, correction may be difficult. Although the patient's main concern may be the appearance of the teeth, the requirements of function and stability must not be sacrificed to this. Where these three requirements are not mutually compatible, priority should usually be given to function and stability. It is important to recognize that a large number of malocclusions do not require treatment on the grounds of dental health. Hence, should the patient be unconcerned about his or her malocclusion it is acceptable in many instances to advise that no treatment be undertaken. This is particularly true of the mild malocclusoin where to effect any real improvement requires that almost ideal occlusion is obtained (Fig. 8.1). This is really possible only with skilful use of fixed appliances and assumes that the patient will cooperate fully

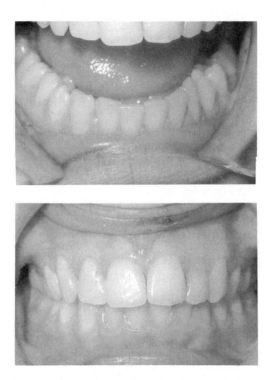

Figure 8.1 Minor malocclusions should be accepted. In this case perfection would need to be achieved to effect any real improvement in what is already a very acceptable occlusion. This patient requested treatment to align her mildy crowded lower incisors!

with treatment. Such cases will be successful in the long term only if there is neglible relapse after appliances are withdrawn.

Only in exceptional circumstances should permanent retention of an unstable occlusal result be planned as the culmination of orthodontic treatment. Permanent retention is acceptable in malocclusions associated with clefts of the lip and palate, and in other cases where a denture or bridgework that would be required to replace missing teeth can be used as an orthodontic retainer. In the adult, a deep and traumatic overbite that cannot readily be treated in any other way, or the drifting of teeth affected by periodontal disease and bone loss, may reasonably be stabilized with a permanent retainer. It may also be acceptable to apply permanent retention to the lower labial segment by means of a bonded lingual wire to preserve alignment of the lower incisors. This is because, even in the most expert hands, crowding in this region almost always returns (Little, Wallen and Reidel, 1981; Little, Reidel and Årtun, 1988). However, in general the problems of long-term appliances should not be underestimated. If plaque control is not of a high order, there will be a deterioration in oral health; and if the retainer is abandoned by the patient, rapid relapse of the corrected tooth positions can be expected.

Where permanent retention is to be employed and the treatment has been provided by an orthodontist it is essential to clarify who is to be responsible for checking and maintaining this. It may well be more convenient for the patient if the general practitioner is prepared to undertake this as part of routine care. The dentist will probably wish to have a set of post-treatment models and must understand the need to see the patient as a matter of urgency should the need arise. Otherwise it seems to us that the management of the retainer remains the responsibility of the orthodontist.

Timing of treatment

The age of 10–14 years is usually regarded as the optimal time for most orthodontic treatment. By this time the greater part of facial growth has taken place and the relationship of the arches is established and will be unlikely to change significantly. It is an advantage that at this age most children still have some facial growth to take place, which will assist in overbite reduction and spontaneous tooth movement. Increasing social awareness leads to good motivation, although by 14 years cooperation may become less certain.

After 14 years, treatment becomes progressively more difficult and it may be better to delay it until cooperation can be secured. In late adolescence the parents have limited influence over their children, who are particularly sensitive to the fads and fashion of teenage peer pressure. Oral hygiene may deteriorate and appliance wear become unsatisfactory for many months. From a technical point of view, growth is limited by this time. Cooperation tends to be rather less of a problem with fixed appliances but headgear and intraoral elastic wear may be far from satisfactory.

By the age of 18 or 20 years it will usually be clear from discussion whether or not the patient is prepared to wear the necessary appliances. However, treatment has to be undertaken without the benefit of facial growth. Overbite reduction in particular can be a problem. It is our view that except where very minor tooth movement is being undertaken (for example, before prosthetic or crown and bridge work), adult orthodontics should be seen as the province of the specialist.

An approach to treatment planning

There are really three stages in treatment planning, each containing several steps. These are:

1 *Treatment aims*
   a A decision on whether to treat or accept the malocclusion.
   b Determining whether the objective should be an ideal or compromise.

2 *Treatment details*
   c Estimation of the space requirement:
      i   lower arch (choice of extractions if required),
      ii upper arch (choice of extractions if required).
   d Indentification of the tooth movements required and appliances necessary to achieve these.
   e Determination of the final buccal occlusion desired and how this is to be obtained.
   f Estimation of the anchorage requirements and a decision on how this is to be obtained.

3 *Treatment time and prognosis*
   g An estimate of the overall treatment time (including an allowance for breakages, holidays and other untoward but inevitable delays in treatment).
   h The choice of retention regimen.
   i An estimate of prognosis for stability once appliances are withdrawn.

These steps are all to some extent linked and are not necessarily always carried out in this order. For example, having arrived at an estimate of prognosis for stability one might find that it is so poor that one decides to accept the malocclusion. Similarly, if a patient is not prepared to accept the need for fixed appliances at step (e) one could return to (b) and adopt a compromise treatment using removable appliances alone. The decisions for each of these three stages should be recorded and it must be emphasized that treatment planning must always be preceded by a thorough clinical examination, the findings of which should also be recorded as described in Chapter 5.

Ideal or compromise objectives?

It is often better to achieve limited treatment objectives that offer some significant improvement in a reasonable time rather than aim for the ideal and fail to achieve an acceptable result. There are some patients who, for example by reason of the distance thay have to travel or unwillingness to undergo fixed appliance treatment, may not be suitable candidates for ideal specialist treatment. For these a simpler treatment carried out by a general practitioner may be a suitable alternative. However, it is essential that a compromise treatment does confer benefit and does not leave the patient worse off in the long term; and such a decision must be by informed consent of the patient and parent and not influenced by a lack of skill on the part of the clinician. If there is any doubt as to whether such treatment offers a good prospect of improved social or dental health, it should not be undertaken.

Space requirements

The lower arch

It is good practice to consider the lower arch first. In most cases the size and form of the lower arch has to be accepted because teeth are in a position of balance between the labial and lingual musculature (Frölich, Thüer and Ingervall, 1991). This zone of soft tissue balance appears to be narrow and hence changes in lower arch form produced by orthodontic treatment are very liable to relapse.

In general the initial labiolingual position of the incisor teeth gives the best indication of their position of long-term stability and an attempt to alter this should not be made without good reason (Mills, 1968; Houston and Edler, 1990). Where a significant amount of space is required it will usually be necessary to extract permanent teeth; but with mild degrees of crowding there are several alternatives. First, the crowding can be accepted, although it should be borne in mind that it is sometimes difficult to align upper teeth satisfactorily around an irregular lower arch. Alternatively, where there is mild imbrication confined to the lower labial segment, the size of individual teeth can be reduced interdentally. This can be an acceptable solution in a caries-resistant mouth where the incisors or canines have broad crowns, the reduction of which will not pose a threat to the supporting interdental bone. Finally, where lower incisors are mildly imbricated and their alignment is to be part of the proposed treatment, it may be felt that permanent retention by means of a bonded lingual retainer is the only way of ensuring this in the long term (Little, Reidel and Årtun, 1988; Little, 1900). If such a course is to be followed and the crowding is only mild, such alignment can be achieved by proclination provided that there is no local deficiency in the labial attached gingiva, which might precipate gingival recession. It must be understood by all concerned (the patient, the parent and the referring dentist) that the teeth will always be in an inherently unstable position and therefore retention must be continued indefinitely.

Choice of extraction of teeth in the lower arch

Some teeth are inherently more suitable for extraction as part of orthodontic treatment. For example, it is usually undesirable to remove upper anterior teeth because of the effect on the appearance of the dentition. In many cases premolars will be the teeth of choice for extraction, both because their location in the middle of the arch is suitable for the relief of anterior and posterior crowding and because there are two premolars in each quadrant having very similar shapes. Thus there is little detriment to the contact of the remaining premolar

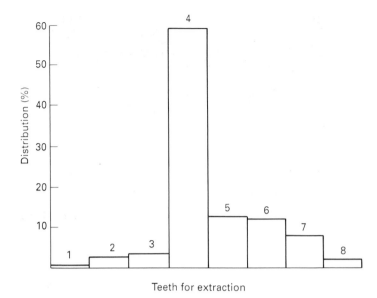

Teeth for extraction

Figure 8.2 The distribution of the choice of teeth for extraction as part of orthodontic treatment (after Bradbury (1985)).

with adjacent teeth. This preference for premolar extractions is clearly seen in Fig. 8.2.

There are, however, particular circumstances that justify the extraction of almost any other tooth.

Incisors and canines

The temptation to relieve lower labial segment crowding by extraction of an incisor or canine should be resisted except in a few well-defined circumstances. After loss of a lower canine, the contact relationship between the lateral incisor and first premolar is rarely satisfactory because of the shape of the crowns (Fig. 8.3). In general a lower canine should be extracted only when it is ectopic.

Loss of a lower incisor is often followed by a gradual decrease in lower intercanine width, with reappearance of crowding in the remaining lower incisors. To some extent, upper intercanine width is buttressed by the lower arch and so secondary reduction in upper intercanine width and upper incisor crowding may follow, particularly in the child whose face is still growing.

The circumstances in which a lower incisor may be extracted are where:

1 A lower incisor is of poor prognosis because of trauma, caries or gingival recession.
2 The lower labial segment is fanned with distal inclination of the canines and it would technically be very difficult to correct this by extractions further back in the arch. The most upright incisor should

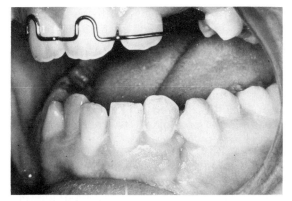

Figure 8.3 The contact relationship between a lower lateral incisor and first premolar is rarely satisfactory because of the shape of the teeth.

usually be selected for extraction so that the other teeth can be tipped into the correct positions.

3 Previous orthodontic treatment involving extraction of upper premolars has left a well-aligned upper arch and a good buccal segment intercuspation but unacceptable crowding of the lower incisors (Fig. 8.4) (in these cases, the lower incisors may be large relative to the uppers).

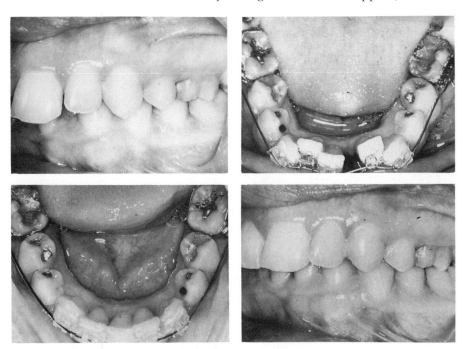

Figure 8.4 This adult patient had been treated by extraction of upper first premolars but the lower incisor crowding had subsequently become worse. Treatment involved the extraction of a lower incisor and use of a fixed appliance. The upper incisor spacing was closed with a removable appliance. Note that the overjet is still increased at the end of treatment.

4 A mild Class III incisor relationship with an acceptable upper arch, and lower incisor crowding: this is still usually better treated by extraction of the lower first premolars.

In all these circumstances, treatment should, if possible, be delayed until the patient has stopped growing and generally fixed appliance treatment will be required to align the lower teeth. Arranging four upper incisors around three lowers is often difficult and may necessitate the extraction of an upper premolar so that one canine can be positioned to occlude between the lower premolars. This in turn can mean that the upper centre line is displaced.

These difficult cases should, whenever possible, be referred to an orthodontic specialist because of the complexities of planning treatment, the technical difficulties and the uncertainty about long-term stability.

Premolars

First premolars are the teeth of choice for extraction to relieve lower labial segment crowding that is moderate to severe. Where the canines are mesially inclined, spontaneous improvement in lower incisor alignment will usually follow (Fig. 8.5). Space closure occurs most rapidly during the first 6 months (Berg and Gebauer, 1982) and will continue gradually for a number of years provided the occlusion allows this (Cookson, 1970; Persson, Persson and Skagius, 1989). In the growing child, with sufficient crowding, an acceptable contact will usually be

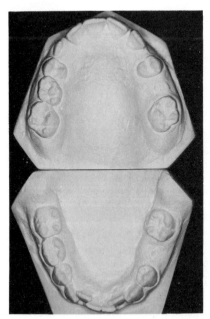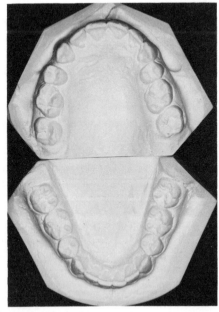

Figure 8.5 Where lower first premolars are extracted at the optimal time in a child and there is moderate crowding with favourably inclined teeth, alignment of incisors and closure of the extraction space may occur spontaneously to a satisfactory extent.

established between the canine and second premolar. Often there is some tipping of the canine and second premolar towards one another but, unless food packing occurs, there is no evidence that this is detrimental to periodontal health (Persson, Persson and Skagius, 1989).

Active alignment and space closure with a fixed appliance will usually be required (a) where lower canines are not mesially inclined; (b) where space requirements are minor; and (c) in adults. If an appliance is to be fitted, it is best not to delay this for too long after the extractions, because alveolar process resorption at the extraction site may delay tooth movement and there may be a permanent constriction of the process at that place (Fig. 8.6).

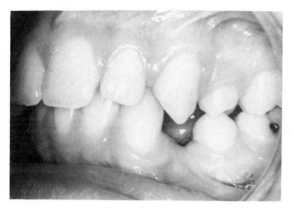

Figure 8.6 Where space closure has not rapidly followed extraction, alveolar bone resorption produces a constricted alveolar process, and space closure, even with a fixed appliance, is liable to be slow and more difficult.

Second premolars should be extracted when they are excluded completely from the arch. This may happen after early loss of the second deciduous molars, and the premolar will usually erupt lingually. Where there is more than 2–3 mm of residual space at the second premolar site, spontaneous space closure after extraction is usually rather unsatisfactory, with mesial tipping of the first permanent molar and disruption of the occlusion. Spontaneous alignment of the lower incisors is much less satisfactory than where first premolars have been removed.

On the other hand, with mild lower incisor crowding that is to be treated with fixed appliances, second premolars can be a good choice for extraction. Space closure can be completed by controlled forward movement of the lower molars, without the danger of unwanted retraction of the labial segment, which can occur in such cases where first premolars have been extracted. The presence of the first premolar anterior to the extraction site alters the anchorage balance in a way that favours closure from behind.

Second premolars should be extracted only where controlled tooth movement is to be undertaken with fixed appliances; except where they are completely excluded from the arch after early loss of deciduous molars, in which case they can be removed without affecting other teeth.

Molars

First permanent molars are seldom teeth of choice for extraction for orthodontic reasons because even when they are removed at the optimal time, the contact relationship between the second premolar and the second permanent molar is rarely ideal (Fig. 8.7) and can be poor (Fig. 8.8) (Richardson, 1983). The guidelines for management of cases where at least one first permanent molar is of poor prognosis are discussed in Chapter 9.

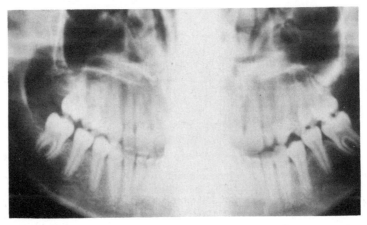

Figure 8.7 A good result after extraction of first permanent molars at an early age.

The extraction of lower second permanent molars has been advocated for a number of reasons, as follows:

1 *To relieve impaction of the second premolar.* Where the second premolar is slightly short of space due to forward drift of the first permanent molar after premature loss of the second deciduous molar, extraction of the second molar will allow the distal movement of the first molar (Fig. 8.9). This may occur spontaneously if a vertically impacted premolar forces its way in, or an appliance may have to be used to assist this tendency. Little, if any, relief of incisor crowding is to be expected in these circumstances; indeed the crowding may worsen as a second premolar erupts.

2 *To relieve impaction of lower third molars.* While the removal of a lower second permanent molar will usually allow the third molar to erupt, it will rarely come into an ideal position (Fig. 8.9) (Dacre, 1987). Guidelines

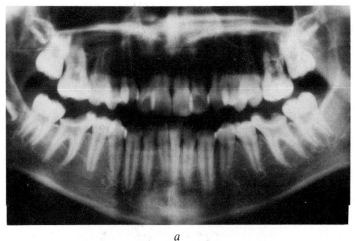

a

b

Figure 8.8 A poor result after late extraction of lower first permanent molars.

have been given based upon the radiographic appearance in the sagittal projection, which avoid the worst results (Cryer, 1967) but these are not to be relied upon (Dacre, 1987). The buccolingual and mesiodistal inclinations must be checked. The cuspal pattern on the radiograph will indicate whether there is an unfavourable lingual inclination of the tooth (Fig. 8.10). If the tooth is inclined mesially at more than 30° to the long axis of the second molar, the prospects of satifactory eruption are likely to be poor and extraction of the third molar is advisable. Spacing between the developing third molar and the second molar is a further unfavourable sign (Lawlor, 1978). However, even in the apparently ideal case, the third molar may undergo surprising changes in its inclination after extraction of the second molar (Fig. 8.11) and it may be necessary to institute local fixed-appliance treatment after it erupts to attain as good a position. For this reason practitioners carrying out lower second molar extractions should be well trained in the use of appliances that can derotate, upright and bodily advance lower third molars should this become necessary (Bishara and Burkey, 1986).

Thus, if the only problem is an impaction of the third molar, it is preferable either to leave matters as they are or to think in terms of removing the third molar itself (see below).

3 *To relieve minimal lower incisor crowding.* Occasionally minimal lower incisor alignment takes place spontaneously after the loss of second molars but the effect is almost always transient. As it is not generally practical to retract entire lower buccal segments, because of the difficulties of applying extraoral traction to the lower arch, it is unwise to rely upon any such improvement.

4 *To prevent lower incisor crowding.* There is evidence to show that patients who have had lower second molars removed suffer less lower arch shortening (and hence incisor imbrication) than those who have not (Richardson, 1983).

When, in spite of the problems mentioned, it is decided to extract the second molar, timing is important. If premolar crowding is to be relieved, the second molar should be extracted before the premolar becomes deflected lingually, which generally means as soon after eruption of the second molar as is convenient. If the extraction is delayed until after the third molar roots are more than one-third formed, the prospects for its satisfactory eruption are reduced.

Third molars are commonly impacted and have to be removed (Von Wowern and Neilsen, 1989). This can happen even when other teeth have been extracted. Impacted third molars have been implicated in the late crowding of lower incisor teeth, although the evidence is not clear-cut (see Chapter 3). If they are left until pericoronitis develops, not only may the patient be inconvenienced, but permanent bone loss and pocket formation may occur distal to the second molar. The conventional timing of extraction of a third molar is when two-thirds of its root has formed. Later than this, there is the danger of root dilaceration, which may make removal more difficult and may risk damage to the mandibular nerve if the roots are close to the canal. Earlier removal by a conventional approach is technically difficult because the tooth is almost spherical and rotates when attempts are made to elevate it.

It has been argued that if there is the risk that pressure from third molars may accentuate mesial drift of buccal segments and aggravate incisor crowding, they should be removed before root formation commences. Enucleation at a very early stage, when only the cusps have calcified, was suggested by Henry (1938). This has fallen into disfavour because it commits the child to surgery at an early age before it is possible to assess whether other extractions for orthodontic reasons would avoid the need, and even before third molar impaction can be predicted with confidence. Subsequently, Henry (1969) pioneered the technique of lateral trepanation, in which the completed crown of the tooth is removed by lateral approach. When undertaken by an oral surgeon experienced in this technique, it is safe and relatively atraumatic (Burgess, Houston and Howe, 1971) but it is not simple and has not been adopted widely. It is indicated only when it is quite certain that third molars will have to be removed at some stage and there are positive indications for early removal, for example a low impaction against the second molar where any root development could involve the mandibular canal. There is no evidence at the present time that removal at this rather than at a more conventional time prevents crowding of the lower incisors.

The upper arch

The upper arch should be built up around the lower. The aim in most cases will be to align the upper teeth with a normal overbite and overjet of the incisors. Provided that the lower labial segment is well aligned and matches the upper incisors in size (see p. 69), this should be possible if the upper canines occlude in the correct relationship with the lowers. In planning treatment, it is easy to estimate how much space will be required to permit this relation of the canines, allowing for any distal movement of the lower canine teeth required to relieve lower incisor crowding. If crowding in the lower labial segment is to be accepted, or if the upper incisors are large relative to the lowers, then either corresponding upper incisor crowding or an increase in overjet will have to be accepted. Conversely, if the lower incisors are spaced or the upper incisors are small, or if they are retroclined (see Fig. 12.3), it is not necessary to retract the upper canines as far as Class I to obtain sufficient space for the upper incisors to be correctly aligned.

As a general rule, in Class I and Class II cases, if lower buccal teeth are to be removed, teeth at least as far forward should be removed from the upper arch. Thus, if lower first premolars are to be removed, it will usually be appropriate to extract upper first premolars, but if lower second or third molars are to be extracted, there is a greater freedom of choice in the upper arch. The removal of lower second premolars should be accompanied by extraction of upper first or second premolars, the latter choice usually giving a situation that is easier to manage, at least with fixed appliances. These are guidelines only and should not be adhered to rigidly. Clearly they do not apply when a lower incisor or canine is extracted. In Class III cases, the reverse applies and it will usually be appropriate to remove teeth from the lower arch at least as far forwards as from the upper.

Spontaneous space closure afer extractions will usually take place only if the buccal teeth can come forward together (Persson, Persson and Skagius, 1989). Therefore, it is usually desirable in such cases to match extraction sites in the lower arch by similar extractions in the upper arch. Where fixed appliances are to be used, other factors such as the needs of anchorage may be more important considerations than the tendency for unopposed teeth to overerupt.

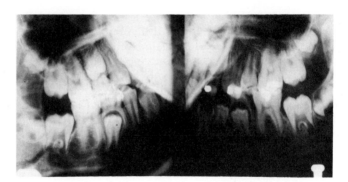

a

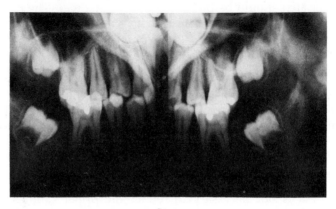

b

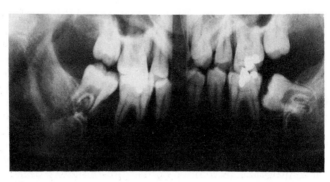

c

Figure 8.9 In this case it was considered that the slight lower buccal segment crowding could best be relieved by extraction of the second molars. One third molar erupted satisfactorily, the other failed to do so.

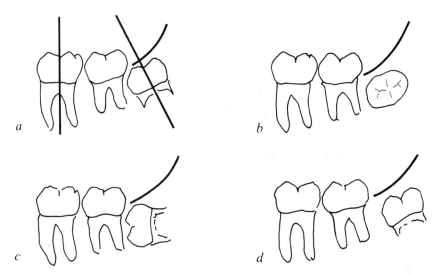

Figure 8.10 Different developmental positions of lower third molars. (a) This would be considered favourable for satisfactory eruption after second molar removal. A transversely positioned third molar (b) and a horizontally impacted tooth (c) should be removed surgically before root formation is complete. Where the third molar is spaced from the second molar (d), the prognosis for its satisfactory eruption after loss of the second molar is not good.

Choice of extraction of teeth in the upper arch

Incisors and canines

If an upper central incisor has been lost or irretrievably damaged, the space may be used to relieve crowding elsewhere and the lateral incisor on the side of loss can be crowned to simulate a central incisor (Fig. 8.12). It will not be possible to obtain an ideal result as the neck of the tooth is rather narrow, but this may sometimes be preferable to extracting another tooth to relieve crowding and fitting a prosthetic replacement for the lost incisor (see Chapter 9).

Where lateral incisors are peg-shaped or badly displaced and there is crowding in the labial segment, their extraction may allow alignment of the teeth with a reasonable appearance, provided that the canines are recontoured, just as can be done where lateral incisors are developmentally absent (see Chapter 9). This can offer a simple solution to the case where the upper lateral incisors are palatally displaced and the canines are erupting labial to them and are vertical or inclined distally (Fig. 8.13). The more conventional solution of extracting first premolars and using a fixed appliance to align the teeth may give an aesthetic result that is only marginally better in spite of the long and difficult course of treatment. Lateral incisors should not be removed where the canines would look unsightly adjacent to the central incisors because of their colour or form.

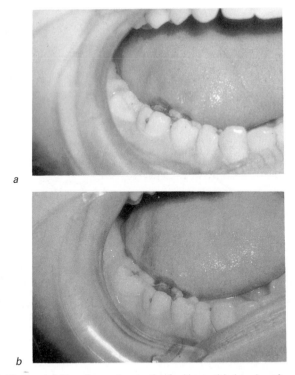

a

b

Figure 8.11 The variability of eruption path of a lower third molar after the elective extraction of a second molar. This patient, who originally had a Class II, division 2 malocclusion that had been successfully treated by removal of all four second molars and distal movement of the upper buccal segments (see Chapter 12), returned at 19 years with an impacted lower third molar. (a) At presentation; (b) after 9 months fixed-appliance treatment to upright the third molar.

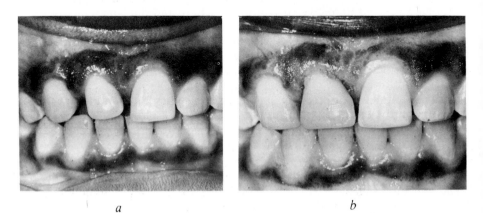

a   *b*

Figure 8.12 (a) After the loss of a central incisor, the remaining teeth were aligned and the lateral incisor moved into the centre of the residual space. (b) A temporary composite restoration suffices until a jacket crown can be made. Note that before the permanent crown is made the gingival level should be adjusted for a good aesthetic result.

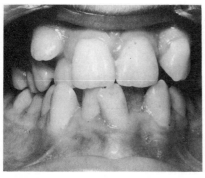
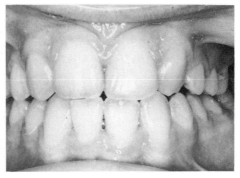

Figure 8.13 Very occasionally, the extraction of a poorly positioned upper lateral incisor provides a simple solution to an orthodontic problem. Note that in this patient there were originally only lower incisors and the lower central incisor was removed because of its poor position and lack of labial plate of bone.

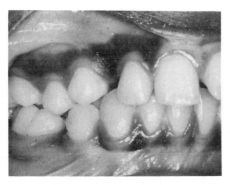
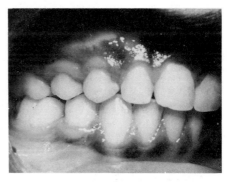

a   *b*

Figure 8.14 The extraction of a poorly positioned upper canine and closure of any residual space can give a good result.

The permanent canines are important teeth, and where possible should be retained. However, the upper permanent canines are not uncommonly ectopic and their alignment with orthodontic appliances can be difficult or even impossible. Sometimes transplantation of the canine is feasible (see Chapter 19), but if the situation is not favourable, the solution may be to extract the canine itself. Provided that the first premolar has erupted or can be moved adjacent to the lateral incisor so that its palatal cusp does not show and does not interfere with lateral excursions of the mandible, the result may be very good (Fig. 8.14). Certainly, it is a mistake to remove a well-positioned first premolar and then achieve only partial alignment of the permanent canine.

Premolars

First premolars are the teeth most commonly extracted to relieve appreciable upper labial segment crowding or to allow reduction of a

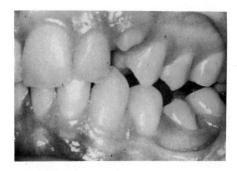
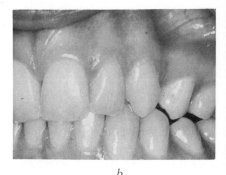

a   *b*

Figure 8.15 Removal of an upper first premolar at the optimal time allows satisfactory spontaneous alignment of a buccally crowded canine. In this case the canine became slightly more upright than the ideal but was quite acceptable without active treatment.

moderate or large overjet. Where upper canines have to be retracted by more than 3–4 mm, good results can be obtained after the loss of first premolars, more readily than by any other extractions. This also applies in Class I and Class II cases where space requirements are less but where it is necessary to extract lower first premolars to relieve lower arch crowding. The optimal timing of extraction of these teeth in crowded cases is as the upper canine teeth start to emerge (Fig. 8.15). Maximum spontaneous alignment and dropping back of the canines will follow. If the premolars are extracted earlier, it is difficult to be confident that the canines are mesially inclined, and unplanned space loss may occur. Delayed extraction of the premolar may well mean that the canine erupts along a forward path so that the position of the apex is less favourable, and spontaneous improvement and the ultimate position of the tooth may be prejudiced. On average, it takes 9 months from the emergence of the canine until it reaches the occlusal level. If space requirements are critical, a space-maintaining appliance should be fitted. If this is not done, the situation should be reviewed at 3-monthly intervals.

When upper second premolars are excluded completely from the arch due to forward drift of the first permanent molars after breakdown or early loss of deciduous molars, it will usually be best to extract them when they erupt palatally. The removal of upper second premolars to provide space for canine retraction with removable appliances is often rather unsatisfactory because the first premolar tilts and the first permanent molar rotates around its palatal root (Fig. 8.16). Generally, where removable appliances are to be used it is better to extract first premolars if an appreciable amount of space is required, or to retract buccal segments if space requirements are small. However, where fixed appliances are to be used and less than half a unit of space is required, excellent results can be obtained after loss of second premolars. Adequate space is provided for correction of the mild crowding and closure of residual space can be obtained without the risk of excessive

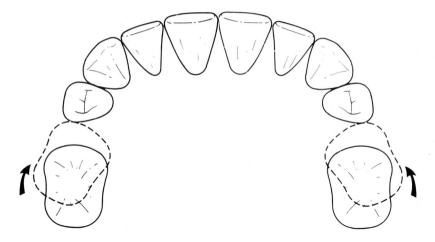

Figure 8.16 The extraction of upper second premolars should be reserved for cases where either this tooth is totally excluded from the arch or where fixed appliances are to be used to control the position of the adjacent teeth. Uncontrolled loss of the second premolar produces tipping and rotation of the first molar and first premolar.

retraction of the labial segments, which can sometimes happen when first premolars are extracted in mildly crowded cases.

Molars

Although the consequences of loss of first permanent molars in the upper arch are less serious than in the lower, these teeth should rarely be chosen for extraction unless one or more has a poor long-term prognosis. Guidelines for the management of cases where the extraction of first permanent molars is enforced are given in Chapter 9. In mildly crowded cases where less than 3–4 mm of space is required for the labial segments, good results can be obtained after retraction of the buccal segments. This is difficult when upper second permanent molars are erupting or have erupted, and is facilitated by their extraction. The retraction of first permanent molars to make space for crowded second premolars is also simpler when the second molars have been removed., Provided that the upper third molars are of good size and are favourably positioned, they will usually erupt satisfactorily after the loss of the upper second permanent molars. The exraction of upper second per-manent molars is contraindicated when the upper third molars are absent and where lower arch crowding is to be treated by the extraction of premolars. A successful combination can be the loss of lower third molars and upper second molars. This can leave the lower second molars unopposed but they will not overerupt provided that the upper first molars are moved back into the correct occlusal relationship with them. In due course, the upper third molars will erupt into occlusion.

Upper third molars are frequently short of space where no other upper extractions have been undertaken. They rarely give rise to problems but will usually erupt buccally and distally inclined, when they can be extracted. There is generally little advantage in removing them before they erupt and their proximity to the maxillary antrum can make this hazardous.

Coordination of extraction sites

Lower arch first

Look at the lower arch to decide whether extractions are indicated or whether the alignment is acceptable. It is necessary to allow for posterior crowding and for the fact that lower arch crowding may get significantly worse with growth. This change is particularly marked during the pubertal growth of boys between 13 and 16 years. In cases suitable for treatment by the general dental practitioner, the labiolingual position of the lower incisors should not be deliberately altered. Where there is moderate lower incisor crowding in a growing patient, instanding or labially placed incisors can be expected to align spontaneously after extraction of premolar for the relief of crowding. On the other hand, any appliance that might advance the lower labial segment or expand the lower intercanine distance should be avoided because such changes are not stable in the majority of cases.

Upper arch

In order to have enough space to reduce any overjet and relieve crowding, the easiest guide is to ensure that there is enough room (with or without extraction) to retract the upper canines into their correct Class I articulation with their opponents. Allowance has to be made for any pre-existing crowding in the lower labial segment (Fig. 8.17). This means imagining where the lower canines will be when any lower incisor crowding has been relieved before matching the position of the upper canines to these corrected positions. Clearly this guide only applies if all teeth in the labial segments are present and of normal size – i.e. beware of missing lower incisors and small upper lateral incisors.

Tooth movements required

It is best to list the precise movements required and then to determine whether the case requires appliances and whether these are of the fixed or removable type.

Spontaneous changes

Mesially inclined canines will usually spontaneously drop distally to some extent once space is available, provided (a) they are still erupting, and (b) there is no occlusal interference. This tendency is especially marked in the lower arch but declines rapidly in the first few months after extraction of the first premolars. Certainly it is unusual to see any significant change in the alignment of the labial segment beyond 6 months after extraction (Berg and Gebauer, 1982; Stephens, 1983). Although lower incisors tend to align as the canines drift distally, rotated incisors rarely improve (Creekmore, 1982) and it is only labid-lingual displacements that can be relied on to do so. In the upper arch, spontaneous alignment of crowded incisors is minimal.

The only other change that can be relied upon is the tendency for extraction spaces to close (Cookson, 1970; Stephens, 1983). Despite frequent talk of 'dumping' and 'collapse' into extraction spaces, provided a good molar occlusion is established first, the premolar space closure achieved in this way is accomplished with minimal changes in the axial changes of the adjacent teeth. It must be remembered that this is a growth related change (Stephens and Houston, 1985) and that in the postpubertal patient (after 14 years in girls and 16 years in boys), such space closure will be very slow to take place and will usually be incomplete.

Removable appliances (see Chapter 15)

These are suitable for tipping movements so the axial inclination of teeth adjacent to extraction sites should be carefully assessed. Single-rooted teeth tip about points close to the centroid of the root so that an estimate of their likely final angulation can be made from the study models. Upper removable appliances are very effective space maintainers provided they are worn conscientiously and are particularly suitable for the case in which upper premolars have been removed to allow a buccally crowded canine to improve as it erupts. In such cases it is then a simple matter to add a spring to the appliance should complete alignment not be achieved spontaneously.

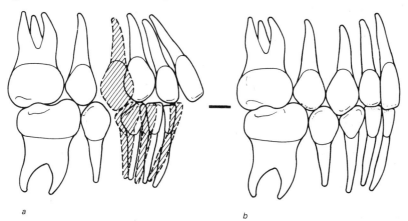

a   b

Figure 8.17 (a) When applying the 'canine rule' to determine space required in the upper arch, allowance must first be made for any lower anterior crowding. (b) In non-extraction cases and 4-unit extraction cases, where it is intended to achieve a Class I incisor relationship the molar occlusion must also remain Class I. This will often require the use of headgear to reinforce the anchorage.

A removable appliance carrying an anterior bite plane is very effective at reducing an excessive overbite in the growing patient; and posterior biteplanes are favoured for the elimination of mandibular displacing ativity concurently with correction of an instanding incisor, or maxillary expansion to eliminate a unilateral posterior crossbite.

Fixed appliances (see Chapter 16)

Rotations, bodily retraction of teeth, space closure, extrusion and intrusion of individual teeth all require fixed appliances. It is also usually advisable to use fixed appliances where there are a large number of individual tooth movements to be undertaken. This is because a succession of removable appliances would be required whereas a fixed appliance can usually achieve all of them, often simultaneously.

Functional appliances (see Chapter 17)

These are useful in the early correction of selected Class II, division 1 cases.

Surgery

Minor surgical procedures may be required in the management of displaced and unerupted teeth. Major orthognathic surgery is now routinely used in the correction of gross vertical and horizontal sheltered discrepancies. In general such treatment will require preparatory tooth alignment using fixed appliances and will not be undertaken until facial growth is complete.

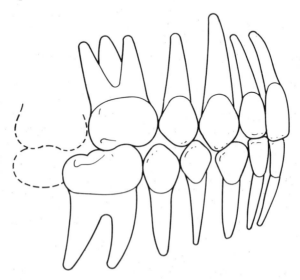

Figure 8.18 If the lower arch is well aligned and upper first premolars are removed to provide space to overjet reduction, the molar occlusion must end up in a full-unit Class II occlusion.

Planning the buccal occlusion

Molar occlusion does not change spontaneously either during or after treatment (Lloyd and Stephens, 1979; Stephens and Lloyd, 1980), hence any desired changes must be included in the treatment plan. In the intact ideal occlusion there is the same number of teeth in each quadrant and both the incisor occlusion and the molar occlusion is Class I. For this reason, if no extractions are planned (or the same number of teeth are to be removed in each quadrant), and a Class I incisor occlusion is to be obtained at the end of treatment, steps must also be taken to obtain or preserve a Class I molar occlusion (Fig. 8.17b). On the other hand, if only upper first premolars are to be removed the molar occlusion must end up a full unit Class II (Fig. 8.18). Rarely will it be desirable to achieve an intermediate molar occlusion, but half-unit Class II and Class III buccal relationships may be necessary where teeth are missing in the labial segment of one arch or are of unusual size, for example small upper lateral incisors.

There are several ways in which the molar or buccal occlusion can be changed. These are:

1 Intramaxillary fixed appliances and to a lesser extent removable appliances operating in one arch can change the molar occlusion. The effectiveness of this approach is limited by the anchorage available. For example, it may be necessary to move buccal teeth forward one at a time in the lower arch to prevent lingual movement of the lower incisors whilst attempting to correct a Class II molar occlusion by this means. Similarly, a maxillary screw plate can correct a half-unit Class II molar relationship on one side of the mouth but there is the danger that the incisor overjet will be increased as this is carried out.
2 Intermaxillary traction is the usual means of correcting molar occlusion in some fixed-appliance techniques, for example the Begg technique, and in most fixed-appliance treatment it is available if required. Intermaxillary forces are also generated by myofunctional appliances.
3 Extraoral force applied to molar bands is one of the most effective ways of obtaining a rapid change in Class II molar relationships. In this form it is the usual way of achieving molar correction in Class II cases treated using the straight-wire technique. Less rapid change can be achieved using extraoral force applied to a removable 'en masse' appliance.
4 Phased extractions: on occasions it may be possible to effect a change in molar occlusion by extracting in one arch only, or a few months earlier than in the other. This effect is particularly marked after premature loss of deciduous teeth and should be borne in mind when considering enforced extraction of these teeth (Joondeph and McNeill, 1971) (see Chapter 9–Compensating extractions).

Estimating anchorage requirements

Anchorage is considered more fully in Chapters 14–16 but must be mentioned briefly here also. Removable appliances rely upon intramaxillary anchorage, which may be supplemented with extraoral anchorage. Fixed appliances use these forms of anchorage and in addition employ intermaxillary anchorage by means of light latex elastics running between the upper and lower appliances (see Fig. 16.18). In addition, fixed appliances can use the greater resistance offered by relatively few teeth that are prevented by the appliance from tipping to provide the anchorage for tipping forces applied to larger numbers of teeth.

It is possible to make an assessment of the anchorage requirement of an individual case only in the broadest terms. This is because the forces being applied cannot always be measured with any great degree of precision and, in the case of fixed appliances, the frictional losses incurred by the archwire/bracket slot remain unknown. In general it is best to be pessimistic about anchorage and to err on the side of providing too much. In the event of this being the case, headgear wear can always be reduced and intermaxillary elastics can be discarded.

Putting the treatment plan into effect

Because the success of any treatment plan is greatly dependent on the active cooperation of the patient and frequently involves the extraction of sound teeth, it is essential for the patient and parent to be fully aware of the implications of embarking on treatment. Colour photographs of appliances should be used at an early stage to demonstrate the type of appliance to be employed. If there is any doubt in the patient's mind they should be asked to go away and come to a decision in their own time. Occasionally it may be helpful to bond anterior brackets to the upper anterior teeth and send the patient away for a week to determine whether they can accept the prospect of such attachments for 2 years or more. Removable appliances should always be fitted and signs of good wear confirmed before extractions are carried out.

It cannot be overemphasized that clear treatment objectives are essential. Occasionally it will be necessary to modify the treatment plan in the light of the treatment response but this is unusual. Except in the case of specific interceptive measures, the temptation to embark upon an initial first stage of treatment before considering the next step should be avoided.

References

Berg, R. and Gebauer, U. (1982) Spontaneous changes in the mandibular arch following first premolar extractions. European Journal of Orthodontics, 4, 93–98

Bishara, S. E. and Burkey, P. S. (1986) Second molar extractions – a review. American Journal of Orthodontics, 98, 415–424

Bradbury, A. J. (1985) A current view on patterns of extraction therapy in British health service orthodontics. British Dental Journal, 159, 47–50

Burgess, P., Houston, W. and Howe, G. (1971) Orthodontic and surgical observations on the removal of mandibular third molars by lateral trepanation. Dental Practitioner, 22, 69–72

Cookson, A. (1970) Space closure following the loss of lower first premolars. Transactions of the British Society for the Study of Orthodontics, 27–32

Creekmore, T. D. (1982) Teeth just want to be straight. *Journal of Clinical Orthodontics*, **16**, 745–764

Cryer, B. S. (1967) Third molar eruption and the effect of extraction of adjacent teeth. *Dental Practitioner*, **17**, 405–416

Dacre, J. (1987) The criteria for lower second molar extraction. *British Journal of Orthodontics*, **14**, 1–9

Fröhlich, K., Thüer, U. and Ingervall, B. (1991) Pressure from the tongue on the teeth in young adults. *Angle Orthodontist*, **61**, 17–24

Henry, C. B: (1938) Prophylactic odontectomy of the developing mandibular third molar. *American Journal of Orthodontics and Oral Surgery*, **24**, 72–84

Henry, C. B. (1969) Excision of the developing mandibular third molar by lateral trepanation. *British Dental Journal*, **127**, 111–118

Houston, W. J. B. and Edler, R. (1990) Long term stability of the lower labial segment relative to the APo line. *European Journal of Orthodontics*, **12**, 302–310

Joondeph, D. and McNeill, R. (1971) Congenitally absent second premolars: an interceptive approach. *American Journal of Orthodontics*, **59**, 50–66

Lawlor, J. (1978) The effects on the lower third molar of the extraction of the lower second molar. *British Journal of Orthodontics*, **5**, 99–103

Little, R. M. (1990) Stability and relapse of dental arch alignment. *British Journal of Orthodontics*, **17**, 235–242

Little, R. M., Reidel, R. A. and Årtun, J. (1988) An evaluation of changes in mandibular anterior alignment from 10 to 20 years post retention. *American Journal of Orthodontics and Dentofacial Orthopedics*, **93**, 423–428

Little, R. M., Wallen, T. R. and Reidel, R. A. (1981) Stability and relapse of mandibular alignment – first premolar extraction cases treated by traditional edgewise mechanics. *American Journal of Orthodontics*, **80**, 349–365

Lloyd, T. G. and Stephens, C. D. (1979) Spontaneous changes in molar occlusion after extraction of all first premolar teeth – a study of Class II division 1 cases treated with removable appliances. *British Journal of Orthodontics*, **6**, 91–94

Mills, J. R. E. (1968) The stability of the lower labial segment. *Dental Practitioner*, **18**, 293–305

Persson, M., Persson, E. and Skagius, S. (1989) Long term spontaneous changes following removal of all first premolars in Class I cases with crowding. *European Journal of Orthodontics*, **11**, 271–282

Richardson, M. E. (1983) The effect of lower second molar extraction on late lower arch crowding. *Angle Orthodontist*, **53**, 25–28

Stephens, C. D. (1983) Factors affecting the rate of spontaneous space closure at the site of extracted mandibular first premolars. *British Journal of Orthodontics*, **10**, 93–97

Stephens, C. D. and Houston, W. J. B. (1985) Facial growth and premolar extraction space closure. *European Journal of Orthodontics*, **7**, 157–162

Stephens, C. D. and Lloyd, T. G. (1980) Changes in molar occlusion after extraction of all first premolars – a follow-up study of Class II division 1 cases treated with removable appliances. *British Journal of Orthodontics*, **7**, 139–144

Von Wowern, N. and Neilsen, H. O. (1989) The fate of lower third molars after the age of 20. A four year follow-up. *International Journal of Oral and Maxillofacial Surgery*, **18**, 277–280

Further reading

Stephens, C. D. and Isaacson K. E. (1990) *Practical Orthodontic Assessment*, Butterworth-Heinemann, Oxford

Chapter 9

Local factors and early treatment

The causative factors of malocclusion may be categorized as follows:

A *General factors* (affecting the all or the greater part of the occlusion)
Skeletal relationships
Soft tissue form
Disproportion between the size of the teeth and the size of the arches

B *Local factors* (affecting one or two adjacent and/or opposing teeth).

General factors are considered to be largely determined genetically and cannot be intercepted to any great extent.

Local factors by their nature produce a local disturbance in dental development that becomes more severe the longer it continues to operate. Such factors can usually be 'intercepted' with advantage.

The local factors may be classified as follows:

1 *Variation in tooth number*
Supernumerary teeth
Hypodontia (oligodontia)
Premature loss of deciduous teeth or unplanned loss of permanent teeth
Retained deciduous teeth

2 *Variation in tooth form*
Macrodont teeth
Microdont teeth
Additional cusps
Invagination
Evagination

3 *Abnormalities in tooth position*
Ectopic crypts (local rotation, misplaced development, impaction not caused by crowding)
Transposition of teeth

4 *Local abnormalities of soft tissue*
Fraena
Sucking habits

5 *Local pathology*
Cysts
Trauma.

As almost all local factors can readily be identified and removed at an early age, it is these that are the target for interceptive measures. Even so, it is true to say that because malocclusions arising from other causes are much more common it is only occasionally that the removal of a local factor at an early age will allow an ideal occlusion to develop without further intervention. Because of this there is always some debate, when both genetically determined and locally operating factors are judged to be contributing to a particular malocclusion, as to whether interceptive measures are appropriate. Estimates of their potential application have ranged from 5 to 15 per cent of malocclusions or potential malocclusions identified at the early mixed dentition stage.

The general practitioner has the major role to play in monitoring the development of the child's occlusion. During the period from birth to the completion of the permanent dentition the practitioner's aims should be threefold:

1 The treatment, or referral for advice, of those malocclusions that might, with advantage, be intercepted.
2 The avoidance of causing a malocclusion or aggravating an existing, developing malocclusion by neglect or through inappropriate dental treatment.
3 The institution of conventional orthodontic treatment, or referral for treatment, at the appropriate time.

Management of the developing dentition

The deciduous dentition

Natal teeth

These are teeth that are present at birth or erupt shortly after. They are rare but are most frequent in the lower incisor region. Only 10 per cent of natal teeth are supernumerary and so they should be removed only if they interfere with feeding or are causing ulceration of the underside of the tongue. The loss of one or two lower deciduous incisors will have little effect on the development of the permanent dentition.

It is well recognized that a lack of spacing between the deciduous incisors just before they are shed is indicative of incipient crowding in the permanent dentition (Fig. 9.1). Indeed, the longitudinal studies of Leighton (1971) have shown that by 3 years of age there must be 6 mm or more space between the teeth of the lower dental arch in order for there to be no chance of incisor crowding in the permanent dentition. Similarly, severe skeletal discrepancies may be apparent at an early age. While some clinicians have advocated treatment of malocclusion in the deciduous dentition, the advantages of this approach have not been adequately demonstrated. Interceptive measures are therefore few and are principally concerned with the institution of good oral hygiene and dietary control, with such restorative care as is necessary.

Gemination in the deciduous dentition is quite rare. Fusion of deciduous incisors, either to an adjacent incisor or to a supernumerary

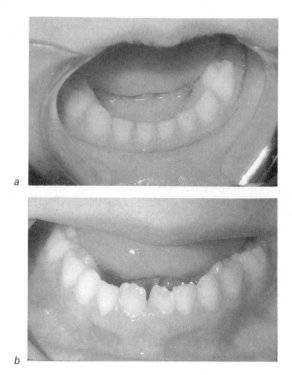

Figure 9.1 (a) A lack of spacing between the deciduous incisors at the end of the deciduous dentition in this 3-year-old indicates insipient crowding. (b) This becomes apparent when the permanent incisors erupt.

incisor, is occasionally seen. There is no indication for treatment. Gemination of deciduous teeth is seldom a cause of any problem and the teeth are invariably shed in the normal manner. However, the condition is frequently followed by a similar disturbance in the permanent dentition.

Enforced extraction of deciduous teeth

The principles governing the indications and choice of extraction of permanent teeth as part of orthodontic treatment are widely agreed and practised. Unfortunately, opinions on the management of enforced extractions of deciduous teeth have varied widely in the past. This has meant that many general practitioners have come to regard the premature extraction of any deciduous tooth as a regrettable and harmful necessity to which the only answer is the fitting of a space maintainer. All too often, patient cooperation makes such a procedure impossible and no further measures are usually undertaken. This is unfortunate for unless space maintainers are to be employed there are many cases where the extraction of a solitary deciduous tooth is inappropriate.

It is therefore important for the general practitioner to have a clear understanding of the principles governing the effects of premature

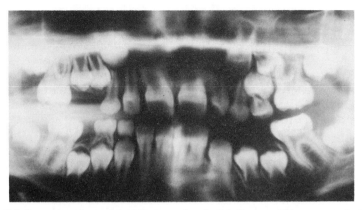

Figure 9.2 Premature loss of deciduous molars in this 9-year-old has concentrated crowding in the premolar region.

deciduous tooth loss in order that the likely effects in the individual patient can be estimated and any undesirable effects minimized.

The effect of loss of a deciduous tooth depends upon the age at which it is lost and the degree of crowding inherent in the developing dentition. There is little adverse effect when the jaws are well developed and the dental arches are large. However, where there is crowding, the premature loss of a deciduous tooth may allow crowded teeth to erupt at the expense of an underlying successional tooth, which thereby becomes partially or totally excluded from the arch (Fig. 9.2). In the intact arch, any crowding of the permanent dentition tends to occur at the front and the back of the mouth (i.e. in the incisor and posterior molar segments). In the premolar region the size of the deciduous molars ensures that their successors have enough space reserved for them. Because of this location of crowding there are two effects of premature loss:

1 mesial migration of posterior teeth;
2 spreading out of crowded anterior teeth.

These occur in varying amounts depending on the tooth lost, the arch in which it is lost, the age of the patient, the degree of crowding and the nature of the occlusion.

Early loss of deciduous incisors

The loss of deciduous incisors through caries does not usually affect the occlusion as they will be shed naturally by 5 or 6 years of age. Traumatic loss may occur at an earlier age but unless there is some damage to the underlying permanent incisor (see Dilaceration below) there is usually no untoward effect.

Early loss of deciduous canines

The deciduous canine is not usually lost early because of caries but because its root is resorbed by a crowded lateral incisor. This is more frequent in the lower arch. The lateral incisor encroaches on space previously occupied by the deciduous canine, and the permanent canine is excluded from the arch (Van der Linden, 1990). With unilateral loss there is a marked shift of the centre line to the affected side. There is merit in balancing the loss of one deciduous canine by extraction of its antimere in order to attempt to minimize the displacement of the centre line, although this is not always successful.

In general terms, extraction of the deciduous canines allows improvement in any crowding of the permanent incisors and this was one of the reasons for the popularity of elective extraction of deciduous canines as the first part of the procedure known as 'serial extraction' (see below).

Early loss of deciduous molars

Where the arches are potentially crowded, it is the buccal segments that are most severely affected by early loss. The deciduous teeth most commonly extracted prematurely because of the effects of dental caries are the first and second molars. With modern preventive care this loss is becoming less frequent, but it is still a factor to be reckoned with. Space will also close if contact areas are lost due to caries or poor restoration. The earlier the extraction of the deciduous tooth and the greater the tendency to crowding, the more severe the effects will be (Breakspeare, 1951; 1960; Lundström 1955; Clinch, 1959; Richardson, 1965). Occasionally the occlusion itself will maintain space, for example due to the intercuspation of the first permanent molars or overeruption of the opposing deciduous tooth. More usually, though, there will be space loss.

Early loss of second deciduous molars

If the second deciduous molar is extracted before eruption of the first permanent molar, the latter tooth will erupt in a more anterior position and total space loss may occur. With later extraction, the upper first permanent molar rotates round its palatal root; while in the lower arch the permanent molar tips mesially with some rotation. The upper second premolar usually erupts into the palate and the lower usually erupts lingually or, with later extraction, may impact vertically between lower first molar and first premolar.

Early loss of first deciduous molars

Where a first deciduous molar is lost prematurely, the second deciduous molar and the first permanent molar drift forwards without rotation or tilting and the anterior teeth spread around the arch. Unilateral loss may cause a shift of the centre line. The consequences depend largely on the sequence of eruption of permanent teeth. In the upper arch, the first premolar usually erupts into the arch but the canine is outlocked (Fig. 9.3); in the lower arch the effect is more variable and sometimes the canine erupts first and the first premolar is short of space.

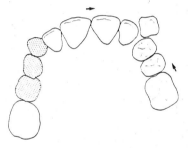

Figure 9.3 The effect of early loss of |D with forward movement of |56 and shift of the centreline, causing |3 to become outlocked.

Space maintenance and balancing or compensating extractions

It is impossible to separate the local problems created by early loss of deciduous teeth from the more general problems of crowding, but some thought has to be given to maintaining space as a local preventive measure.

In view of the fact that many children have potentially crowded mouths and will require extraction of permanent teeth anyway, the use of space maintainers is rarely essential. One situation in which space may be maintained with some advantage is where there is an acceptable alignment of the teeth but with the tendency to mild crowding. In such a case, early loss may produce a localized malocclusion for which it is difficult to plan simple orthodontic treatment.

There are domestic difficulties in inflicting a space-maintaining appliance on young children and their parents, and in persuading them of the need for it to be worn continuously for a number of years, particularly when there is no guarantee that this will avoid the need for later orthodontic treatment. Prolonged use may also hinder good plaque control, with a possible increase in caries. Removable space maintainers fail if not worn adequately, while those that are fixed in the mouth require regular inspection as plaque formation around the appliance and underneath bands, if cement leaches out, is liable to lead to caries.

With improved preventive measures, the number of deciduous teeth that have to be extracted because of caries is diminishing. The natural tooth forms the ideal space maintainer and it is always preferable to root fill an exposed deciduous tooth and to retain it rather than extract it prematurely. Where only one tooth is cariously exposed or giving symptoms, serious attempts should therefore be made to conserve the tooth by conventional methods of pulp treatment.

Where cooperation does not permit root treatment of a deciduous molar, space maintenance by other means is usually not an option for the same reason. In such cases opinion is divided on the desirability of further extractions. A 'balancing' extraction involves the removal of a tooth on the opposite side of the same arch (although not necessarily the antimere) in order to preserve symmetry. A compensating extraction is the removal of the equivalent tooth in the opposing arch to maintain the buccal occlusion.

Where extractions have to be carried out under general anaesthesia, balancing and compensating extractions must be considered. Where contralateral and opposing teeth are of poor prognosis there is little difficulty in applying the principles of balancing and compensating extraction, as all authorities agree on the undesirability of submitting a patient to several general anaesthetics.

Balancing extractions are designed to eliminate centre-line displacements that will require fixed appliances for their later correction. Compensating extractions are a means of preserving interarch relationships by allowing the posterior teeth to drift forward together. It follows that where centre lines are already misplaced or the buccal occlusion is far from ideal, there may be little to be gained by the elective removal of additional deciduous teeth where these are conservable and the patient is sufficiently cooperative to make this possible within a reasonable period.

General rules

Class I cases with mild crowding: if a first deciduous molar has to be extracted on one side of the upper arch, the contralateral tooth should be extracted to prevent centre line shift and allow some temporary improvement in incisor crowding. This is a 'balancing extraction'. If one first deciduous molar has to be extracted in the lower arch it may be desirable to balance, extracting the contralateral tooth, and this may signal the need for compensating extractions in the upper arch, particularly if the teeth are of poor quality and need extensive restoration.

Table 9.1 Anomalies revealed by orthopantomogram in a sample of 9- to 10-year-olds attending a general dental practice (after Neal and Bowden, 1988)

Anomoly	Frequency (%)
Displaced teeth	12.9
Maxillary canines	10.2
Mandibular 2nd premolars	1.4
Maxillary incisors	0.4
Others	0.9
Missing teeth	9.1
Mandibular 2nd premolars	4.8
Maxillary lateral incisors	1.9
Maxillary 2nd premolars	1.9
Mandibular incisors	0.5
Pathology	5.3
Large restorations	3.0
Untreated caries	1.9
Retained roots	0.3
Cysts	0.1
Abnormal teeth	2.2
Peg-shaped incisors	1.4
Crown hyperplasia	0.4
Invaginations	0.4
Supernumerary teeth	0.5

Where there is gross crowding in the lower arch and a Class II malocclusion with deep overbite, extensive active treatment will be required. It is better, therefore, to limit the extraction to the offending deciduous molar and not complicate the problem further by compensating or balancing extractions. The reverse is true if one deciduous molar has to be extracted in a Class II case in a crowded upper arch.

It used to be thought that the loss of second deciduous molars should not be balanced or compensated because the effect on the centre line was minor. Recent evidence suggests that significant centre line movement can occur with the early removal of these teeth before crowded permanent incisors start to erupt.

The mixed dentition

As all teeth of the permanent dentition, with the exception of third molars, have reached at least the stage of crown formation by 8 years of age, routine extraoral radiography at or shortly after this time is desirable for all children undergoing regular dental treatment. It is also an integral part of treatment planning for the casual attender who requires extraction for the relief of pain. Common problems that such films may reveal are given in Table 9.1.

Supernumerary teeth

All teeth extra to the normal complement are given the generic name of supernumerary teeth. They occur in about 1 per cent of the population and result from excessive but organized growth of the dental lamina. Most supernumeraries are found in the upper incisor region (Fig. 9.4) but they can occur anywhere in the jaws (Taylor, 1972).

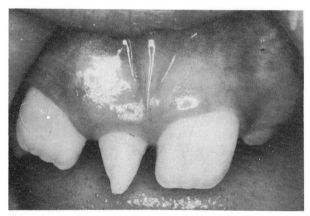

Figure 9.4 Mesiodens erupted between the upper central incisors.

Supplemental teeth

As the name implies, this refers to duplication of teeth in the normal

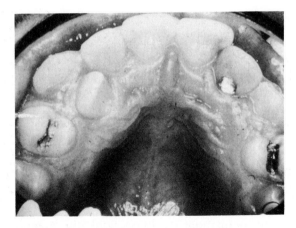

Figure 9.5 Supplemental upper right lateral incisor.

series, the most common being the permanent lateral incisor (Fig. 9.5). It may be difficult to distinguish the true lateral incisor from its supplemental 'twin'. Usually one of them has to be removed because of crowding and where both are equally well formed, the correct extraction is that of the tooth which is most displaced. A supplemental tooth may have a deep cingulum pit and a coronal invagination. It is possible that supplemental teeth are an evolutionary throw-back (atavism) as the primitive mammalian dentition had three incisors, one canine, four premolars and four molars in each quadrant.

Other forms of supernumerary

Other supernumerary teeth differ in shape from the normal series. The term 'mesiodens' is applied to a conical type of supernumerary, which is usually found in the midline (Fig. 9.4). This either displaces or more commonly prevents eruption of the central incisors (Fig. 9.6). The presence of a large central diastema or delayed eruption or displacement of a central incisor indicates the need for a radiographic examination. There is usually only a single supernumerary of this type, but sometimes there is a cluster of two or more. On occasion they are placed high and inverted in the palate and have even been known to erupt into the floor of the nose.

The other principal type of supernumerary is tuberculated and is more often paired. They are most commonly located on the palatal side of the central incisors, thus preventing their eruption (see Fig. 9.8).

Where supernumerary teeth are not deflecting or delaying eruption of the incisors they may be left alone if they are inaccessible; but if there are signs of enlargement of the follicle, with potential cystic formation around the crown, they should be removed. The position of unerupted supernumeraries can be established by the radiographic technique used to locate unerupted canines (see Fig. 9.6), adopting the principle of

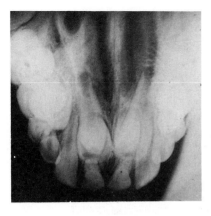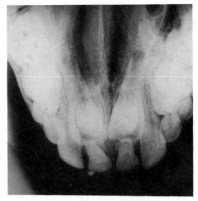

Figure 9.6 Tuberculated supernumeraries palatal to the upper central incisors preventing their eruption. The two films were taken with a shift of the tube. The teeth furthest from the tube appear to move with it (see Fig. 9.7).

parallax (Fig. 9.7). A true lateral radiograph of the incisor region assists in locating those that are lying deeply in the palate and enables a decision to be made as to whether a buccal rather than a palatal approach should be made to remove them. Supernumeraries should not be removed surgically before the patient is 6 years of age because there is a danger of displacing the permanent tooth during the operation.

Space requirements must be considered as part of the general orthodontic treatment plan. In a potentially crowded arch, the lateral incisor

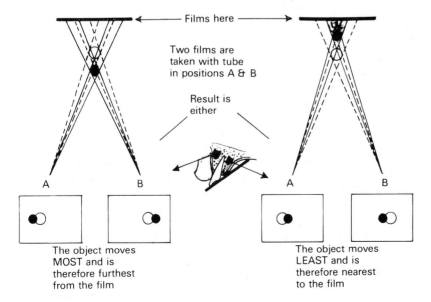

Figure 9.7 Explanation of the parallax system.

may encroach on the space for the unerupted central incisor and so the deciduous canines may have to be extracted to provide temporary space. This can be done at the same time as removal of the supernumeraries (Fig. 9.8).

Delayed incisors may take up to 18 months to erupt. Where eruption is very delayed by a dense mucoperiosteum, an incision has to be made over the incisal edge.

Supernumeraries may also develop either in the premolar or third molar region where they may either be similar in form to other teeth in the region or conical. Development occurs after most permanent teeth have erupted and thus there is little adverse effect on the occlusion. Multiple supernumeraries occur in cleiodocranial dysostosis, an extremely rare condition.

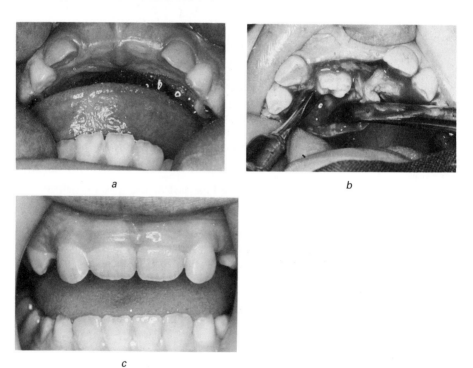

a

b

c

Figure 9.8 A series showing the case involving the supernumeraries in Fig. 9.6: (a) 1|1 unerupted and obstructed by supernumeraries; (b) the stage of surgical removal; (c) eruption of incisors after 1 year (note C|C were extracted to give temporary space to be followed by extraction of 4|4).

Gemination (see Brook and Winter (1970))

Gemination of permanent teeth is not very common. Usually upper or lower incisors are affected. Where this occurs, treatment will depend on the degree of crowding caused. Where there is a normal number of incisors and the gemination appears to be the merging of two of these teeth, no treatment may be required. On the other hand, an actual increase in the number of incisor crowns caused by a true gemination of one of the four incisors will usually cause an unacceptable degree of incisor crowding. When an upper central incisor is geminated it can present a very difficult aesthetic problem (Fig. 9.9). Sometimes the underlying form of the tooth can be camouflaged by restorative measures such as judicious modification of crown form to simulate two adjacent normal teeth. In other cases, extraction and prosthetic replacement by a tooth of normal size and shape will be the only satisfactory solution.

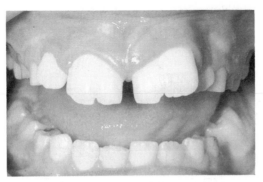

Figure 9.9 Both upper central incisors are partially geminated, presenting a very difficult aesthetic problem (see text).

Hypodontia

Small or missing teeth cause spacing in arches that are of normal or above average size. The prevalence of missing teeth is around 6 per cent (Grahnen, 1956; Davies, 1968). In rare cases of true hypodontia or 'oligodontia', many teeth are missing and those present may be small and abnormal in shape (Fig. 9.10). Anodontia, the total absence of teeth, is rare (Sarnat, Brodie and Kubacki, 1953).

Missing upper lateral incisors

These teeth may be absent unilaterally or bilaterally. If one is absent the other may be of normal size but is often small and conical (Fig. 9.11). An important associated consideration is the effect of the absence of this tooth on the eruptive path of the maxillary canine, which frequently becomes misplaced palatally (Brin, Becker and Shalhav, 1986). Where the canine is unerupted, this possibility should always be eliminated by clinical and radiographic examination.

The local problem caused by a missing lateral incisor varies according to arch size and relationship. In a crowded arch or when the deciduous canine is retained, the permanent canine may erupt into contact with the central incisor. If the canine is not too pointed, a reasonable aesthetic

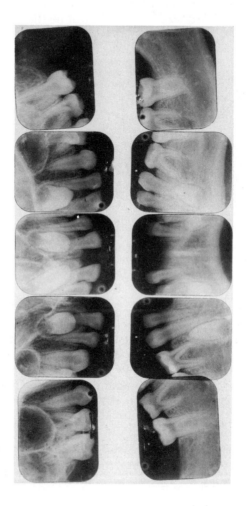

Figure 9.10 The intraoral radiographs of a case of hypodontia showing many teeth missing. The only permanent teeth present are two small upper incisors and two lower caniniform teeth.

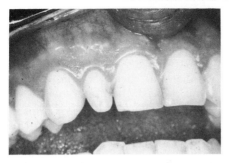

Figure 9.11 Missing upper left lateral incisor with the contralateral tooth small and conical.

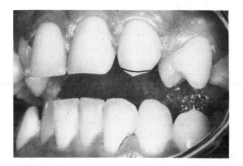

Figure 9.12 Missing upper left lateral incisor with canine erupted next to central incisor. The canine can be stoned to give a better appearance, as indicated by the line.

result may be obtained by reducing its tip (Fig. 9.12). More extensive modification by reshaping is possible but can never overcome the underlying problem of concealing the size of a bulky canine adjacent to a rather small central incisor. Where necessary, the crown can be recontoured using an acid-etch, composite-resin technique.

In the average to large arch, spacing can be dealt with in several ways. Where it is minimal it may be acceptable to the patient. Where this is not the case, sufficient space for a denture or a bridge may be obtained by retracting the canine and approximating the central incisors to concentrate the spacing at the site of the missing tooth (see Fig. 10.8).

Commonly, the space for the upper lateral incisor is too large to be accepted but too small to accommodate a reasonably sized pontic. In such instances there are a number of possible options:

1 Create adequate space for a lateral incisor pontic by distal movement of upper buccal segments after the extraction of upper second or third molars if posterior crowding is present, or by extraction of a premolar in order to create adequate space for a lateral incisor pontic after canine retraction.
2 Closure of the anterior spacing by forward movement of posterior teeth. Fixed appliances and prolonged retention are required.

It should be remembered that opening up space will have to be followed by a lifetime's wear of a prosthetic device with all its attendant problems. Acceptance of a canine next to the central incisor is to be preferred in many cases.

Where there is a Class III incisor relationship and missing upper lateral incisors, advancement of the upper labial segment tends to open up the spaces further so that a pontic may be necessary. Finally, in those few cases in which there is enough crowding elsewhere in the arch to justify the extraction of a premolar, serious consideration should be given to the possibility of transplanting this tooth (see below) into the site of the missing incisor (Andreasen *et al.*, 1990 a, b, c, d).

Missing lower central incisors

Although this is not a common occurrence, when one or more lower incisors are missing their replacement is a difficult technical procedure. At the present time an acid-etch bridge can provide a satisfactory solution to the replacement of a single incisor in a proportion of cases only. Hence, where the arch is of adequate size and the space is unlikely to close, deciduous teeth should be left in place for as long as possible. Unfortunately, they rarely last for long, owing to a combination of occlusal wear and root resorption. If the lower arch is crowded the space can close quite readily, although controlled movement with a fixed appliance may be needed. Absence of teeth in the lower labial segment may have an adverse secondary effect on the upper labial segment because of the difficulty of arranging the six upper anterior teeth around only five (or sometimes four) lower teeth. If the buccal occlusion is good and the lower incisor space is allowed to close, some degree of crowding will appear in the upper incisor region as the upper and lower buccal teeth drift forward. Sometimes, because the overjet is increased or the upper lateral incisors are unusually small, there is no such disturbance. In other cases it may be necessary to accept that a poor buccal occlusion is preferable to upper incisor irregularity.

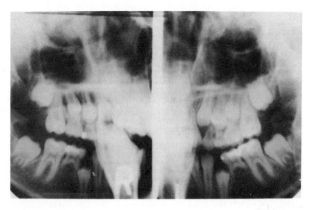

Figure 9.13 Rotated oblique lateral radiographs showing both lower second premolars to be absent.

Missing premolars

The fact that lower second premolars, and less frequently upper second premolars, may be missing makes it essential to take routine radiographs before contemplating the extraction of any permanent teeth for relief of crowding (Fig. 9.13). In many cases where there is potential crowding, absence of lower premolars means that the extraction of permanent teeth can be confined to the upper arch. The lower second deciduous molars are then removed as part of the treatment of lower arch crowding. It should be pointed out, however, that space closure may require a fixed appliance. It is worth remembering that some premolars develop late and they should not be assumed to be missing until 9 years of age. When lower second premolars are missing and the arch is of ample size, second deciduous molars that are not resorbing may remain in place until 30–40 years of age unless they show signs of submergence or are of poor quality. Retention of such teeth does mean that at a later stage there will be more than enough space to fit a pontic (Fig. 9.14).

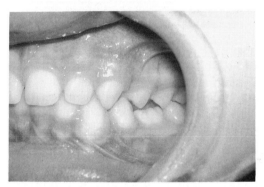

Figure 9.14 A 12-year-old with uncrowded arches where the lower second premolar is absent. The second deciduous molar has good roots and is likely to be retained for many years.

Missing lower third molars

Absence of these teeth has little adverse effect on the developing occlusion and may be of some benefit, as impactions are common and there may be less chance of later deterioration in incisor alignment. Second permanent molars should not be extracted for orthodontic reasons before the presence of third molars has been confirmed. Third molar development is very variable and may start as early as 7 years or as late as 14 years of age.

Teeth of abnormal form

Dens-in-dente (Fig. 9.15)

Where the lateral incisors are small and conical it is important to check

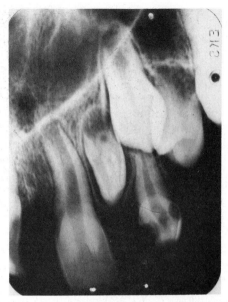

Figure 9.15 A dens-in-dente involving upper left lateral incisor. The pulp may become infected after eruption of the tooth.

with a radiograph whether there is some abnormality. The radiograph may reveal an appearance described as 'dens-in-dente' (tooth within a tooth), produced by a coronal invagination. The deep cingulum pit leads into a cavity with a deficient enamel lining, which allows bacteria to gain ingress to the pulp. The pulp may become infected soon after the tooth emerges into the mouth. If the cingulum pit can be sealed promptly this process may be prevented, but in other cases the tooth may have to be extracted because the difficulties of adequate root treatment after abscess formation or because of the general deformity of the crown (Fig. 9.15).

Dilaceration

This term describes an abnormal angulation between the crown and root of a tooth or within the root (Fig. 9.16). The site of deformation depends on the timing of the disturbance during the tooth's development. It is usually due to a blow to a deciduous tooth, driving it up into the alveolar process. Sometimes the deciduous tooth re-erupts, but the forming permanent incisor is damaged because of its developmental position close and palatal to the root of its predecessor. Little can be done to prevent this type of trauma as young children are liable to falls and other accidents. Occasionally, dilaceration occurs without any history of trauma.

A dilacerated upper incisor may fail to erupt or may remain high in the labial sulcus (Fig. 9.17). In most instances it has to be removed surgically. Only rarely, where there is minimal malformation, can a dilacerated tooth be brought into the arch.

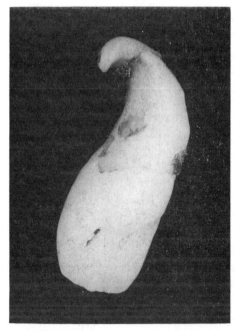

Figure 9.16 An extracted dilacerated central incisor showing distortion of the root.

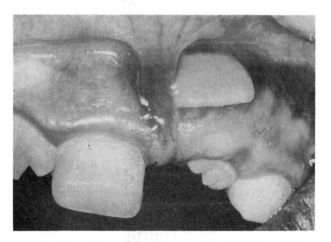

Figure 9.17 Tilting of the adjacent lateral incisor where the dilacerated central incisor was unable to erupt.

Other malformations

Other abnormalities of tooth form may cause a local problem. Lingual cusps on upper incisors and canines are occasionally encountered and may require judiciuous reduction to overcome occlusal interferences. Compound or complex odontomes sometimes replace teeth of the normal series. A complex odontome is a diffuse mass of totally disorganized

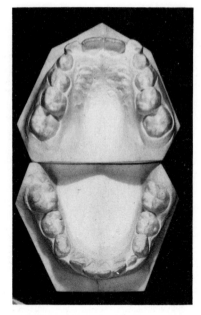

Figure 9.18 Impacted upper first permanent molars.

dental tissue. Compound odontomes may be a collection of denticles. These odontomes have to be removed.

Abnormalities of tooth position

Impacted first permanent molars

The impaction of the first permanent molar under the distal bulge of the second deciduous molar may escape notice during routine inspection (Fig. 9.18). These impactions are quite common, the prevalence being about 0.5 per cent. It is argued that the underlying cause is crowding, although it is difficult to resolve the disparity between the typical distal angulation of crowded maxillary molars with the mesial angulation where first molars are impacted, and it is probable that an abnormal orientation of the crypt is a factor. Management may involve one of the following:

1 *Observation*. Provided that the crown of the tooth is sufficiently exposed to ensure good oral hygiene it is reasonable to keep the area under observation as long as the deciduous tooth remains vital and the permanent molar remains caries free. In mild cases, impaction may be self-correcting.

2 *Disimpaction*. Disimpaction is frequently advocated, using brass wire placed around the mesial contact of the first molar. Such a procedure can be very difficult and is reserved for the more stoical child. It should not be attempted without good local anaesthesia for

initial placement of wire. Several weekly visits are needed for adjustment. Initially 0.5 mm wire should be used and later 0.6 mm will
usually be required to complete the process.

In those cases where there is minimal crowding, and such a course of
early treatment will avoid later appliance therapy, disimpaction may be
worthwhile attempting. For more crowded cases it is generally better to
follow the scheme outlined in 3 below.

Even when such treatment is successful it will often be the case that
the impaction has initiated resorption of the root of the second deciduous molar, which will therefore be lost prematurely. Space maintenance will then be required at once to prevent space loss.

3 *Extraction*. Should the impaction have caused extensive resorption
or pulpal death of the deciduous tooth, it will usually be necessary to
extract the maxillary second deciduous molar. If this happens, or the
tooth is lost by premature exfoliation, it will usually not be worthwhile
considering space maintenance as the first permanent molar will have
already migrated mesially to a considerable extent beneath the resorbed
deciduous tooth. This space loss presents little problem in the long
term. In the uncrowded case the first molar can be quickly and easily
moved distally again to accommodate the second premolar using fixed
or removable appliances (Fig. 9.19). The most appropriate time to
undertake the removable-appliance therapy is when the first premolar
has erupted enough for it to carry a clasp upon which a conventional
appliance can be retained, but before the second molar has descended
enough to impede this movement. The molar can be retracted either
with a screw or, if the first molar is too inclined for clasping, a palatal
spring (0.7 mm) can be used. The tooth, once repositioned, can be held
by conventional clasping during subsequent appliance therapy or until
the second premolar has appeared.

In the more crowded case it may be preferable to remove a premolar
(either the first or the excluded second premolar) as part of conventional
treatment at 12 or 13 years; associated distal movement may also be
required.

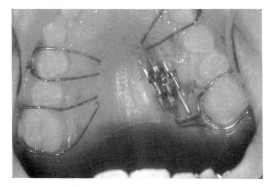

Figure 9.19 Distal movement of a mesially placed first molar, which was formerly
inpacted, to allow the second premolar to align.

Abnormal position of crypts

The crypt of any tooth may be displaced or rotated. Some teeth are very much more commonly affected than others. For example, the lower second premolar quite commonly shows rotation or tipping of its developing crown, which usually corrects in later development and eruption. The lower third molar also shows a wide range of crown orientation, which may improve during development.

In most cases where the crypt of a developing tooth is abnormally placed there is little that early intervention can achieve. However, the maxillary canine is by far the most commonly misplaced tooth (apart from the lower third molar) and ectopia of this tooth is amenable to early intervention.

Ectopic upper canines

The upper canine is particularly liable to be displaced during its long path of eruption from under the orbital floor. The prevalence of ectopic canines is about 2 per cent. The tooth commonly just misses the correct path of eruption and becomes deflected palatally, and the deciduous canine is retained. More rarely it may be grossly displaced and lies horizontally near the floor of the nose or high in the buccal sulcus.

It is now recognized that there is an association between the form of the permanent lateral incisor and the likelihood of ectopic eruption of the canine. Where the lateral incisor is small or absent the probability of a palatal path of eruption is greatly increased (Brin, Becker and Shalhav, 1986). Ectopic eruption of canines is more likely to be seen in children whose parents had palatally misplaced canines or who had anomalous lateral incisors or late developing lateral incisors (Zilberman, Cohen and Becker, 1990)

Early recognition that a canine is erupting ectopically is extremely important. By the age of 8 years the crown of the canine may be detectable as a bulge high in the buccal sulcus. If this is not apparent by 10 years it is likely that the tooth is ectopic and its position should be determined radiographically (Ericson and Kurol, 1986).

The standard occlusal radiograph does not provide enough information to locate a misplaced canine. Some dental surgeons still use a vertex occlusal radiograph (Fig. 9.20) taken with the tube in the region of the vertex of the skull and angled along the long axis of the incisors. This method is to be deprecated because of unnecessary irradiation of the pituitary gland, eyes and other structures. As far as the general practitioner is concerned, two intraoral views taken with different tube positions give a reliable indication of whether the tooth is palatal or buccal to the line of the arch (Fig. 9.21). The tooth furthest from the tube moves in the same direction as the tube according to the principle of parallax (see Fig. 9.7). This method is not always satisfactory because it does not deal with a canine that is very high. However, such cases would, of course, normally be referred for specialist advice.

Where the canine is confirmed as being palatally misplaced, prompt removal of the deciduous canine will usually bring it back on to a

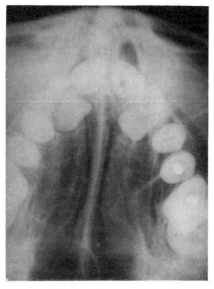

Figure 9.20 Vertex occlusal radiograph. (*Note*: not recommended in view of danger to sensitive areas, because of long exposure and often indistinct picture.)

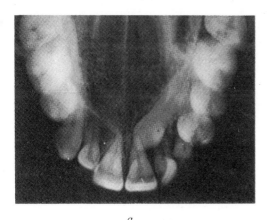

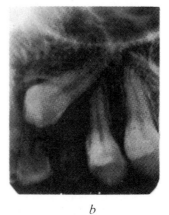

a   *b*

Figure 9.21 Standard occlusal (a) and intraoral view (b) showing how the unerupted canine has moved with the shift of tube from overlapping the central incisor apex to overlap that of the lateral. The unerupted tooth has moved with the tube; by the principle of parallax it is therefore on a palatal aspect. Two periapical views can also be used.

normal course of eruption (Ericson and Kurol, 1988). In making any assessment it is important to note whether there is any resorption of the root of the lateral incisor or, if this tooth is missing, of the upper central incisor. Root resorption takes place rapidly and may be well advanced by 12 years of age but rarely starts after 14 years. The incisors affected may be completely symptomless and early removal of the canine may prevent loss of the adjacent tooth, which may remain vital and firm, even with only one-third to one-half of its root. Where the lateral incisor is a poor risk or surgical removal of the canine might cause further damage, it may be better to extract the lateral incisor and allow the canine to erupt if it is suitably placed.

In the older patient the position of an ectopic canine may be indicated by the position of the adjacent teeth. For example, a labially tilted upper lateral incisor may indicate that the canine is either high and buccal, or low and palatal to its root.

Simple treatment where the canine is not markedly displaced

Where sufficient space is not available for the tooth, space must be made either by extracting the first premolar, which is slightly smaller than the canine, or by distal movement of the buccal segment on that side. The canine may not be very displaced and if its apex is in a good position, it may erupt into the palate without help (Fig. 9.22). If, after a period of observation, it does not appear to be erupting, overlying bone and soft tissue can be removed.

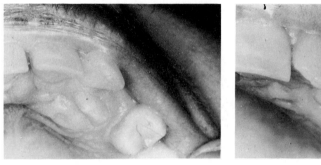 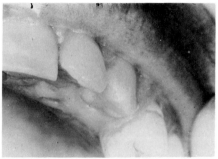

a   *b*

Figure 9.22 A mildly displaced, palatally erupting canine may be moved into the arch with a simple removable appliance following loss of the deciduous canine and local tooth movement to accommodate it: (a) before and (b) after treatment.

Where the unerupted canine is in the line of the arch or slightly buccally placed but with a good axial inclination, it may erupt and require no appliance guidance if adequate space has been created as described previously. The more mesially displaced canine, which may or may not cause resorption of the lateral incisor, can sometimes be allowed to erupt into the position of the lateral if that tooth is extracted or missing.

Treatment when the canine is markedly displaced

In deciding whether a tooth should be brought into the arch from a difficult position, the most important factor is whether the patient is prepared to accept treatment and appreciates the time involved. The procedure should be explained in detail and the patient should not be unduly encouraged as voluntary cooperation over at least 18 months is essential for success. The patient may prefer to accept some form of compromise.

If it is decided to leave the buried canine it should be reviewed by radiographic examination to check that there is no enlargement of the crypt with cystic formation. Its extraction can be delayed and sometimes it is possible to combine this with extraction of third molars if they are impacted. In some cases where the tooth is distant from the arch and where there is considerable crowding, the first premolar and the lateral incisor may be in contact and give an acceptable appearance and function. In other cases the deciduous canine may be left in place for many years if its crown is intact and it is aesthetically acceptable (Fig. 9.23).

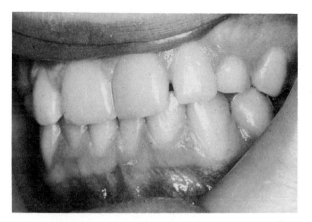

Figure 9.23 Retention of deciduous canine may be aesthetically pleasing when permanent canine is grossly displaced.

Where the deciduous canine is not viable or its crown has been subjected to considerable attrition or caries, space will usually need to be recreated before replacement. A small amount of additional space can often be obtained by local anterior tooth movement but some distal movement of the buccal segment will usually be required to make adequate space for a pontic of reasonable size.

Treatment of the established palatal maxillary canine

Where there is a reasonable prognosis for bringing the fully developed palatally misplaced canine into the arch (Fig. 9.24), and the patient is prepared for a prolonged course of treatment, the first requirement is to provide adequate space. Where space requirements are minimal, some distal movement of the buccal segments may be carried out. Usually there will have been a shift of incisor centre line that will also require correction as part of the space-gathering procedure. Where crowding is more severe the first premolar may need to be extracted. Once space has been provided the position of the tooth will need to be reassessed.

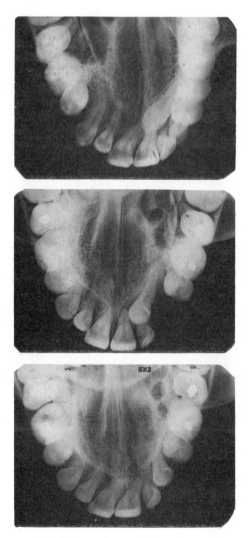

Figure 9.24 Radiographs showing displaced canine brought into position by traction following the extraction of |C̲ and |4̲.

Occasionally a minimally displaced tooth will show considerable improvement as space is made available, and it may erupt without further intervention. However, in most cases, the alternatives are simple surgical exposure or surgical exposure with the attachment of a bracket and gold chain to enable traction to be applied. This can be tied to the attachment and when the flap is sutured the chain can be left curled up until healing has taken place, when it can be unwound and attached to the appliance.

Traction will be necessary if the tooth is markedly displaced palatally, or is buccally displaced, and most operators prefer routinely to bond an attachment when the tooth is exposed. The essential feature of the appliance used to apply traction is a long arm, which can be soldered either to the bridge of an Adams clasp on a removable appliance or to a palatal arch of a fixed appliance. The patient must be able to attach the spring to the protruding links of chain. In many ways a removable appliance, which can be taken out to clean the mouth, is preferable. As the tooth erupts, links of the chain can be removed. It may take 12–18 months to align a difficult canine and during this time other aspects of treatment may have to be deferred. Almost always fixed-appliance treatment will be necessary for final alignment and the patient should understand this when treatment is being outlined (Ferguson, 1990).

Surgical transplantation

Maxillary canines that are surgically accessible and of a crown size that will fit the available space in the dental arch may be transferred from their impacted position into the definitive site by repositioning or transplantation.

Transplantation of a displaced canine is an extension of the repositioning technique, and the same general principles of assessment and the preparation of space in the arch should be adopted. In repositioning, there is usually room to move the canine into a suitable position within the existing space in the alveolar process. Immobilization of the transplanted tooth may be achieved by attaching it to an existing fixed upper arch or splinting with a removable appliance. The period of fixation is generally limited to 2–3 weeks after transplantation: early return to functional forces enhances the establishment of a normal periodontal attachment.

Vitality in transplanted teeth is less important in the assessment of success than viability; while there may be some darkening of the crown and little or no response to electrical or other pulp tests for a considerable period, the transplant that is firm, showing no radiological signs of apical rarefaction and little or no root resorption should not be subjected routinely to endodontic therapy.

After 2 years a degree of root resorption is evident in about half of cases. The overall success rate of canine transplantation depends on many factors, not least of which is the age at which transplantation is carried out. Teeth with patent apices are obviously likely to achieve a new pulpal blood supply more rapidly than those with closed apices. Nevertheless, canine transplants in adolescents and young adults have success rates in the region of two-thirds of cases after 5 years, but only one-third after 10 years (Moss, 1972). With results of this order, the procedure must be given serious consideration when all other treatment avenues appear closed. Recently, modification of the standard transplantation technique, incorporating a two-stage endodontic treatment, has allowed successful results to be achieved in adults into late middle age (Sagne and Thilander, 1990). Transplantation of premolars is also highly successful provided this is undertaken before root growth is completed (Andreasen et al., 1990 a, b, c, d).

Total transposition

On rare occasions there is a total transposition of teeth, such as the lower canine and lateral incisor, or upper canine and first premolar (Fig. 9.25). Orthodontic treatment to correct the transposition is not indicated and the position has to be accepted unless crowding makes the extraction of one or other tooth necessary.

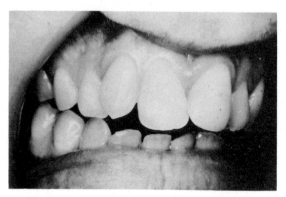

Figure 9.25 Total transposition of upper canine and lateral incisor.

Sometimes the lower lateral incisor is observed erupting lingual to the line of the arch, with a marked distal angulation. If left untreated this will develop into a full transposition once the canine has erupted. In such a case a local fixed appliance may be used to correct the problem. In the past this was rather an ordeal for the average 7-year-old but nowadays the advent of bonded brackets makes this a realistic intervention. Removal of the deciduous lateral incisor may be required, and where crowding is present both the deciduous canines may need to be extracted. Treatment takes only a few weeks but retention should be continued until the permanent canine has appeared unless the oral hygiene precludes this desirable precaution.

Sucking habits

In the infant various digit- and dummy-sucking habits are extremely common (see Chapter 2). They usually produce an anterior open bite or an incomplete overbite and increased overjet (Fig. 9.26). The upper arch may be narrowed by pressure from the cheeks on the buccal teeth, which are not supported by the tongue or by occlusion with the lower arch. As both arches are then of equal width, there is often a lateral mandibular displacement into the position of maximum occlusion, causing a unilateral crossbite. These defects may disappear quite rapidly if the habit ceases by 7–8 years and it is the sole causative factor. It is wrong to underestimate the effects of prolonged and persistent sucking habits. The degree of disturbance in the incisor region is in proportion to the amount of time, force and manner in which the digit is sucked.

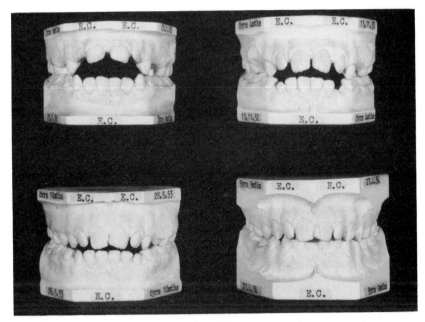

Figure 9.26 The effects of finger sucking and the spontaneous reduction of the resultant open bite after withdrawal of the habit.

Few children persist in the habit to the point where the behaviour justifies psychological investigation; and drastic measures to break it are inappropriate. Parents should be discouraged from nagging, as this is often counterproductive.

Early active intervention

Cooperation of patients is finite. In most cases it is usually limited to about 2 years of appliance wear. Hence interceptive measures that involve the prolonged use of appliances should usually be avoided because in most cases this will prejudice the success of later conventional orthodontic treatment, which is almost always required. However, there are specific instances where there is general agreement that an early course of treatment should be undertaken; these are now considered.

Planned extraction of deciduous teeth

In some circumstances the timely extraction of deciduous teeth can simplify later treatment: this is known as 'guidance of eruption'. Clearly the extraction of deciduous teeth can, at best, only relieve crowding temporarily and there is the danger of space loss due to forward drift of the first permanent molar teeth. Extraction of a deciduous tooth is, of course, indicated where it is deflecting or interfering with the eruption of its permanent successor.

Crowding of the permanent incisors can sometimes be relieved by extraction of deciduous canines at the expense of space for the permanent canines. An important indication for this is where upper lateral incisors are trapped in a palatal position. The removal of the upper deciduous canines just before or as the permanent lateral incisors are emerging can allow them to escape labially. This is advantageous because if they are allowed to erupt fully in a palatal position it will usually be found that their apices are palatally positioned and a fixed appliance may be required to move them labially. In the lower arch, a labially crowded incisor may have a very thin mucoperiosteal covering with little or no bony labial plate. Rapid gingival recession may occur with poor plaque control, tooth-brushing trauma or even without any obvious explanation. The extraction of lower deciduous canines allows the crowded incisors to align, with improved prospects for their periodontal health. The removal of deciduous canines to relieve incisor crowding in either arch almost always means that the first premolars in that arch have to be extracted at a later date to provide space for the permanent canines. The ideal timing for the premolar extractions is just as the permanent canines are emerging through the alveolar mucosa.

Serial extractions

This approach, of the planned extraction of certain deciduous teeth followed by the removal of first premolars, in order to encourage spontaneous correction of incisor irregularities, was given the name 'serial extraction' by Kjellgren (1948), although the technique is much older and was described by Bunon in 1745. Kellgren recommended three stages:

1 All deciduous canines are extracted just as the upper permanent lateral incisors are emerging, at about 8½–9½ years of age in a child with average dental development. The objective of this stage, as described above, is to promote incisor alignment. In suitable cases, this is usually successful.

2 All first deciduous molars are extracted 1 year later, ideally when the first premolar roots are about half formed. The objective of this stage is to encourage the eruption of the first premolars in advance of the canines. In fact, upper first premolars usually erupt before the permanent canines, without any stimulus from the extraction of their deciduous predecessors. The lower permanent canine may still erupt before the first premolar and, if the first deciduous molar has been extracted, the premolar will become impacted between the canine and second deciduous molar. It may then be necessary to remove the second deciduous molar to allow the first premolar to erupt, with the risk of mesial drift of the first permanent molar unless a space maintainer is fitted. It is obvious that the extraction of the first deciduous molar is of doubtful benefit and it may result in loss of space from forward drift of the buccal segment. This stage is not recommended.

3 The first premolars are extracted as the permanent canines are emerging to provide space for them to erupt into the line of the arch. Before extracting these teeth it is essential to re-evaluate the case and in particular to assess the conditions and positions of the other permanent teeth. It is particularly important to check that the upper canines are favourably placed: they should be mesially inclined and should be palpable buccally. The first premolars must not be extracted too early because the inclinations of the canines cannot be assessed reliably before they are about to emerge. Moreover, undue space loss may follow too early an extraction. If on re-evaluation it is decided that the extraction of first premolars is not the most appropriate course of action, then treatment must be replanned.

Serial extraction as described by Kjellgren has little place in modern orthodontics. It was developed at a time when orthodontic appliances were crude and when appliance treatment was not widely available. However, the concept of guidance of eruption to simplify orthodontic treatment is still important and can be used to advantage in some cases.

We now never practise serial extraction as originally described. However, the extraction of deciduous canines alone is a useful measure in certain instances:

1 To provide space so that a crowded but unerupted maxillary lateral incisor may erupt without being held lingually and thus deflected into linguo-occlusion. Once a positive overbite has been obtained such teeth will not correct spontaneously even when space is made available.

2 To provide space for crowded maxillary incisors which are already in linguo-occlusion to be corrected in the early mixed dentition.

3 To provide severely crowded lower incisors with space in which to spontaneously align. This can be justified only if the periodontal health of lower teeth is held to be at risk.

4 To ensure that incisors which have been delayed by the presence of a supernumerary tooth have sufficient space to ensure their eruption (see below).

5 To encourage a palatally misplaced maxillary canine to align (see above).

The problem of the first permanent molars with a poor long-term prognosis

Enforced extraction of first permanent molars poses a number of problems for the orthodontist, particularly where these are delayed until the normal orthodontic age (Fig. 9.27). The options are to rely upon improvement by spontaneous alignment or to treat actively.

Spontaneous alignment

Spontaneous alignment of crowded teeth after extractions is most effective when first premolars are removed. In particular, buccally displaced canines and crowding in the lower labial segment show a marked tendency to improve when first premolars are removed.

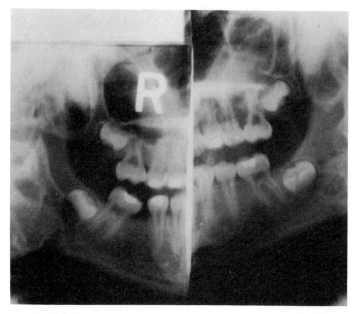

Figure 9.27 The effects of extraction of first permanent molars at differing ages. Note satisfactory positions of the upper second molars (despite some slight rotation of these teeth) but that in the lower right quadrant the later extraction of the right first permanent molar has led to an unsatisfactory position of the second molar.

In contrast, after extraction of first molars there will generally be:

a little spontaneous alignment of lower anterior teeth;
b limited alignment of buccally displaced canines (usually limited to those cases in which the canine is actively erupting and where no more than 1 or 2 mm of space is required);
c poor space closure if the second molar has erupted with tipping of the lower second molar and rotation of the upper (Fig. 9.27);

Active treatment

If fixed appliances are used skilfully most problems caused by enforced extraction of first permanent molars can be overcome. However, treatment usually lasts somewhat longer than with first premolar extractions; and headgear reinforcement of the anchorage will be required in most Class II, division 1 cases. Problems with such treatment are:

1 Fixed appliance treatment may be contraindicated in patients who present with poor first molars caused by inadequate oral hygiene and poor dietary control unless this can be changed.
2 This group of patients includes an appreciable proportion of socially deprived children who may not be able to attend regularly, particularly if this involves a journey to a distant hospital unit.
3 Anchorage may be a problem in cases with severe crowding or a

marked Class II skeletal pattern. In these cases, good headgear wear will usually be required.

While many patients for whom the first molars must be extracted have neither the interest nor the oral hygiene to permit lengthy fixed-appliance therapy, less ambitious removable appliance treatment does not always provide an alternative. Removable appliance treatment tends to be protracted and the adage that the treatment time is doubled and the prognosis halved compared with premolar extraction cases is sadly only too true. This has led to the policy, (widely agreed throughout the UK) of identifying as early as possible those crowded cases in which loss of the first molars is thought to be unavoidable in the long term, and removing these teeth as soon as possible after 8 years of age.

Treatment principles

The lower arch

Where first molars are extracted between the ages of 8½ and 9½ years (or where root development of the second molar has not exceeded one third), the second molar will usually achieve an acceptable position with respect to the second premolar (Fig. 9.28). If extractions are delayed beyond this time, the second molars will have an increasingly mesio-angular path of eruption. Fortunately the chances of an acceptable out-come are enhanced in cases with mild crowding where this has been localized to the premolar region by premature loss of deciduous molars (Fig. 9.29).

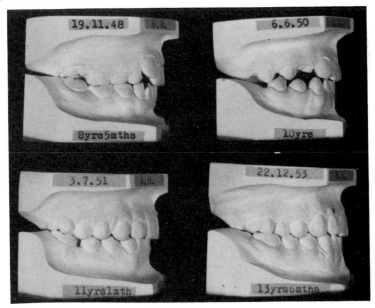

Figure 9.28 Models showing mildly crowded arches where the extraction of all first permanent molars in a Class I case at the age of 9 years has allowed a satisfactory result and some relief of incisor crowding.

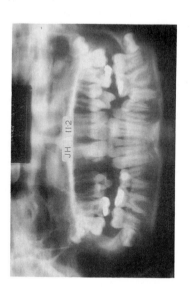
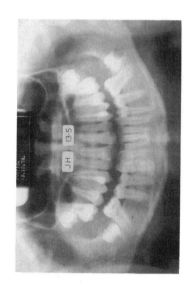
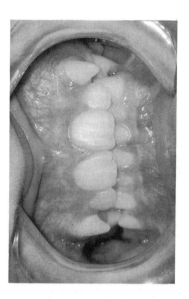
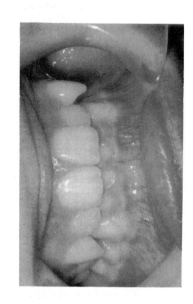

Figure 9.29 Early loss of deciduous molars has allowed a good result where loss of the first molars was carried out at 11½ years – well beyond the ideal age: (a) before extractions; (b) at 13 years 5 months.

The upper arch

The pre-eruptive distal inclination of the second molar generally allows this tooth to achieve a reasonably upright position after mesial migration, even when the extraction of the first molar has been delayed beyond the optimum time by as much as a year or so.

Exceptions to the general rule of early extraction

Mildly excluded canines will usually drop into place after first molar extractions in the upper arch; but where it is evident that significant space will be required for anterior alignment there may be a case for preserving the first molars until the second molars erupt. Controlled use can then be made of the available space (Fig 9.30). Unfortunately this frequently means that treatment cannot begin until the patient has reached the age of 13 or 14 years and may then be unwilling to wear appliances. For this reason some prefer to extract the first molars early and regain the necessary space by means of headgear applied to second molar bands. This is because these teeth usually erupt no later than 12 years where first molars have been removed.

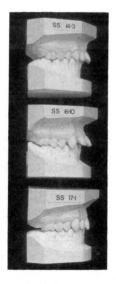

Figure 9.30 Retaining the upper first molars until the second permanent molars can be clasped to allow the space to be used for the correction of an overjet. Whilst this appears logical it results in a very prolonged course of removable-appliance treatment started at a relatively late age. This patient needed to wear extraoral anchorage throughout the 3-year treatment.

Postponed extraction in the lower arch is seldom indicated, as mesial movement of the lower second molar occurs less readily here. The exception is where there is a severe malocclusion present for which fixed appliances are to be used.

Early use of appliances

As extraction of the upper first molar severely limits the use of upper removable appliances until the second molar can be clasped, extractions should be deferred until any lingually occluding incisors have been proclined. Unfortunately this is not the whole story for there are frequently situations where these guidelines will prove to be inadequate. In many cases expert advice will be needed. These include:

a a substantial malocclusion superimposed on the complication of enforced first molar loss;
b severely crowded cases – where further extractions may be required;
c mildly crowded cases – where there may be large residual spaces.

Specialist advice will also be required to determine the need for balancing and compensatory extractions. The routine application of a simple dogma is not good practice here because the individual case will have many factors to be considered or predicted. Where only one molar has a poor prognosis, decisions on balancing and compensating are best taken one quadrant at a time. It may be, for example, better to extract first molars on one side of the mouth and first premolars on the other. On the other hand, in mild cases it may be best to confine the extractions to first molars on one side of the mouth only and accept some centre-line displacement rather than produce excess space in all four quadrants.

Traumatic loss of an upper central incisor

The traumatic loss of a central incisor is extremely distressing for both the child and parent. Emergency treatment is crucial to the long-term outcome (Andlaw and Rock, 1982). Wherever possible the avulsed incisor should be reimplanted even when the period out of the mouth has been too long to assure success. Where this is not possible, provision should be made for immediate maintenance of the space – that is to say the space should be retained initially by temporary means and within a few days by a clasped denture carrying spurs to ensure that no migration of adjacent incisors can occur. Subsequently, when the trauma of the event has passed, the long-term treatment can be planned. There are always a number of considerations to be taken into account (Andlaw and Stephens, 1987). In general it will be preferable to think in terms of maintaining the space. This is because crowning of an adjacent lateral seldom provides a satisfactory long-term solution. Adhesive bridges have a high success rate where the occlusion is favourable but this is greatly reduced in the developing mouth. In almost all cases, therefore, a denture will be required at least initially until conventional bridgework or an intraosseous implant can be considered. In some cases, autotransplantation of a premolar may be possible.

Where initial orthodontic treatment has been carried out to align the maxillary incisors, or to regain lost space, it is necessary to retain the anterior teeth for at least the usual period of 6–9 months before replacing the retainer with a bonded pontic.

Incisors in linguo-occlusion

It is universally agreed that anterior teeth in linguo-occlusion should be corrected as early as possible. In this way the associated displaced path of mandibular closure will be discontinued and the risk of gingival damage to the lower incisors will be avoided (see Fig. 1.5). The self-use of wooden spatulas has been advocated in the past but, although these can be effective for a single tooth in crossbite, the method requires a particularly stoical 7-year-old for it to be successful. Conventional upper removable appliances are therefore recommended (see Chapters 10 and 12).

Where upper central incisors are in linguo-occlusion treatment should not be delayed until the lateral incisors have erupted. The mandibular displacement will almost certainly ensure that at least one lateral incisor will erupt into crossbite if the central incisors remain uncorrected. Where central or lateral incisors are short of space, both upper and lower deciduous canines should be removed. The lower extractions ensure that the lower labial segment will be well aligned, without one lower incisor being crowded labially, which makes the upper correction more difficult. It is worthwhile remembering that sometimes lateral incisors are held palatally through lack of space and thereby erupt into crossbite. Prompt removal of the deciduous canines before an overbite has been established almost always ensures that the problem will be self-correcting. Where the overbite is established and active treatment is required it is important not to delay. By the time the patient reaches 10 years of age the permanent canine will be fairly low in the ridge and can often impede labial movement of a lateral incisor before a satisfactory overbite has been obtained. In these circumstances, alignment will have to be delayed until relief of crowding and retraction of the erupted canine can be undertaken.

Treatment of posterior crossbite (see also Chapter 10)

Where a persistent thumb habit has produced narrowing of the inter-canine distance there may well be cuspal interference in the canine region and a displacement in the mandibular path of closure. It is generally preferable to correct displacements before a unilateral cross-bite becomes fully established in the permanent dentition. This may not be possible if the habit continues; but where it has been largely abandoned, careful grinding of the cusps of the deciduous canines may eliminate the interference and allow non-displaced closure to be regained in the cuspal position. Failing this, the crossbite should be corrected by conventional means. There is still considerable argument about the most appropriate timing of such treatment. Some advocate early treatment in the mixed dentition; others point out that there may be no real advantage to be gained by early intervention, particularly where later orthodontic treatment is required.

Early intervention in cases of skeletal discrepancy

Opinions differ widely as to the desirability of early intervention for cases that show a severely abnormal facial form. On the one hand such treatment can be justified if it is likely to produce even a modest improvement and if this results in better chance of success in later orthodontic treatment. On the other, the extent to which facial pattern can be modified by treatment is at best very limited and will seldom be sufficient to make the difference between a surgical and an orthodontic approach. There is also the additional problem of declining cooperation, caused by embarking on protracted treatment at an early age, which make a worthwhile outcome even less certain.

The use of myofunctional appliances in the early correction of sagittal discrepancies is discussed in Chapter 17. In the vertical dimension, excessive face height can be the cause of a 'skeletal' open bite but there is no evidence that early treatment is of any great advantage. On the other hand, reduced lower face height can be increased by treatment aimed at encouraging a posterior mandibular rotation (see Chapter 7). Where a marked anterior growth rotation is the cause of a deep overbite that is causing trauma to the soft tissues the early use of a simple anterior bite plane may be indicated. It should be emphasized, though, that traumatic overbite is rare. The overwhelming majority of overbites that are complete against the palatal soft tissue cause no damage and hence their treatment should be left to conventional means at the usual time.

Summary

The general practitioner plays the key role in instituting prompt interceptive measures. Although the practitioner may not have the experience to plan treatment it is his or her responsibility to identify abnormal dental development in the child and refer patients for advice where this appears to be necessary. The investigations required are surprisingly few. These are:

1 Routine radiography at the age of 8–10 years for all patients who are regular attenders to determine the presence of all successional teeth and eliminate the possibility of undetected supernumerary teeth and other pathology.
2 A consideration of the need for balancing and/or compensating extractions when undertaking removal of unsaveable deciduous teeth.
3 The prompt correction of permanent incisor teeth that erupt into crossbite.
4 A conscious consideration of the long-term prognosis of the first permanent molars at an early age (by 10 years at the latest).
5 Routine palpation for maxillary canines from 8 years onwards and the use of localizing radiographs where the canine cannot be detected clinically at 10 years and over.

References

Andlaw, R. J. and Rock, W. P. (1982) *A Manual of Paedodontics*, Churchill Livingstone, Edinburgh

Andlaw, R. J. and Stephens, C. D. (1987) Prevention and the avulsed anterior tooth. In *Positive Dental Prevention* (ed. R. J. Elderton) Heinemann, London

Andreasen, J. O., Paulsen, H. U., Yu, Z., Ahlquist, R., Bayer, T. and Schwartz, O. (1990a) A long term study of 370 autotransplanted premolars. Part 1 – Surgical procedures and standardised techniques for monitoring healing. *European Journal of Orthodontics*, **12**, 3–13

Andreasen, J. O., Paulsen, H. U., Yu, Z., Bayer, T, and Schwartz, O. (1990b) A long term study of 370 autotransplanted premolars. Part 2 – Tooth survival and pulp healing subsequent to transplantation. *European Journal of Orthodontics*, **12**, 14–24

Andreasen J. O., Paulsen, H. U., Yu, Z. and Schwartz, O. (1990c) A long term study of 370 autotransplanted premolars. Part 3 – Periodontal healing subsequent to transplantation. *European Journal of Orthodontics*, **12**, 24–37

Andreasen, J. O., Paulsen, H. U., Yu, Z. and Bayer, T. (1990d) A long term study of 370 autotransplanted premolars. Part 4 – Root development subsequent to transplantation. *European Journal of Orthodontics*, **12**, 38–50

Breakspeare, E. K. (1951) Sequelae of early loss of deciduous molars. *Dental Record*, **71**, 127–135

Breakspeare, E. K. (1960) Further observations on early loss of deciduous molars. *Dental Practitioner*, **11**, 233–250

Brin, I., Becker, A. and Shalhav, M. (1986) The position of the maxillary permanent canine in relation to anomalous or missing lateral incisors: a population study. *European Journal of Orthodontics*, **8**, 12–16

Brook, A. M. and Winter, G. B. (1970) Double teeth: a retrospective study of 'geminated' and 'fused' teeth in children. *British Dental Journal*, **129**, 123–130

Clinch, L. M. (1959) A longitudinal study of the results of premature loss of deciduous teeth between 3–4 and 1–15 years of age. *Dental Practitioner*, **9**, 109–126

Davies, P. L. (1968) Agenesis of teeth of the permanent dentition. A frequency study in Sydney school children. *Australian Dental Journal*, **13**, 146–150

Ericson, S. and Kurol, J. (1986) Radiographic assessment of maxillary canine eruption in children with clinical signs of eruption disturbance. *European Journal of Orthodontics*, **8**, 133–140

Ericson, S. and Kurol, J. (1988) Early treatment of palatally erupting maxillary canines treated by extraction of the primary canines. *European Journal of Orthodontics*, **10**, 283–295

Ferguson, J. W. (1990) Mangement of the unerupted maxillary canine. *British Dental Journal*, **69**, 11–17

Grahnen, H. (1956) Hypodontia in the permanent dentition. *Odontologisk Revy*, **7** (Supplement 3)

Kjellgren, B. (1948) Serial extraction as a corrective procedure in dental orthopaedic therapy. *Acta Odontologica Scandinavica*, **8**, 17–43

Leighton, B. C. (1971) The value of prophecy in orthodontics. *Transactions of the British Society for the Study of Orthodontics*, 1–14

Lundstrsöm, A. (1955) The significance of early loss of deciduous teeth in the aetiology of malocclusion. *American Journal of Orthodontics*, **41**, 810–826

Moss, J. P. (1972) The unerupted maxillary canine. *Dental Practitioner*, **22**, 241–248

Neal, J. J. D. and Bowden, D. E. J. (1988) The diagnostic value of panoramic radiographs in children aged nine to ten years. *British Journal of Orthodontics*, **15**, 193–197

Richardson, M. E. (1965) The relationship between the relative amount of space present in the deciduous dental arch and the rate and degree of space closure subsequent to the extraction of a deciduous molar. *Dental Practitioner*, **16**, 111–118

Sagne, S. and Thilander, B. (1990) Transalveolar transplantation of maxillary canines: a follow-up study. *European Journal of Orthodontics*, **12**, 140–147

Sarnat, B. G., Brodie, A. G. and Kubacki, W. H. (1953) Fourteen year report of facial growth in a case of complete anodontia with ectodermal dysplasia. *American Journal of Diseases of Children*, **86**, 162–169

Taylor, G. S. (1972) Characteristics of supernumerary teeth in the primary and permanent dentition. *Dental Practitioner*, **22**, 203–208

Van der Linden, F. P. G. M. (1990) *Problems and Procedures in Dentofacial Orthopedics*, Quintessence, Chicago, pp. 27–38

Zilberman, Y., Cohen, B. and Becker, A. (1990) Familial trends in palatal canines, anomalous lateral incisors, and related phenomena. *European Journal of Orthodontics*, **12**, 135–139

Chapter 10

Class I malocclusions

Class I malocclusions include all those anomalies where the antero-posterior relationship of lower and upper arches is within normal limits. There may, however, be transverse or vertical arch malrelationships. Crowding and local irregularities (see Chapter 9) are common causes of Class I malocclusion. Generalized spacing is unusual. All of these irregularities may be found in association with the other classes of malocclusion.

Occlusal features

The incisor relationship is Class I (Fig. 10.1). This does not imply an ideal incisor relationship because the category of Class I comprises a range of incisor relationships. Hence there may be an anterior open bite or a bimaxillary proclination with an increase in overjet and a reduction

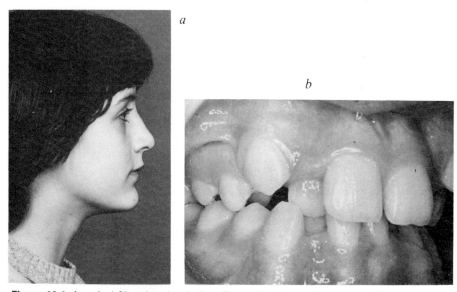

a

b

Figure 10.1 A typical Class I malocclusion. The patient has a Class 1 dental base relationship and a pleasing profile.

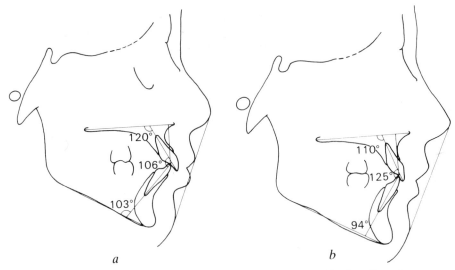

Figure 10.2 (a) A Class I malocclusion with bimaxillary proclination. Note that although the overjet is somewhat increased it cannot be reduced satisfactorily by simple retroclination of the upper incisors because the incisor occlusion is already Class I. (b) The bimaxillary proclination has been reduced and is now stable: the soft tissues have adapted to the new position of the teeth. Although the bimaxillary proclination was reduced completely during treatment, the incisors have come forward slightly since appliances were withdrawn; however, the lower incisor edge is still in advance of the upper root centroid.

in overbite (Fig. 10.2). The buccal segment relationship is often Class I, but there may have been drift of first permanent molars following premature loss of deciduous teeth; and if the canines are crowded they may not be in a Class I relationship. It may be difficult to decide how to classify a borderline case. For example, if several of the upper incisors are instanding, should the patient be described as having a Class III malocclusion? It is probably reasonable to be guided by the general features: if at least two upper incisors are in a Class I relationship and if the other occlusal features are compatible with a Class I occlusion the case should be classified as such. It should be remembered that classification is merely an aid to description and the treatment of a borderline case should not be affected by its categorization.

Skeletal relationships

Although the skeletal pattern will usually be Class 1, mild skeletal malrelationships accompanied by dentoalveolar compensation are often seen, and occasionally a Class I malocclusion will be found associated with moderate Class 3 or Class 2 skeletal pattern. With a Class 2 skeletal pattern, compensation is usually by lower incisor proclination. Where there is a Class 3 skeletal pattern, upper incisors will usually be slightly proclined and the lowers retroclined to some degree.

Vertical and transverse skeletal malrelationships may be associated with anterior open bites and crossbites, respectively, although these are found more commonly where there is a Class III malocclusion.

Facial growth

In Class I cases, the anteroposterior jaw relationship is generally favourable and this does not usually change appreciably with facial growth: any minor changes are absorbed by dentoalveolar adaptation. Skeletal open bites tend to become more severe because dentoalveolar compensation for the increased anterior intermaxillary height is already at its limits and vertical dentoalveolar growth may not keep pace with any further facial growth.

Soft tissue form and behaviour

The soft tissue pattern is favourable in the great majority of Class I cases and does not impose limitations on treatment objectives. Incomplete overbites associated with digit-sucking habits tend to improve, unless they are maintained by an adaptive swallowing pattern. In cases of bimaxillary proclination, the lips are full and everted, and this is a major factor in determining the tooth positions (Fig. 10.2).

Mandibular position and path of closure

There are no characteristic mandibular postures. However, occlusal irregularities such as instanding incisors and unilateral crossbites are frequently associated with mandibular displacements, and so it is important that the path of closure is checked during the initial assessment.

Dentoalveolar

In the majority of Class I malocclusions the underlying problem will be one of tooth/arch discrepancy. Usually this will be dental crowding but occasionally spacing will be the main concern. Local or general spacing may be the result of developmental absence of teeth, loss of permanent teeth or, more rarely, small teeth in well-formed arches (Fig. 10.3).

Perhaps 5 per cent of malocclusions arise from the effects of 'local factors' (see Chapter 9). If this is the sole cause of a Class I malocclusion, it will usually be appropriate to institute early treatment. Where local factors act in conjunction with other more general causes of malocclusion the case for early intervention will be less clear-cut.

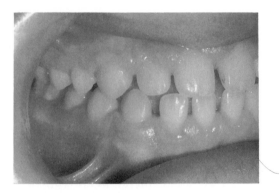

Figure 10.3 An example of generalized spacing.

Treatment objectives

Clearly the primary objective is to deal with the patient's main concern, which will usually be irregularity of the incisors. However, it is important to deal with any other aspect of the malocclusion that might subsequently give problems, and to leave the patient with a healthy, functional occlusion. Particularly where removable appliances are to be used, treatment objectives are limited by the tooth movements that can be achieved. An overambitious treatment plan may leave the patient worse off than before, with excessive, unclosed extraction spaces, tilted teeth and a disrupted occlusion. This can be a major problem in the milder cases where only a small amount of the extraction space is required for tooth alignment and where residual spaces are difficult to close unless fixed appliances are employed in competent hands. The potential benefit of orthodontic treatment to the patient may be minimal and it is a serious matter if they are left with a poorer occlusion than before. Good results can be obtained with removable appliances in carefully selected cases. Severe problems requiring complex tooth movements, and minor irregularities where near perfection must be achieved if any significant benefit is to be obtained, should be treated with fixed appliances.

Treatment

In a significant proportion of Class I cases the only feature of the malocclusion is crowding; while in others only a local factor may be responsible. The management of local irregularities is discussed in Chapter 9. In general, local factors should be treated as early as possible, although where there are other superimposed causes it may be preferable to delay treatment until the conventional time rather than subject the patient to two courses of treatment. Where dental crowding alone is responsible for the malocclusion it may be possible to treat without appliances through the timely extraction of teeth (Fig. 10.4). In others,

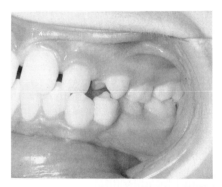
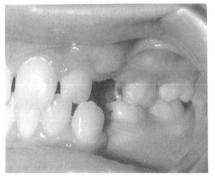
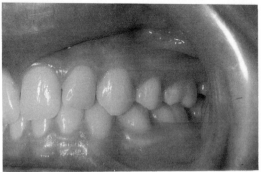

Figure 10.4 A case treated by extraction of all four first premolars. No appliances were used.

some form of space-maintaining appliance will be required to ensure that the anterior teeth and erupting canines have adequate space to align (Fig. 10.5). However, such cases always require a measure of luck and patients should be told that appliances are likely to be required even where all indications for spontaneous alignment are present (see below).

a   *b*

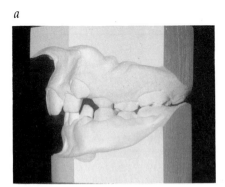
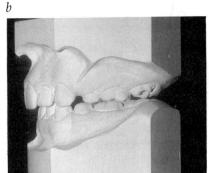

Figure 10.5 A case with more severe crowding that required an upper removable and lower fixed space-maintaining appliance in conjunction with first premolar extractions: (a) before treatment; (b) after treatment.

Crowding

This is due to disproportion between tooth size and arch size. Expansion of arch size to relieve crowding was recommended by Angle but all the long-term studies that have been published have found that relapse is very common (Little, 1990). Expansion of lower intercanine width and labial movement of lower incisors are particularly unstable. Thus, in general, crowding has to be dealt with either by distal movement of buccal segments (which gives limited space in the upper arch and almost none in the lower) or by extractions (see Chapter 8).

Crowding is often first apparent on eruption of the incisors, but may sometimes improve with arch growth and by utilization of the leeway space. Moorrees (1958) found that many cases with a good occlusion in the permanent dentition had previously shown some signs of crowding. On the other hand, there is little hope that moderate to severe crowding in the mixed dentition will improve to any appreciable extent; and in the permanent dentition the tendency is for crowding to become more severe rather than to improve (see Chapter 2).

Where crowding is confined to labiolingual irregularity in the incisor and canine regions, treatment may be achieved by means of first premolar extractions alone. For this to be appropriate the degree of anterior crowding must be such as to require at least half the space provided by the extractions, and the canines must be mesially inclined to facilitate their spontaneous distal movement (see Fig. 10.4). Where more than half a premolar unit of space is required anteriorly, space maintenance will almost always be required. In the upper arch this can be provided by means of a simple Hawley retainer but in the lower a lingual arch is more reliable (Fig. 10.5).

Even in these carefully defined cases, spontaneous improvement cannot be relied upon to achieve a fully corrected malocclusion; and if a satisfactory improvement has not taken place during the six months after extraction, active treatment will be required. As removable appliances are poorly tolerated in the lower arch it will be appreciated that even in these 'simple' cases the general practitioner who has no knowledge of fixed appliances is at a considerable disadvantage.

When mild crowding is seen in the permanent dentition it may well be best to accept this. Premolar extractions will provide a large amount of excess space, the closure of which will require fixed appliances and is likely to be accompanied by retraction of the upper and lower labial segments. The alternative of extracting teeth at the back in the arch (for example, second or third molars) does nothing to relieve anterior crowding unless active measures are employed to move the buccal teeth distally (Fig. 10.6). In the upper arch, extraoral traction can be used to achieve this, but an additional headgear in the lower arch is not well tolerated. Class III elastic traction from a lower fixed appliance to the upper molars can be employed, provided additional headgear wear is forthcoming to overcome this undesirable mesial component of force. Some authorities advocate the use of a lower lip bumper (see Chapter 17). Whichever mechanism is used it is almost inevitable that there will be some reciprocal proclination of the lower incisor teeth.

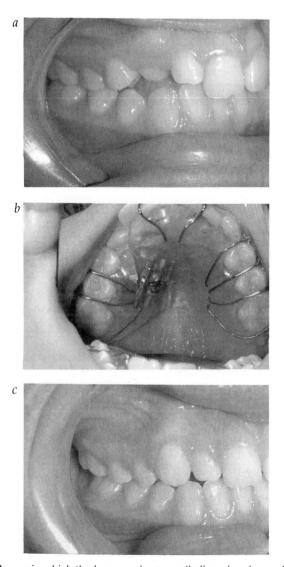

Figure 10.6 A case in which the lower arch was well aligned and crowding in the upper arch was treated by distal movement of the upper right quadrant in order to accommodate the misplaced canine: (a) before treatment; (b) the first upper appliance – because only one side required retraction, no extraoral anchorage was used; (c) after treatment.

If the mildly crowded case is to receive treatment, fixed appliances in both arches will be required, and it will usually be best to think in terms of extracting four second premolars in order to provide adequate anchorage mesial to the extraction site to permit space closure to be achieved without affecting the labiolingual position of the lower incisors (Fig. 10.7).

a

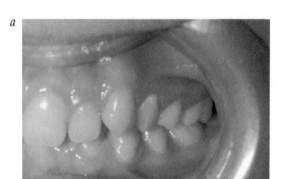

b

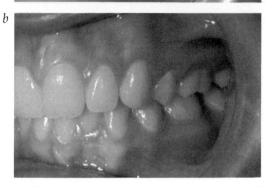

Figure 10.7 A case with mild crowding in both arches that required fixed appliances to close excess extraction space. For that reason four second premolars were removed to improve the anchorage in the anterior segment. (a) Before treatment with the Begg appliance; (b) one year after all retainers had been removed.

Spacing

Spacing may occur because the teeth are small in relation to the size of the arch or because teeth are missing (see Chapter 9). Sometimes this is acceptable to the patient but where this is not the case it is important to discuss fully the implications of treatment. Complete closure of appreciable spacing may not be possible and it is often best to concentrate it at appropriate sites and to fit bridges or prostheses as necessary. In these circumstances, patients are usually keen to avoid a denture but the cost of maintaining expensive bridgework for life should not be underestimated and technical considerations may make bridgework undesirable.

Where lateral incisors are missing it will usually be best to collect available space at this site and use adhesive bridges where the occlusion permits this (Fig. 10.8). For most other cases it will often be best to collect space in the premolar region (Fig. 10.9)

Bimaxillary proclination

Bimaxillary proclination may be a feature of Class II, division 1 malocclu-

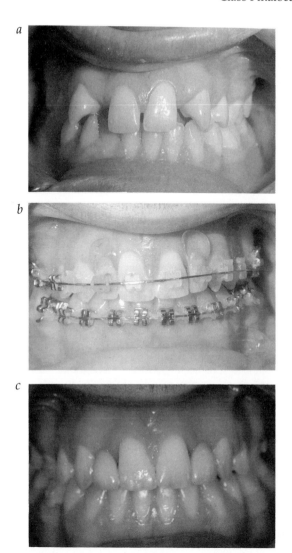

Figure 10.8 (a) A young adult who presented with four missing second premolars and missing maxillary lateral incisors. (b) A straight-wire fixed-appliance technique was used with ceramic upper brackets to close space posteriorly and increase the space at the lateral incisor site. Note that the archwire carries temporary prosthetic replacements for the missing incisors that are retained by acrylic bonded brackets. (c) After fitting of acid etch-retained pontics.

sion, but quite often the incisor relationship is Class I, which may mistakenly be diagnosed as Class II division 1 because of the increase in overjet (see Fig. 10.2). The distinction is very important because the overjet cannot satisfactorily be reduced in Class I cases with bimaxillary proclination unless the lower incisors are also retracted (Fig. 10.10).

The proclination of the upper and lower incisors is due to the soft

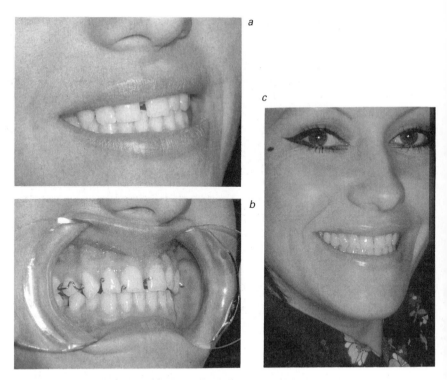

Figure 10.9 (a) This patient had lost the upper right first molar in what had been an uncrowded Class I occlusion; (b) a removable appliance was used to open space at the first premolar site; (c) after fitting of a one-unit bridge.

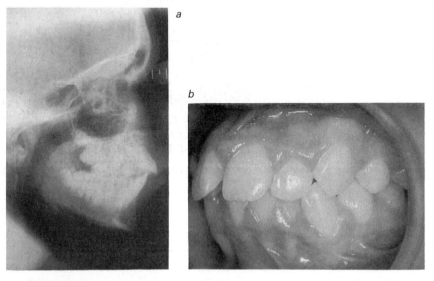

Figure 10.10 A case of bimaxillary proclination: (a) the cephalometric film; (b) the clinical presentation showing an increase in overjet despite there being a Class I incisor relationship.

tissue pattern. Usually the lips are full and everted, and the tongue acts to mould the dental arches as they erupt. Occasionally the tongue itself is very large and is the primary cause of the bimaxillary proclination, although this is unusual.

A mild degree of bimaxillary proclination can be pleasing, and it should be remembered that the lower face fullness will often become less marked in the adult because growth of the nose and increased prominence of the chin change the character of the face. In some racial groups, the incisors are typically more proclined than the Caucasian norms (see Table 6.2). The individual must be compared with the appropriate norms and even having done so, treatment should not be suggested solely because of a deviation from these average values. Treatment is justified only if the individual would be considered to be facially disadvantaged within their own racial group because of the malocclusion. Even if this is the case, it may still not be possible to achieve a stable improvement in the occlusion because of the soft tissue pattern.

It is sometimes suggested that bimaxillary proclination should not be treated because of its potential instability. This is too sweeping a conclusion, because in some cases the soft tissues adapt to the corrected incisor positions. It should be remembered that to a large extent the position of the incisors reflects the soft tissue pattern at the time they erupted, and this may subsequently have matured.

If the tongue is very large and appears to fill the oral cavity as far as can be judged clinically or from a lateral skull radiograph, incisor retraction will probably not be stable, or at least not without a surgical reduction in tongue size, which is justifiable only in the most severe cases. The fundamental question is whether the lips will drop back with the retraction of the incisor teeth, establishing a new position of soft tissue balance. This is most likely to happen where the patient has to make an appreciable effort to obtain a lip seal over the proclined incisors but could be expected to achieve a habitual lip seal after they had been retracted. If the lips are very full and are long enough to obtain a seal easily in spite of the bimaxillary proclination, they may drop back less when the incisors are retracted and so stability is problematical.

The lower incisors have to be tipped back far enough to allow an acceptable inclination of the upper incisors. If there is a Class II skeletal pattern, the lower incisors will still have to compensate for this. The correct position of the lower incisor edge is readily assessed from the edge–centroid relationship: the lower edge in these cases should be positioned to lie directly below the upper incisor centroid (Houston, 1989) (see Fig. 10.2). The need for extraction of teeth in the lower and upper arches can then be evaluated. It is important to allow enough space for full retraction of the upper and lower incisors because if the bimaxillary proclination is reduced only partially, relapse is more likely. The height of the upper incisor edge is also important: the lower lip should cover at least the incisal third of the labial surface of the retracted upper incisors when a lip seal is obtained. If this is not the case, some relapse may occur.

Although the incisors will be tipped lingually, this is best achieved with fixed appliances, which can give more precise anteroposterior and vertical control of tooth positions, and are well tolerated in the lower arch.

Vertical anomalies

By definition, deep overbites are not found in Class I incisor relationships. They are discussed in the chapters on Class II malocclusions. An anterior open bite is present when there is no incisor contact and no vertical overlap of the lower incisors by the uppers. An incomplete overbite is a minor variant of an anterior open bite. Isolated posterior open bites are rare and there is seldom any obvious cause. They are usually attributed to localized failure of alveolar process development.

Anterior open bite

An anterior open bite may be caused by digit-sucking habits (see p. 192); perhaps by atypical swallowing patterns (see p. 21); or by skeletal factors (Fig. 10.11). Atypical swallowing patterns are commonly associated with anterior open bites, but they are often secondary: the tongue tends to come forwards to seal off the gap between the incisors. Such an adaptation commonly perpetuates an anterior open bite caused by digit sucking, even after the habit has been discontinued. Adaptations in swallowing behaviour to obtain an anterior oral seal in Class II, division 1 cases are associated with an incomplete overbite rather than an anterior open bite; but a primary tongue thrust can be a rare cause of anterior open bite (see p. 22).

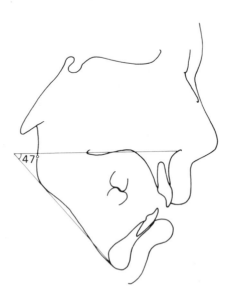

Figure 10.11 A skeletal open bite: the height of the intermaxillary space is increased anteriorly and there is an associated anterior open bite.

These are usually due to an increase in anterior intermaxillary height but can occasionally be attributed to a localized failure of maxillary dentoalveolar development. The latter can occur in patients with clefts of the lip and palate, and rarely in other cases for no apparent reason.

When the anterior intermaxillary height is excessive, the teeth and alveolar processes may grow to their full extent but fail to achieve an overbite (Fig. 10.11). This is more common in Class III cases but can be found with Class I malocclusions. In mild cases the open bite may be confined to the maxillary lateral incisor region because these teeth have shorter crowns than their immediate neighbours. In the more severe cases, the open bite includes all incisors and extends into the buccal segments where only the most distal teeth may meet in occlusion. There is generally a posterior mandibular growth rotation and the open bite tends to become worse with growth.

A skeletal open bite is often of little concern to the patient and it may be the dental practitioner who is the first to draw attention to it. Occasionally the patient will complain of difficulty in incising food but this is rarely a serious problem. There are no periodontal problems typically associated with an anterior open bite and there have been reports of a slightly increased prevalence of tenderness in the muscles of mastication.

It is important to recognize that in cases of skeletal open bite, the posterior teeth are not 'propping open' the bite: these teeth have succeeded in establishing an occlusion at a position where the inter-maxillary height is less, without encroaching on the rest position of the mandible. Thus grinding or extraction of posterior teeth is not helpful – it merely means that the patient has to overclose to obtain an occlusion and is even more liable to suffer from muscle pain. Extrusion of anterior teeth is also ill-advised: the alveolar bone will not usually grow with the teeth and so tooth support is reduced; and the incisors are already at a reasonable height relative to the lips and may look very unsightly if they are extruded.

The only satisfactory treatment of a skeletal open bite is by surgery (see Chapter 19). However, because a skeletal open bite is in itself rarely of serious concern to the patient, surgery may not be indicated unless there is some coexisting anomaly, such as a Class III skeletal pattern, to be dealt with at the same time. It should be noted that surgical correction of skeletal open bite is particularly liable to relapse, owing to the action of the musculature, and careful presurgical planning and postsurgical fixation are essential.

Soft tissue open bite

Open bite caused by the action of the tongue is extremely rare. More commonly the tongue may maintain an open bite caused by a digit habit (see Chapter 9). This is more likely where the habit is discontinued only after growth has ceased. A primary atypical swallowing behaviour (endogenous tongue thrust) is usually associated with a marked anterior sigmatism and a degree of bimaxillary proclination. To all intents and purposes the condition should be regarded as untreatable.

Posterior open bites

A posterior open bite affecting all the teeth in one or both posterior segments is an extremely rare condition of obscure aetiology. More commonly a lateral open bite is seen in which premolars and canines fail to reach full occlusal height. This condition is said to be caused by premature loss of deciduous molars where the tongue spreads into space so provided and fails to vacate this position when the permanent successors erupt. Clinical observation suggests that this is not the whole story. Early loss was, until recently, extremely common but lateral open bite is a rare finding that has not reduced in prevalence as the need for the enforced removal of carious deciduous teeth has declined. Fixed appliances can be used to close a lateral open bite by employing intermaxillary elastic traction. However, even after prolonged retention, such treatment frequently relapses, suggesting some other aetiology than a passive tongue spread (Fig. 10.12).

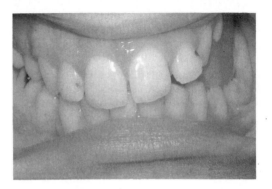

Figure 10.12 A severe lateral open bite.

Transverse anomalies – crossbite

Crossbites are anomalies in the radial relationships of posterior occluding teeth such that the palatal cusps of the upper teeth do not occlude in the central fossae of their lower opponents. Crossbites may be local or segmental. Segmental crossbites, particularly scissors bite and bilateral crossbites, are found most commonly in Class II and Class III cases, respectively, in part because of the anteroposterior discrepancy, but they do arise in Class I cases and will be included here.

Local crossbites

These affect only one pair of occluding teeth and are almost always the result of crowding. The two most common local crossbites are:

1 Where early loss of a maxillary or mandibular second deciduous molar has caused the second premolar to become lingually displaced (Fig. 10.13).

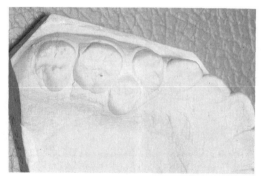

Figure 10.13 A local crossbite of an upper second premolar that has been caused by space loss after early removal of the deciduous second molar.

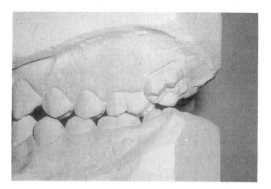

Figure 10.14 A crowded upper second molar that has erupted in local crossbite

2 Where severe posterior crowding in the upper jaw causes the second or third molar to be buccally displaced (Fig. 10.14).

Such conditions are easily treated by local tooth movement after the relief of dental crowding.

Segmental crossbites

These affect most if not all of the buccal teeth in one quadrant. Segmental crossbites may be unilateral or bilateral and often reflect some discrepancy in the widths of the dental bases. The clinician's primary concern should be not with the crossbite itself but with any displacement in the path of closure of the mandible, which is frequently found to accompany crossbites – particularly unilateral crossbite

Unilateral crossbite with lateral displacement (Fig. 10.15)

Where the arches are symmetrical and of equal width, the mandible will usually be displaced to one side or the other in order to obtain maximal intercuspation, producing a crossbite. This type of crossbite may be due

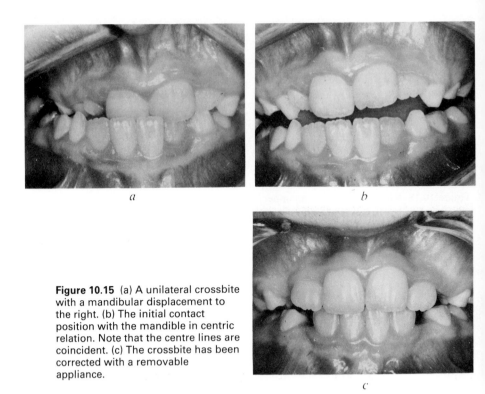

a

b

Figure 10.15 (a) A unilateral crossbite with a mandibular displacement to the right. (b) The initial contact position with the mandible in centric relation. Note that the centre lines are coincident. (c) The crossbite has been corrected with a removable appliance.

c

to a mild discrepancy in dental base widths, but commonly is associated with a digit-sucking habit: when the finger or thumb is being sucked, the teeth are parted, the tongue is low and the contraction of the buccinator muscles narrows the upper arch slightly.

Unilateral crossbites with displacement should be treated by maxillary arch expansion in order to eliminate the cuspal contact in the retruded arc of closure that induces the displacement. A removable appliance with posterior bite planes has the merit that secondary expansion of the lower arch, through intercuspation of the teeth, is avoided. Expansion can also successfully be achieved with a fixed palatal arch (Fig. 10.16).

In some cases where the buccal inclination of the upper teeth is already partly compensating for the underlying dental base discrepancy, further buccal tipping would not give a satisfactory or stable occlusion and rapid maxillary expansion may be indicated. The objective is to widen the maxillary base by expanding the midpalatal suture. The maxilla hinges around its other sutural attachments with the upper facial skeleton and so this procedure is not feasible after the late teens, when some of these sutures may have started to fuse. Bone is laid down at the expanded sutural margins in the usual manner and the dental base expansion is stable. However, the teeth tend to relapse partially under the influence of the facial musculature, and so a degree of overexpansion is desirable.

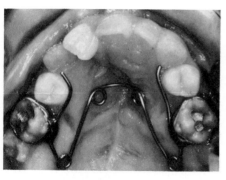
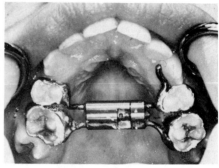

a   *b*

Figure 10.16 (a) A quadhelix appliance for expansion of the maxillary arch; (b) a Hyrax screw for rapid maxillary expansion.

The appliance used is a heavy screw attached to bands or splints (Fig. 10.16). The parent is instructed to turn the screw twice a day over a period of about 2 weeks, producing an expansion of up to 7 mm. The key should be attached to a length of thread so that there is no risk of it being dropped down the patient's throat. Rapid maxillary expansion is indicated in only a few cases and must not be used indiscriminately. Where the maxilla is very narrow, the patient's nasal airway may be improved but treatment is not indicated for this reason alone.

Unilateral crossbite without lateral displacement

These usually display an underlying skeletal asymmetry. This may be pathological in origin (e.g. unilateral cleft palate, unilateral condylar hyperplasia). Correction of the crossbite is seldom indicated: in the first place there may be no functional or aesthetic advantage to the patient; and stability of correction is doubtful.

Bilateral crossbite (Fig. 10.17)

This is always associated with a maxillary dental base that is narrow relative to the mandibular base. Usually there is no displacement and so the patient suffers no functional or aesthetic problems. A danger of treatment is that correction followed by partial relapse could give rise to a unilateral crossbite with an associated mandibular displacement, which in turn might lead to muscle and joint dysfunction. Where there are special circumstances that make upper arch expansion desirable, rapid maxillary expansion is generally to be preferred; but even with overcorrection and prolonged retention, stability cannot be assured.

Scissors bite

This occurs when the upper arch is too broad relative to the lower, and usually reflects an underlying skeletal mismatch. The milder cases

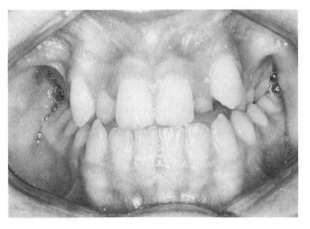

Figure 10.17 A bilateral crossbite.

involve only a few teeth. Complete unilateral scissors bite is seldom found and bilateral cases are very rare.

A scissors bite can cause mandibular displacement on closure into occlusion. If only a few teeth are involved, correction may be straight-forward. A complete unilateral scissors bite with a displacement can be treated by expansion of the lower arch and possibly some contraction of the upper arch, using removable appliances or fixed arches. Stability depends on a good intercuspation of the teeth. A complete unilateral scissors bite without displacement, and the bilateral condition, are very rare and may require surgical intervention.

References

Houston, W. J. B. (1989) Incisor centroid relationships and overbite depth. *European Journal of Orthodontics*, **11**, 139–143

Little, R. M. (1990) Stability and relapse of dental arch alignment. *British Journal of Orthodontics* **17**, 235–241

Moorrees, C. F. A. (1958) Growth changes of the dental arches – a longitudinal study. *Journal of the Canadian Dental Association*, **24**, 449

Chapter 11

Class II, division 1 malocclusions

Class II, division 1 malocclusions are the most common of arch mal-relationships. The prominence of the upper incisors is frequently a cause of concern to the patient and parents; and the risk of incisor fracture is appreciably greater than in other cases (Todd and Dodd, 1985).

Occlusal features

There is a Class II incisor relationship with an increased overjet (Fig. 11.1). The upper incisors are usually proclined but may sometimes be

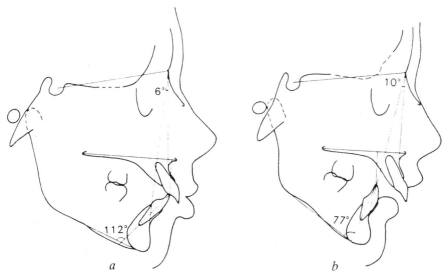

a *b*

Figure 11.1 Typical Class II, division 1 cases showing dentoalveolar compensation and exacerbation. (a) In this case the Class II skeletal pattern is more than compensated by the proclination of the lower incisors so that the lower incisor edge lies in advance of the upper root centroid. Indeed establishment of a Class I incisor relationship by palatal tipping of the upper incisors will leave a mild bimaxillary proclination and a slightly increased overjet. (b) The rather severe Class II skeletal pattern together with the retroclination of the lower incisors makes this a very difficult case to treat (see Fig. 11.7).

of average inclination. The overbite is frequently deep and is often incomplete because of an adaptive pattern of swallowing behaviour or where there is a digit-sucking habit.

Where there has been no early loss of deciduous teeth, the buccal segment relationship is usually Class II, indicating the underlying skeletal pattern. However, it can be Class I if there has been early loss in the lower arch or where the underlying skeletal bases are normally related.

Where the skeletal relationship is Class 1 (18 per cent) or Class 3 (6 per cent) (James, 1963), the incisor malrelationship is likely to have been produced by a digit-sucking habit or by an unusual soft tissue pattern. Crossbite and scissors bite may occasionally be found in association with Class II, division 1 malocclusions.

Skeletal relationships

The skeletal pattern is generally Class 2 (Fig. 11.1), the severity of the arch malrelationship being associated with the degree of the skeletal discrepancy. The anterior facial height is generally average or reduced. In some cases, there is a rather high maxillary–mandibular planes angle (Fig. 11.2).

Dentoalveolar compensation produced by a favourable soft tissue environment may produce proclination of the lower incisors, which has the effect of making the malocclusion less severe than the skeletal pattern would have led one to expect (Fig. 11.1a). In some Class II, division 1 cases, there is a receding chin, which gives a poor facial

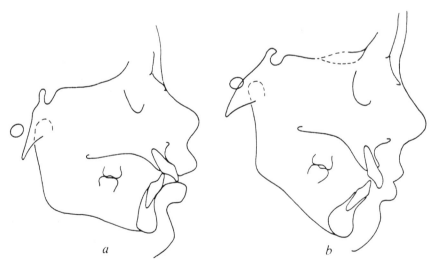

a   b

Figure 11.2 (a) In this case the maxillary–mandibular planes angle is low, the anterior intermaxillary height is reduced and there are signs of an anterior pattern of growth rotation. (b) A rather high maxillary–mandibular planes angle and signs of a posterior pattern of growth rotation indicate that the patient will probably have a trend towards a vertical growth pattern.

profile. This is usually the result of a marked skeletal Class II antero-posterior jaw relationship and an increased facial height, which has the effect of reducing the mental prominence (see below and Fig. 11.2b)

Class II, division 1 cases associated with a Class I skeletal pattern are usually rather mild and are due either to a local factor, such as a digit-sucking habit, or to the relationship of the teeth and alveolar processes to their dental bases.

Facial growth

The wide range of facial morphology that can be associated with Class II, division 1 malocclusions (Fig. 11.2) is a reflection of the varying patterns of facial growth. An anterior direction of mandibular growth with signs of an anterior mandibular growth rotation (Fig. 11.2a) is generally favourable because the skeletal relationship will tend to improve as will the soft tissue pattern. Cases with signs of vertical growth and a posterior mandibular rotation present many difficulties (Fig. 11.2b). The lips are often already incompetent and this may not improve appreciably with maturation. The facial appearance is also poor, with a receding chin, and this may not be helped by treatment directed towards retracting the upper labial segment. The skeletal pattern and facial appearance may deteriorate if treatment encourages further posterior mandibular rotation by allowing extrusion of molar teeth. This tends to occur if cervical-pull headgear is applied to the upper molars.

Soft tissues

Lip pattern is important because stability of overjet reduction depends upon the patient maintaining a lip seal, with the lower lip controlling the upper incisor positions. Many patients with a mild Class II, division 1 incisor relationship can obtain a lip seal without undue effort, or could do so but for the interposition of the upper incisors (Fig. 11.3). At the other extreme, the lips are grossly incompetent and there is little pros-pect of obtaining a lip seal, even after reduction of the overjet (Fig. 11.6).

Swallowing behaviour

In all occlusions, swallowing behaviour is related to lip morphology. Where it is possible for an individual to obtain a lip seal without undue effort this is usually done and swallowing is normal. In some Class II cases, the mandible is postured forwards habitually, which facilitates a lip seal, and swallowing takes place with the teeth parted (see p. 21). Where undue muscular effort is required to obtain a lip seal, either because of the degree of lip incompetence or because of the size of overjet, an anterior oral seal is obtained between the lower lip, the tongue and the alveolar mucosa (Fig. 11.3). When the tongue habitually lies above the lower incisor edges, the overbite is incomplete, although often only to a minor extent.

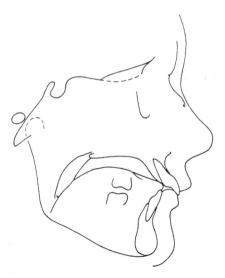

Figure 11.3 The lower lip falls behind the upper incisors and an anterior oral seal is formed by contact between the tongue, palate and lower lip. Note there is also a posterior oral seal between tongue and soft palate.

Atypical swallowing is particularly common in Class II, division 1 cases. Usually these adaptations are necessitated by variations in the incisor relationship. For example, when there is a tongue-to-lower lip seal, swallowing will normally take place with the teeth parted, as is the case when there is a forward posture of the mandible to allow a lip seal. In cases where the overbite is markedly incomplete due, for example, to a digit-sucking habit, the tongue will again come forward into contact with the lower lip. These adaptive patterns are generally of little clinical importance because they are modified spontaneously when the overjet is reduced and the patient is able to achieve a lip seal. The major exception is where the lips are too short to obtain a lip seal even after the overjet has been reduced: a tongue-to-lower lip seal will persist, and the overjet will relapse.

It is important to distinguish an adaptive pattern, which is common Class II, division 1 malocclusions, from a primary (endogenous) tongue thrust, which is rare. Primary tongue thrust has been discussed in Chapter 2: there is often an associated lisp and the overbite is always substantially incomplete and the circumoral contraction during swallowing is greater than would be expected from the degree of lip incompetence. This pattern does not modify on retraction of the incisors, and so it is prudent not to attempt to change the incisor relationship. Any treatment should be directed towards relief of crowding and alignment of the teeth.

The soft tissues and incisor position

The upper incisors will generally lie outside the lower lip and can be *a* 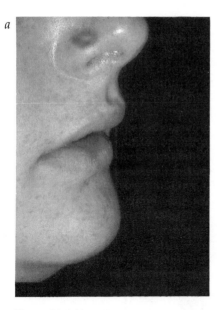   *b*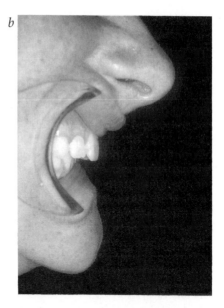

Figure 11.4 Here the overjet is increased due to the underlying Class II skeletal pattern but the incisors have remained within the control of the lower lip because this is rather everted in form. Stability after reduction of such an overjet is always in question. (a) With the lips relaxed there is an acceptable appearance; (b) when the lips are retracted the marked increase in incisor overjet is apparent.

brought into an acceptable position inside the lower lip by orthodontic means. In a few cases the overjet will be increased but the upper incisors will be retained inside the lower lip, which will be rather everted in form. In such cases, reduction of the overjet will almost certainly prove to be unstable. Fortunately such cases usually present quite an attractive appearance (Fig. 11.4).

Where the tongue is involved in producing an anterior oral seal this behaviour will usually be replaced by a lip-together resting posture and seal once the overjet has been reduced. In a few cases this change in behaviour will not take place and the overjet will relapse to some extent (Fig. 11.5). Where the overbite is incomplete, and in the absence of a digit-sucking habit, the lower incisors reflect the position of soft tissue balance.

If the overbite is deep and complete, it is possible that the occlusion of the lower incisors may have held them back during favourable mandibular growth so that their true position of muscle is further forward. This is much less common in Class II, division 1 than in Class II, division 2 (see p. 249).

For similar reasons, in cases where the lower lip lies between the upper and lower incisors before treatment, a small amount of lower incisor advancement may be stable because the muscle balance changes once the overjet has been reduced. When this occurs spontaneously it reduces the difficulty of the case and will often pass unnoticed until the post-treatment cephalometric film is examined. Some clinicians feel that

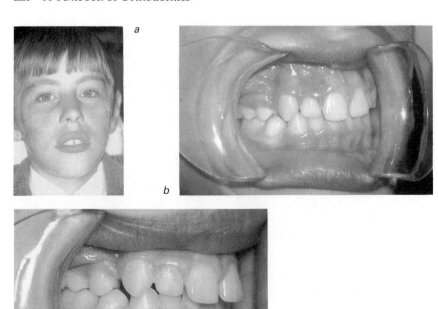

Figure 11.5 A case where relapse of the overjet was almost certainly due to the everted form of the lower lip: (a) before treatment; (b) immediately after treatment with an upper removable appliance; (c) 1 year out of retention.

it is justifiable to procline lower incisors in these circumstances. However it is always difficult to be confident that the deliberate proclination of lower incisors will be stable (Mills, 1968; Houston and Edler, 1990). Where the choice has been inappropriate, post-treatment overjet increase will be accompanied by lower incisor crowding (unless there is residual space in the lower arch). For these reasons many clincians will attempt lower incisor proclination only on the understanding that permanent retention will be used at the end of treatment to maintain the new lower incisor position. Whilst this prospect is generally undesirable it may be justified when the severity of the case precludes any other method of achieving a satisfactory result without resorting to orthognathic surgery.

Bimaxillary proclination

This has already been discussed in Chapter 10. Where there is a Class II, division 1 incisor relationship but marked lower incisor proclination, the achievement of a Class I incisor occlusion will still leave the patient with an increase in overjet. As was pointed out in Chapter 10, a mild degree of bimaxillary proclination in a Class I case can be pleasing and it can be mutually agreed in such circumstances to accept this part of the malocclusion. However, where the patient has a Class II, division 1 incisor occlusion it is difficult for the clinician to be certain how satisfactory the patient will find the end result of treatment confined to retracting the upper incisors alone. Furthermore, because of the everted form of the lower lip, stability of such incisor retraction is less certain than in cases with more usual lower incisor angulation (see Fig. 11.5).

Mandibular position and path of closure

A number of individuals with Class II, division 1 malocclusions posture the mandible forward habitually. In mild to moderately severe cases, this enables a lip seal to be obtained without undue circumoral contraction. In other cases, the posture may have been adopted initially for aesthetic reasons and has become habitual. Cases like this generally swallow with the mandible in the postured position, and some have an anterior position of occlusion. It is important to determine true centric relation and to recognize that these patients do have an upward and backward path of closure to true centric occlusion. It is also important not to mistake this for a distal displacement of the mandible with overclosure, which is very unusual in an unmutilated dentition. Treatment must be planned to centric relation, not to the postured position, because this will be lost when the upper incisors are retracted.

Correction of the incisor position and the establishment of centric relation reveals the true severity of the skeletal pattern, and this may result in a deterioration in facial appearance. The patient, and parents of a child patient, must be warned of this. Acceptance of postures is not recommended because they may be lost later in life as the patient ages.

Treatment

Objectives

In Class II, division 1 malocclusion the major objectives of treatment are to relieve crowding and irregularity of the teeth and to establish a stable Class I incisor relationship in harmony with the other facial features. If the lips are grossly incompetent, a stable reduction in overjet may not be attainable (Fig. 11.6). Where there is an appreciable incisor edge–centroid discrepancy (Fig. 11.7), it may not be possible to obtain a stable overbite reduction because there is insufficient bone to allow the required amount of palatal movement of the upper incisor roots; and the lower incisors cannot be advanced far enough to compensate for the skeletal pattern. In these circumstances a combined surgical and orthodontic approach may be the best way to provide an acceptable result (see Chapter 19). Nowadays orthognathic surgery can give predictable results with a minimum of post-surgical fixation. In severe Class II cases where facial appearance after orthodontic treatment would still be poor, surgical correction of the jaw relationship should be considered as part of the treatment, even where it is possible to reduce an overjet by orthodontic means.

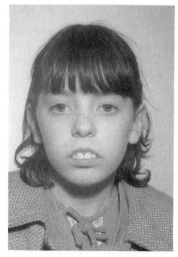

Figure 11.6 Gross lip incompetence and a low lower lip line make the prognosis for a stable incisor relationship after overjet reduction rather poor.

Early mixed dentition

Treatment of a Class II, division 1 malocculsion may be sought in the early mixed dentition, because of the unsightly facial appearance or the vulnerability of the upper incisors to trauma.

While it may be feasible to correct the incisor malrelationship in the early mixed dentition, a number of problems may arise and so this should be attempted only where there are strong indications for doing so. Unless the overjet is corrected fully at this time, there is little prospect of stability. Although the incisors may be spaced, there is rarely enough room to retract them fully. Sometimes it is possible to create space by extraction of the upper deciduous canines, provided that the upper permanent canines are high and buccal, and are well clear of the lateral incisor roots, which will move labially as the teeth are tipped back. In other cases, correction of the arch malrelationships with a functional appliance may be possible and this may be particularly valuable in cases where the severity of the malocclusion necessitates early intervention in order to obtain the maximal help from facial growth (see Chapter 17).

When contemplating early intervention of this kind, two further points should be considered and discussed with the parents. First, in many younger children the lips are parted habitually and so overjet reduction may not be stable. Prolonged retention while waiting for the soft tissues to mature is undesirable, both for dental health and for patient cooperation. Secondly, in most cases treated early, a further course of active appliance treatment is required in the late mixed or early permanent dentition, and thus treatment is liable to extend over many years.

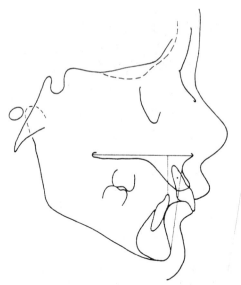

Figure 11.7 A severe Class II, division 1 incisor malrelationship. The incisor edge is 6 mm behind the upper centroid; for a stable reduction in overbite, it should be 2 mm in advance of it. It would be neither possible nor aesthetically acceptable to retract the upper centroid by this amount. Some advancement of the lower incisor edge should occur with growth in this 9-year-old boy, and with a change in the lower lip position some proclination could be stable. However, if growth were not favourable, orthodontic correction of this malocclusion would not be possible.

Late mixed and permanent dentition

The difficulty of correction of the incisor malrelationship is directly related to the severity of the incisor edge–centroid discrepancy. However severe the skeletal malrelationship may be, if there is full dentoalveolar compensation by lower incisor proclination so that the lower incisor edges lie 2–4 mm in advance of the upper incisor root centroid (see Fig. 11.1a), the upper incisors can be tipped back to achieve a Class I incisor relationship with a stable overbite. There may still be other difficulties, for example inclinations of other teeth may be unfavourable, or the overbite may be difficult to reduce, but in general treatment is comparatively straightforward.

Where the lower incisor edges lie behind the upper centroid (see Fig. 11.7), this relationship must be corrected to avoid the risk of creating a Class II, division 2 incisor relationship with a deep overbite.

Favourable incisor edge–centroid relationship

Treatment with removable appliances

Many of these mild cases can be treated with removable appliances.

The lower arch. The best results are obtained where the lower arch can be accepted without extractions, except perhaps of third molars (Fig. 11.8) or where there is moderately severe crowding with favourable

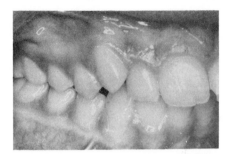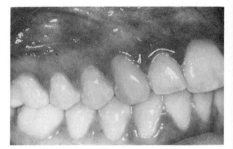

Figure 11.8 A Class II, division 1 malocclusion treated by distal movement of the upper buccal segments using an 'en masse' removable appliance. This was followed by retraction of canines and then the upper incisors. There were no extractions in the lower arch.

a

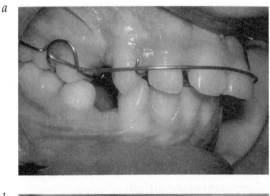

b

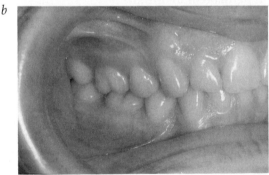

Figure 11.9 A mild Class II, division 1 case with crowding in the lower arch treated by the removal of all four first premolars and the use of an upper removable appliance: (a) showing the upper removable appliance 2 months after extraction of the premolars; (b) 2 years after completion of treatment.

inclinations of the teeth so that spontaneous alignment and space closure can occur after extraction of lower first premolars (Fig. 11.9). If possible, the teeth should be extracted before the second permanent molars have erupted, and certainly while the face is still growing, when spontaneous alignment and space closure are more satisfactory. Where

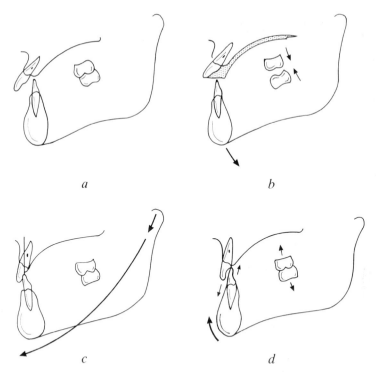

Figure 11.10 Effects of an anterior bite plane (a,b); the immediate effect is to rotate the mandible posteriorly so that the molars are free to erupt. (c) In the growing child, growth in posterior face height catches up and so the mandible rotates anteriorly again. Thus there is no net increase in the anterior intermaxillary height and provided a satisfactory inter-incisor relationship has been achieved, the overbite should be stable. (d) In the adult, the intermaxillary height is liable to regress towards its original value, with gradual intrusion of buccal teeth. The occlusal stop on the incisor will rarely be secure enough to prevent them from sliding past one another as the face height reduces, and the overbite tends to deepen.

maxillary removable appliances are used, overbite reduction depends on accelerated eruption of the buccal segments while the lower incisors are restrained by the bite plane. If this is to be stable, sufficient growth in facial height must occur to restore the relationship of the mandible to the upper face (Fig. 11.10c). It has been pointed out that the posterior rotation of the mandible produced by a biteplane (and by many fixed appliances, particularly when Class II elastics are used) exaggerates the Class II skeletal tendency and increases lip incompetence, both of these changes being particularly unfavourable in Class II, division 1 cases. However, provided the face is still growing, these ill effects are transient (Fig. 11.11).

In adults, overbite reduction with a bite plane is always unsatisfactory. In some patients who have had a tendency to posterior mandibular rotation and a high maxillary mandibular planes angle, a permanent opening of the intermaxillary space may be achieved, with long-term

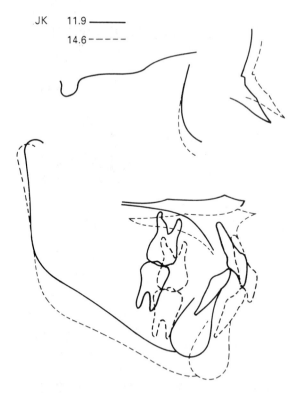

JK   11.9 ————
      14.6 – – – –

Figure 11.11 The cephalometric tracing of a typical Class II, division 1 case successfully treated by means of an upper removable appliance that carried an anterior bite plane (the same case as shown in Fig. 11.9).

undesirable effects on the skeletal pattern and lip incompetence. In others, and particularly where there has been an anterior growth rotation, the maxillary mandibular planes angle will gradually close after treatment, with intrusion of the buccal teeth. However, in these cases, the incisors may not intrude but rather slide past one another with some increase in overjet and overbite (see Fig. 11.10d). For these reasons, active intrusion of the lower labial segments with fixed appliances is indicated in adults.

The upper arch. As a general rule in Class II cases, teeth should be removed from the upper arch at least as far forward as from the lower. When the lower arch is treated without extractions, or where lower second or third molars are to be removed, upper arch treatment depends to a great extent on the amount of space that is required to relieve crowding and reduce the overjet. Retraction of upper buccal segments with headgear (see Fig. 11.8) may be appropriate where less than one-half premolar width of space is needed. This is achieved more readily before the second permanent molars have erupted, or following their extraction. On the other hand, if more space is required in the upper arch, or if lower premolars are to be removed, extraction of upper first premolars is the simplest way of providing the space necessary to

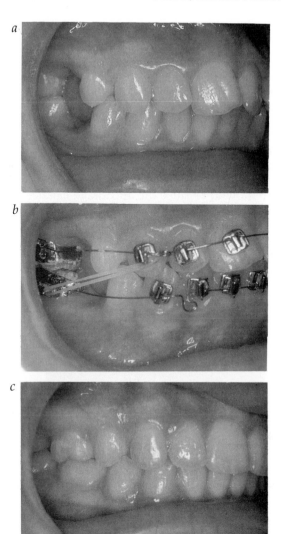

Figure 11.12 A mild Class II, division 1 case treated by removal of all four second premolars and the use of upper and lower fixed appliances: (a) pretreatment; (b) showing the Begg appliance in stage 1; (c) 2 years out of retention.

establish a Class I canine relationship. Provided that the upper canines are mesially inclined and there are no incisor rotations, good results can be obtained with removable appliances where the skeletal relationship is Class I or only mildly Class II.

Treatment with fixed appliances

Mild cases present few difficulties when fixed appliances are used. Where there is no crowding, the lower arch is accepted and the upper arch is retracted. This can often be done with removable appliances but incisor rotation or other dental irregularities may necessitate the use of a fixed appliance. Choice of extraction in the lower arch depends on the degree of crowding, the severity of the anteroposterior discrepancy, and on the type of mechanics to be employed. Mild to moderate crowding is best dealt with by extraction of second premolars (Fig. 11.12) unless intermaxillary anchorage demands are sufficient to require first premolar extractions (so that both first molars and second premolars provide anchorage for incisor retraction).

It is particularly important not to retract lower incisors in Class II cases, and the risk of doing so is less when second rather than first premolars are removed, because the anchorage balance favours closure of residual space by forward movement of the molars rather than by undue retraction of the labial segments. Cases with severe crowding are treated more readily with loss of first premolars (Fig. 11.13), and it should be remembered that reduction of a deep overbite also requires some space. Extractions in the upper arch generally correspond to those in the lower.

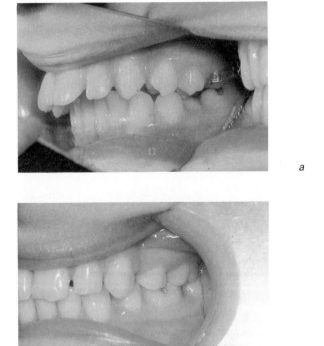

a

b

Figure 11.13 A more severe case than that shown in Fig. 11.12. Here all four first premolars were removed. The post-treatment photographs show the case 10 years after the removal of all retainers. Note that the proclination of the lower incisors,

Overbite reduction, even with fixed appliances, is obtained at least in part by elevation of the buccal segments. This is of little consequence in the child where the face will grow, but every attempt should be made to achieve as much incisor intrusion as possible in the adult. This is difficult. It is essential that the apices of the lower incisors are clear of the lingual cortical plate of the mandibular symphysis, (Fig. 11.13) otherwise intrusion will be almost impossible. Intermaxillary elastics favour molar extrusion.

In some Class II, division 1 cases there is excessive vertical development of the upper labial segment and the patient displays an undue amount of gingiva, especially when smiling. In these cases, if the upper labial segment is merely retracted, the patient will be left with a 'gummy smile' at the end of treatment (Fig. 11.14). Provided that they will still be controlled by the lower lip, some intrusion of the upper incisors during their retraction is desirable: this is best achieved using high-pull headgear to the labial segment during its retraction. Once again, Class II elastics should be avoided because they tend to extrude the upper labial segment.

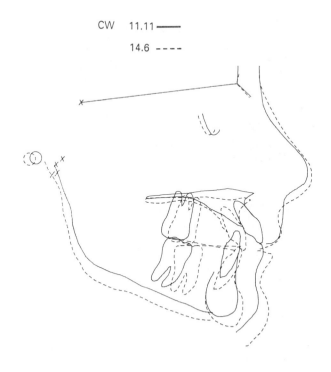

CW   11.11 ——

14.6 - - - -

c

which was unintentional, has remained stable. This has been a major factor in determining the long-term success of the treatment: (a) pretreatment; (b) 1 year out of retention; (c) the cephalometric tracings.

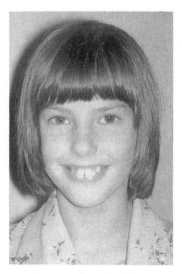

Figure 11.14 A gummy smile. For a good aesthetic result the upper incisors would have to be intruded as well as being retracted.

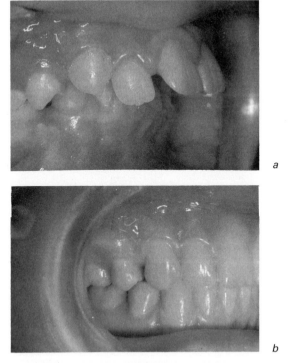

a

b

Figure 11.15 (a) An extremely severe case that did not respond to early treatment with myofunctional appliances and for which surgery provided the only answer. (b) While there is an excellent occlusal result the facial profile (c) leaves something to be desired despite a 10-mm advancement of the lower jaw.

Unfavourable incisor edge–centroid relationship

The incisor edge-centroid relationship must be corrected if a stable reduction in overbite is to be obtained, and these cases are not suitable for treatment with removable appliances (see Figs. 11.7 and 11.14).

By far the simplest method of correcting the edge–centroid discrepancy would be to advance the lower incisor edges, but even where there are signs that the lower incisors have been restrained, or where it is expected that favourable growth of the mandible will reduce the skeletal discrepancy, the amount of advancement of the lower incisors that will be stable is questionable. Thus the incisor edge–centroid relationship should be corrected where possible by palatal movement of the upper incisor roots, using a fixed appliance (Fig. 11.13).

In more severe cases, it is not feasible to correct the incisor edge–centroid relationship completely by palatal movement of the upper incisor roots. This may be because there is insufficient bone palatal to the upper incisors, and little alveolar bone remodelling can be expected at apical level (Fig. 11.13). A further factor may be that extensive palatal movement of the upper incisors might result in an unacceptable facial appearance, with the dentition set too far back relative to the upper face. In these cases it is necessary to explore the possibility of lower incisor advancement. If this is not feasible, surgical correction of the skeletal malrelationship will be necessary (Fig. 11.15).

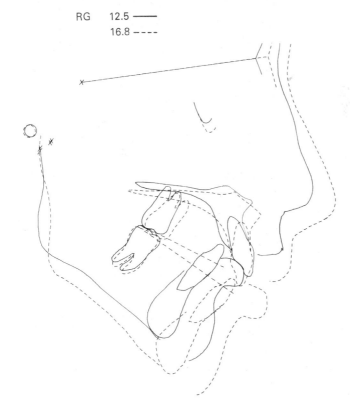

RG   12.5 ——
      16.8 - - - -

c

Some stable advancement of the lower incisor edge can be obtained in the following circumstances:

1 If there has been persistent finger or thumb sucking, the lower labial segment may have been retroclined. Some spontaneous correction may follow cessation of the habit but, particularly if the power lip falls between the upper and lower incisors, full recovery may not occur.

2 Some lower incisor proclination may be stable in cases with a tongue-to-lower lip anterior oral seal, when a lip seal can be established after upper incisor retraction and the soft tissue balance changes.

3 In cases with a deep, complete overbite and the morphological signs of an anterior mandibular growth rotation, full dentoalveolar adaptation may have been prevented by contact of the lower incisors with the palate and some advancement may be stable. Particularly in cases showing signs of a forward mandibular growth rotation, the skeletal relationship may be expected to improve with further growth and this in turn may enable the lower incisor edges to be advanced relative to the upper face.

Lower incisor advancement should be undertaken only where there are no reasonable orthodontic alternatives and where there are signs indicating that the teeth have been held back. The problem for the clinician is that all these signs are fallible and there are no secure guidelines as to how much advancement will be stable. This is discussed in more detail with Class II, division 2 malocculsions (p. 249).

After evaluation of the possibilities of dealing with the incisor mal-relationship, attention can be focused on relief of crowding and correction of other aspects of the malocculsion. The principles here are identical with those discussed previously for the milder cases, except that fixed appliance treatment will always be required.

References

Houston, W. J. B. and Edler, R. (1990) Long term stability of the lower labial segment relative to the APo line. *European Journal of Orthodontics*, **12**, 302–310

James, G. A. (1963) Cephalometric analysis of 100 Angle Class II division 1 malocculsions with special reference to the cranial base. *Transactions of the British Society for the Study of Orthodontics*, 39–50

Mills, J. R. E. (1968) The stability of the lower labial segment. *Transactions of the British Society for the Study of Orthodontics*, 11–24

Todd, J. E. and Dodd, T. (1985) *Childrens Dental Health in the United Kingdom, 1983*, HMSO, London

Chapter 12

Class II, division 2 malocclusions

Class II, division 2 malocclusions (Fig. 12.1) occur in about 10 per cent of children. In milder forms they may be perfectly acceptable function-ally, and the facial appearance can be pleasing. In severe cases the overbite is very deep, possibly associated with periodontal trauma palatal to the upper and labial to the lower incisors. A Class II, division 2 incisor relationship is generally the result of dentoalveolar compensa-tion for a Class II skeletal pattern by retroclination of the upper central incisors (Fig. 12.1). The more severe the anteroposterior skeletal malre-lationship and the more that compensation occurs by retroclination of the upper rather than by proclination of the lower incisors, the deeper the overbite will be.

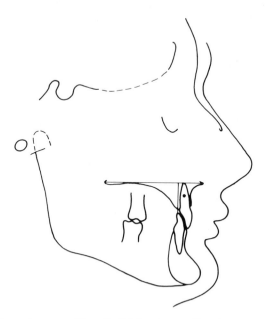

Figure 12.1 A moderately severe Class II, division 2 case. The deep overbite is in part due to retroclination of the upper incisors which is compensating for the mild skeletal II dental base relationship. The lower incisor edge lies behind the upper central incisor root centroid. The lips are competent with a typical high lip line and prominent labiomental fold.

Occlusal features

Class II, division 2 malocclusions are characterized by a Class II incisor relationship with retroclination of the upper central incisors. The upper lateral incisors may also be retroclined, but in crowded cases they are typically proclined, mesially inclined and mesiolabially rotated (Fig. 12.2). The overbite is deep and complete; and the overjet is average or only slightly increased.

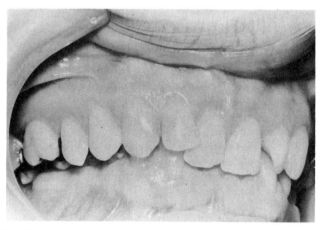

Figure 12.2 A Class II, division 2 malocclusion with a scissors bite. The overbite is deep and potentially traumatic.

Overbite depth is strongly associated with the anteroposterior relationship between the lower incisor edges and the upper incisor root centroid (Fig. 12.1): the greater the discrepancy, the more difficult is stable correction of the overbite. In many cases, there is an increased crown–root angle of the upper incisors (Nicol, 1963; Williams and Woodhouse, 1983) so that although the inclination of the tooth is within average limits, the crown is retroclined and the overbite is correspondingly deep. Sometimes the lower incisors are proclined, helping to compensate for the skeletal pattern, but in other cases they are retroclined (Ridley, 1960).

The anteroposterior buccal-segment relationship is usually mild Class II, although it can be Class I in cases of bimaxillary retroclination. A full unit, Class II buccal-segment relationship is not common. Transversely there may be a scissor bite (buccal crossbite) (Fig. 12.2), which is often confined to the premolars. A bilateral complete scissor bite is rare, which is fortunate because correction is difficult.

Skeletal relationships

The skeletal pattern may be Class I, but is generally mild Class II. A severe Class II skeletal pattern is rarely found because this would

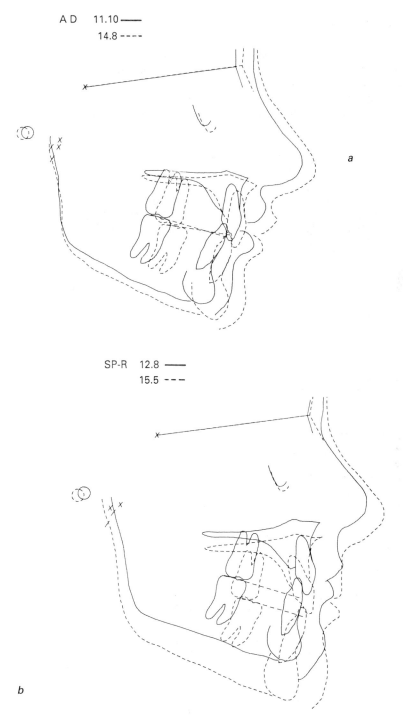

A D   11.10 ———
       14.8 - - - -

SP-R   12.8 ———
        15.5 - - -

Figure 12.3 Showing how (a) horizontal or (b) vertical growth is of assistance in correcting a deep overbite in Class II, division 2 malocclusion.

usually lead to a Class II, division 1 incisor relationship. The lower anterior face height is often smaller than average and characteristically the maxillary–mandibular planes angle is low, with a well-developed mandibular angle. There is usually an underlying forward rotation pattern of mandibular growth and, because of this, the chin appears to be well developed so that the facial profile is good (see Fig. 12.1).

Transversely the maxillary base may be broad relative to the lower, but this is usually compensated for by the angulation of the teeth, although a scissor bite involving the premolars is not rare.

Facial growth

In many patients with Class II, division 2 malocclusion, facial growth is favourable, and there is an anterior mandibular rotation as has been mentioned (see p. 135). Even where the skeletal pattern improves with growth, the malocclusion will generally not change because dentoalveolar adaptation maintains the pre-existing incisor relationship. However, favourable growth in both a horizontal and vertical direction is very important in helping the orthodontic correction of a severe Class II, division 2 incisor malrelationship (Fig. 12.3).

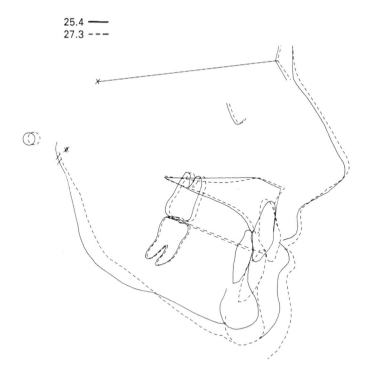

25.4 ——
27.3 – – –

Figure 12.4 The 'unfurling' of the lower lip in a severe Class II, division 2 malocclusion treated by orthognathic surgery to correct the underlying Class II skeletal pattern and increase the lower facial height.

Soft tissue pattern

The lips are almost always of adequate length to meet without strain. Frequently the lip line is high relative to the upper incisor crown, and the higher the lip line the more retroclined the upper incisors are liable to be (Nicol, 1955; 1963).

In the past, some have described the lips as being hypertonic or hyperactive but there is absolutely no basis for this (Rix, 1960). What is being observed is a rather everted form of the lips due to their length relative to a reduced lower face height. In fact Class II, division 2 lips show less electomyographic activity than those of other incisal groups (Marx, 1965). Moreover, when treatment is undertaken to correct the horizontal and vertical skeletal discrepancy of the severe Class II, division 2 case (see below), there is frequently a dramatic 'unfurling' of the lips, which thereafter appear quite unremarkable (Fig. 12.4).

There is often a well-developed labiomental fold (see Fig. 12.1), which is due to a combination of lip abundance and a marked mental eminence. Rix (1948) described a tooth-apart swallowing behaviour in Class II, division 2 cases, but this is rarely of clinical importance.

Mandibular function

Mandibular posture and path of closure are generally normal. The deep overbite may prevent free lateral excursion of the mandible, but symptoms of muscle or facial pain seldom result from this. If many posterior teeth have been lost, there may be a posterior displacement of the mandible and overclosure, which are associated with muscle and joint pain; and the development of a traumatic overbite (see Fig. 1.6).

Treatment objectives

In mild cases, the occlusion may be aesthetically and functionally satisfactory and so treatment is not indicated. On the other hand, the position of the upper lateral incisors may be very unsightly if they are proclined, and this is the most common of these patient's complaints. Where the overbite is not very deep, it may be accepted and treatment directed towards alignment of the lateral incisors. A deep and potentially traumatic overbite must be corrected, although this can be difficult, particularly in the adult.

Treatment

If the overbite is to be accepted

The lower arch

In these cases, treatment is directed toward relief of crowding and alignment of the teeth, particularly of the upper lateral incisors. If the lower arch is well aligned or only mildly crowded, it should be accepted in spite of the fact that crowding may well increase during the later stages of facial growth (see p. 39). The extraction of lower premolars in these cases may be followed by a small amount of lingual tipping of the most outstanding lower incisors as they align, and this can be enough to lose the anterior occlusal stop and precipitate a serious deepening of the overbite.

Severe lower arch crowding is not common but when it is found, extraction of first premolars is required; provided that all the lower permanent teeth are present, sound and in favourable positions, spontaneous alignment of the lower labial segment and closure of the extraction spaces may be expected. However, if the overbite is already deep, there is the risk of it becoming worse and these cases are better treated with fixed appliances as described below.

Where the lower arch is completely uncrowded a functional appliance may be indicated (see Chapter 17). Such treatment requires initial

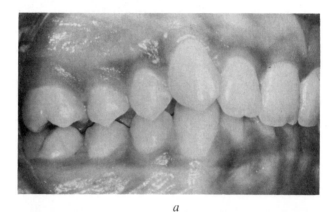

a

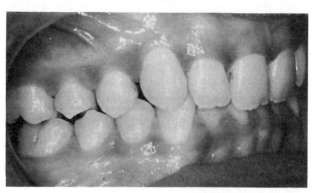

b

Figure 12.5 A mild Class II, division 2 malocclusion treated by retraction of upper buccal segments with headgear: (a) start of treatment; (b) completion of treatment. The buccal segment relationship has been corrected and the prominence of the lateral incisors and canines has been reduced.

proclination of the upper incisors to allow the sagittal correction to be made. However, because of the tendency of lower arch crowding to increase during growth and because most functional appliances encourage the posterior teeth to move forward, such treatment does run the risk of producing significant (and occasionally unacceptable) lower arch crowding by the end of treatment.

The upper arch

Distal movement of the upper buccal segments after the removal of second permanent molars is generally the best approach to treatment (Fig. 12.5) where the buccal segments are less than one-half premolar width in disto-occlusion and provided that lower premolars are not to be extracted. With a more severe Class II buccal segment relationship or when lower first premolars are to be lost, upper first premolars should be removed. In many cases, adequate alignment of the upper arch can be obtained with removable appliances. The lateral incisor position is particularly liable to relapse to a small extent but this can be quite acceptable. Where these teeth are rotated severely, fixed appliances are necessary and all possible measures should be taken to prevent relapse to an unacceptable degree. Over-rotation, pericision and prolonged retention are all helpful (see Chapter 17).

Because the upper incisors are retroclined, they need less space than would be the case if they had average inclinations. The reason is that the contact areas are positioned more labially, and if the teeth were at average inclinations with these contact positions, the overjet would be increased (Fig. 12.6). Thus, even if the lower incisors are slightly crowded, it may still be possible to align the upper incisors around them with the canines in a Class I relationship.

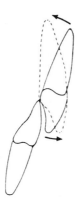

Figure 12.6 In a Class II, division 2 incisor relationship the contact areas of the upper central incisors lie too far forward relative to the lower incisor edges but this is masked by their retroclination. If the inclination of the upper incisors were to be corrected by rotating them around their contact areas, this would be revealed by the increase in overjet.

If the overbite is to be corrected

The first step is to consider how the incisor relationship is to be dealt with, and then decisions can be made about other aspects of treatment.

Overbite control

In a growing child, the overbite may be corrected by restraining the lower labial segment while allowing growth of the buccal segments, so levelling the curve of Spee. The mandible is rotated posteriorly but, with growth, posterior facial height catches up (see Fig. 11.7). In many Class II, division 2 cases, the upper labial segment also has to be prevented from erupting in order to correct the relationship between the incisor edges and the lower lip (see Fig. 12.1). In adults, active intrusion of the labial segment is required, and this is difficult. Class II, division 2 cases do not often tolerate a permanent increase in inter-maxillary height and if this happens, through elevation of the buccal segments in an adult, the buccal teeth will be intruded gradually by the forces of the occlusion. The incisors are liable to slide past one another, rather than to intrude, with consequent deepening of the overbite. Because of the importance of avoiding excessive molar extrusion during overbite reduction, a high-pull headgear to the upper incisors may be favoured as an alternative to Class II elastic traction to achieve this objective (Fletcher, 1981). However, Mills (1973) believes that such intrusion is rare and overbite reduction is invariably related to the amount of vertical growth taking place in the lower part of the face.

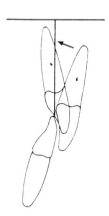

Figure 12.7 A stable reduction of the overbite requires correction of the edge–centroid relationship.

The crucial factor in overbite stability in all treated cases is correction of the incisor edge–centroid relationship (Fig. 12.7). Stability can be ensured by sufficient retraction of the upper centroid using fixed appliances with palatal root torque but in severe cases the alveolar process may not be thick enough to allow full correction in this way, because little periosteal bone remodelling occurs on the palate at the level of the incisor apices. Thus, in severe cases, it may be necessary to advance the lower incisor edges. This is achieved much more simply than is upper palatal root torque, but stability is uncertain. If the lower incisors drop back again through soft tissue imbalance, the overbite will deepen and the lower labial segment will become crowded. A further danger is that the alveolar bone labial to the lower incisors is thin and with injudicious or rapid proclination of these teeth, crestal bone loss and gingival recession may occur.

Before the decision is taken to advance the lower labial segment, there must be a definite indication that this will be stable. In many Class II, division 2 cases, mandibular growth following eruption of the incisors has been favourable, with improvement in the skeletal pattern, but this has not been reflected in a change in the incisor relationship because of dentoalveolar adaptation resulting from the incisor contact. Where the incisor overbite is to be reduced by upward and forward movement of the upper incisor edges, it is reasonable to assume that the lower incisors will be freed to adopt a new, more labial, position of balance (Fig. 12.8).

Favourable growth may occur during and after orthodontic treatment. Indications of earlier favourable growth are those of anterior growth rotation (see p. 135). Retroclination of the lower incisors may also point

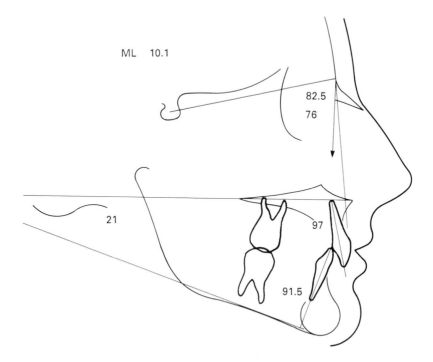

Figure 12.8 In this case it is reasonable to assume that the lower incisors might adopt a more labial position once they are freed from occlusion with the upper incisors/palate.

to previous dentoalveolar adaptation due to occlusal factors, which could reasonably be reversed in conjunction with a change in the level of the upper incisors relative to the lower lip. The problem is that even when the indications for lower labial-segment advancement are favourable, there is no reliable guide to the amount that will be stable. Some clinicians use an anterior bite plane in the hope that the lower incisors will then adopt a position of muscle balance, but the occlusion of the incisors on the bite plane may impede their movement, particularly if they are retroclined. Others rely on the A–Pog line to indicate a position of lower incisor stability, but there is no sound biological basis for this because stability depends on soft tissue, not skeletal, balance. Clinical experience does suggest that in Class II cases, the lower incisors will not be stable if they are moved forward further than the A–Pog line and so it does provide some guide to the reasonable limits of labial advancement.

In this area of uncertainty, a reasonable approach is to advance the lower incisors only as far as is necessary to obtain a secure edge–centroid relationship. If this can be done in the mixed or early permanent dentition, using a functional appliance (see p. 328), there is the opportunity to test the stability of the incisor position by leaving the appliance out for some months before detailed finishing with a fixed appliance if this is necessary. Should the lower incisors start to drop back during this period, it is an indication that bodily retraction of the upper incisors with the fixed appliance will be required.

In the older patient where treatment is started with a fixed appliance, it may be advisable to retain any advancement of the lower incisors with a lingual retainer until facial growth is virtually complete. This ensures that, if there is favourable facial growth during the retention period, dentoalveolar adaptation will occur with labial movement of the upper rather than lingual movement of the lower incisors. In all cases where the lower labial segment has been advanced during treatment, there is the risk of some relapse and so there is the increased likelihood of the development of lower incisor crowding after treatment. The patient should be warned of this.

Treatment of the cases with minimal space requirements

Uncrowded cases, or those where there is only mild crowding and a moderately deep overbite, may be treated without extractions; or possibly with extraction of second or third permanent molars. In some cases a functional appliance fitted after the retroclined upper incisors have been proclined to an average inclination can give a good result (Fig. 12.9). Functional appliances should not be used in mild cases where there is a degree of lower incisor crowding unless there is reason for believing that the inevitable reciprocal labial movement of the lower incisors will remain stable (see above).

Where there is slight lower arch crowding, the lower buccal segments can be retracted. This may be done with a lip bumper (see p. 323) or with headgear to the lower arch, either before the second molars have

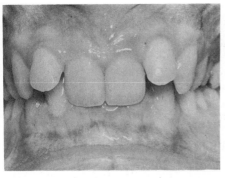

a

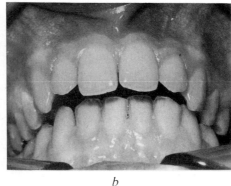

b

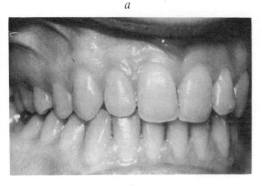

c

Figure 12.9 A Class II, division 2 malocclusion before treatment with a functional appliance: (a) the malocclusion before treatment; (b) the upper incisors have been proclined using a removable appliance; (c) the arch relationship has been corrected with a functional appliance.

erupted or after their extraction. However, headgear to the lower arch is often not well tolerated. Distal movement of lower first permanent molars is best undertaken just before exfoliation of the second deciduous molars so that the leeway space is not lost by forward drift. The anterior teeth may align spontaneously but if they do not, and certainly if there is an appreciable curve of Spee, a lower fixed appliance is required. Overbite reduction requires space and it is very difficult to reduce a deep overbite in even a mildly crowded lower arch without proclining the lower incisors.

Distal movement of the upper buccal segments can be undertaken using headgear to an 'en masse' appliance or to bands on the upper first permanent molars, either before eruption of the upper second molars or subsequent to their extraction if third molars are favourably positioned.

After the creation of adequate space by buccal segment retraction, the interincisor relationship must be corrected. This involves overbite reduction and palatal root torque of the upper incisors and will normally require fixed appliances (Fig. 12.10). The latter movement in particular requires good anchorage and this is provided most reliably by headgear. High-pull headgear to the upper labial segment helps to control its vertical level as well as supplementing anchorage.

a

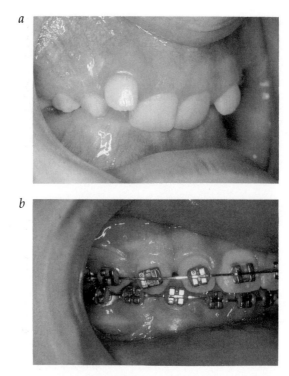

b

c

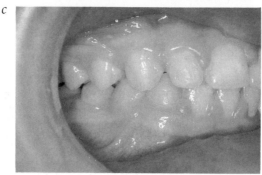

Figure 12.10 A severe Class II, division 2 malocclusion successfully treated without extractions: (a) pretreatment; (b) showing the straight-wire fixed appliance; (c) 1 year out of retention.

Crowded cases

Where there is definite crowding, extraction of premolars and treatment with fixed appliances is required (Fig. 12.11). With severe crowding, and particularly where the overbite is very deep so that appreciable palatal root torque is needed, loss of first premolars will be indicated in both arches.

Where crowding is only moderate, the choice of extraction depends

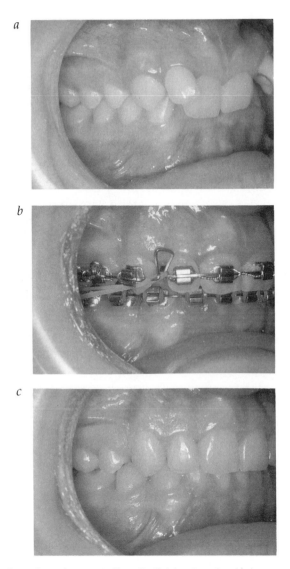

Figure 12.11 A moderately severe Class II, division 2 malocclusion treated by fixed appliances after extraction of first premolars: (a) pretreatment; (b) showing the edgewise appliance; (c) 1 year out of retention.

partly on the type of technique to be employed. For example, where there is moderate lower arch crowding and Begg mechanics with Class II intermaxillary anchorage are to be used, first premolars may still be the teeth of choice. On the other hand with the straight-wire technique, where headgear rather than Class II anchorage is used, care must be taken not to retract the lower labial segment during lower arch space closure because this would exaggerate the tendency to dental retrusion

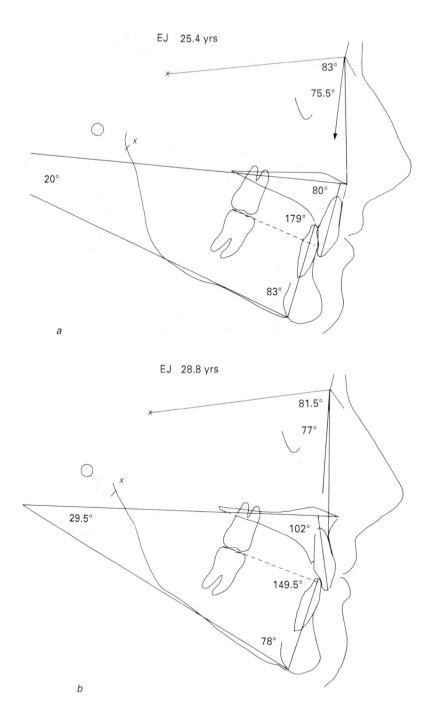

Figure 12.12 A very severe Class II, division 2 case treated by a combined orthodontic and orthognathic approach in which the upper incisors were proclined and the mandible then advanced surgically to correct the Class II skeletal pattern: (a) pretreatment; (b) 1 year after surgery. Superimposed tracings are shown in Fig. 12.4.

and would increase the amount of palatal movement of the upper incisor apices that is required for overbite stability. Hence, in such a case, the clinician might feel that the second rather than first premolars would be a better choice for extraction, because the anchorage balance then favours closure of excess space by mesial movement of the molars rather than by retraction of the labial segment.

Regardless of the technique employed, ideally the overbite should be reduced as far as possible by intrusion of the upper and lower incisors. This depends on there being enough cancellous bone above the incisor apices, and the inclination of the teeth may have to be adjusted (see Fig. 12.1) to allow intrusion to occur. Almost invariably some extrusion of premolars and molars will occur as the curve of Spee is flattened, but provided that the anterior intermaxillary height is not opened up excessively, growth in posterior face height should catch up. In patients in whom growth is nearly completed, or in adults, overbite reduction is a major problem and any increase in anterior intermaxillary height is very liable to close up, with possible overbite deepening. In severe Class II, division 2 cases, intrusion of upper incisors is as important as is depression of the lower incisors, because unless they are elevated relative to the lower lip, the crowns will be held back and it will be almost impossible to obtain a stable incisor edge–centroid relationship.

Functional appliances

Because myofunctional appliances such as the Harvold activator encourge vertical development of the posterior teeth as well as correction of a Class II arch relationship, their use has been advocated in the early treatment of Class II, division 2 malocclusion. For this to be undertaken it is necessary to procline the maxillary incisors either before or during the period of functional appliance wear. With good cooperation such treatment may be very successful in achieving gross correction of the malocclusion in the actively growing patient but it will usually need to be followed by conventional fixed-appliance treatment to complete tooth alignment (Isaacson, Reed and Stephens, 1990).

Surgical treatment

For the severe case, and for the adult who has an unacceptable overbite, a combined surgical/orthodontic approach is required (Fig. 12.12, and see also Chapter 20).

References

Fletcher, G. G. T. (1981) *The Begg Appliance and Technique*, Wright, Bristol, pp. 131–132

Isaacson, K. G., Reed, R. T. and Stephens, C. D. (1990) *Functional Orthodontic Appliances*, Blackwell Scientific, Oxford, p. 51

Marx, R. (1965) The circumoral muscles and incisor relationship: an electro-myographic study. *Transactions of the European Orthodontic Society*, 187–202

Mills, J. R. E. (1973) The problem of overbite in Class II division 2 occlusion. *British Journal of Orthodontics*, **1**, 34–38

Nicol, W. A. (1955) The relationship of the lip line to the incisor teeth. *Transactions of the British Society for the Study of Orthodontics*, 75–81

Nicol, W. A. (1963) The lower lip and the upper incisor teeth in Angles Class II division 2 malocclusion. *Transactions of the British Society for the Study of Orthodontics*, 81–84

Ridley, D. R. (1960) Some factors concerned with the reduction of excessive incisor overbite in Angles Class II division 2 type of malocclusion. *Transactions of the British Society for the Study of Orthodontics*, 118–138

Rix, R. E. (1948) Deglutition. *Transactions of the European Orthodontic Society*, 191–198

Rix, R. E. (1960) Some problems for consideration – 1. *Transations of the British Society for the Study of Orthodontics*, 101–107

Williams, A. and Woodhouse, C. (1983) The crown root angle of maxillary incisors in different incisor classes. *British Journal of Orthodontics*, **10**, 159–161

Chapter 13

Class III malocclusions

In Class III malocclusions, the lower incisor edges lie anterior to the cingulum plateau of the upper incisors (Fig. 13.1). Class III malocclusion is found in about 3 per cent of children. Almost invariably there is an underlying skeletal malrelationship and the prominence of the chin as much as the malocclusion is frequently of concern to the patient and their family.

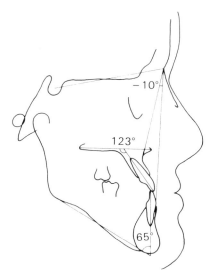

Figure 13.1 A Class III malocclusion. The incisor malrelationship is milder than would have been expected from the skeletal pattern, owing to dentoalveolar compensation.

Occlusal features

The severity of the incisor malrelationship varies greatly. In mild cases the incisors meet in an edge-to-edge relationship, when there may be an anterior mandibular displacement to obtain a posterior occlusion (Fig. 13.2). This exaggerates the severity of the incisor malrelationship. In more severe cases there is an appreciable reverse overjet. Frequently,

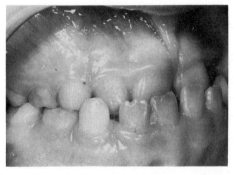

a

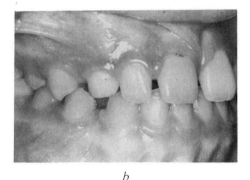

b

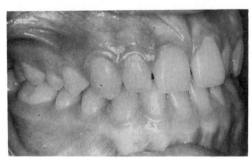

c

Figure 13.2 (a) Although an edge-to-edge incisor contact can be obtained, the mandible is displaced forwards to obtain maximum occlusion. (b) Correction of the reverse overjet by proclination of the upper incisors eliminates the mandibular displacement. (c) The occlusal correction has been stable, owing to the good overbite and a favourable pattern of facial growth.

there is some degree of dentoalveolar compensation for the skeletal malrelationship and so the malocclusion may be less severe than would have been expected from the skeletal pattern (Fig. 13.1). The buccal segment relationship may be Class I and it is unusual to find a full premolar width of mesio-occlusion.

The upper arch is often narrow as well as being short, and the lower arch is broad. Thus crossbites are common. This tendency is exacerbated by the anteroposterior arch malrelationship in that a broader part of the lower arch opposes a narrower part of the upper. Because of this, where the arch widths are equal, there is generally a displacement of the mandible to one side, producing a unilateral crossbite. Sometimes, a unilateral crossbite is a reflection of asymmetry of one of the arches. Where there is a more severe discrepancy in arch widths, there is a bilateral crossbite (Fig 13.3).

There are wide variations in intermaxillary height. Quite frequently the anterior intermaxillary height is increased and there is a skeletal open bite (Fig. 13.4a). In moderately severe cases where the lower incisors lie anterior to the uppers and the intermaxillary height is reduced, the overbite may be deep (Fig. 13.4b). When the incisors meet edge to edge, the overbite is, of course, reduced regardless of the anterior intermaxillary dimensions.

The upper arch is frequently crowded because it is short and narrow, while the lower arch may well be spaced. Severe lower arch crowding is not common.

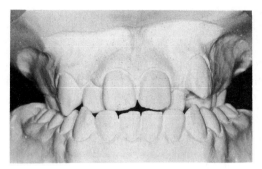

Figure 13.3 A Class III malocclusion with a bilateral crossbite.

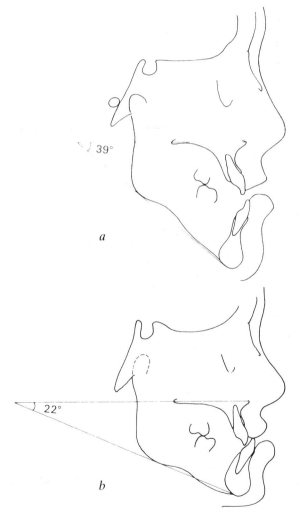

Figure 13.4 Different facial types associated with Class III malocclusions. (a) The anterior intermaxillary height is large and there is an associated skeletal open bite. This type of facial pattern can be expected to grow primarily vertically. (b) The anterior intermaxillary height is reduced and the overbite is deep.

Skeletal relationships

There is usually a Class III skeletal pattern and its severity is reflected in the arch malrelationship. Particularly when measurements are made from a cephalometric radiograph taken with the teeth in maximum occlusion, it is important to check clinically for a mandibular displacement that would exaggerate the prognathism.

It is often assumed that in Class III cases, it is only the mandible that is at fault. Frequently there is an element of maxillary retrusion; and the mandibular prominence may be due not only to its length but to some shortness of the cranial base. Where surgical correction is planned, it is very important to evaluate the different components of the skeletal malrelationship so that the appropriate surgical procedures are undertaken. In some cases, a degree of maxillary advancement, instead of or in conjunction with a mandibular set-back, is necessary for the best facial appearance.

Facial growth

In Class III cases, facial growth is usually unfavourable: the usual tendency for the mandible to become more prognathic relative to the upper face is adverse. Dentoalveolar adaptation may maintain the occlusal relationship but in many of the more severe cases this is at its limits by the commencement of the pubertal growth spurt and further adaptation is not possible. Thus, any reverse overjet tends to become worse and incisor relationships that are just edge to edge may drop into lingual occlusion.

Vertical facial growth increases any tendency to skeletal open bite, particularly where there is a high maxillary–mandibular planes angle and a tendency towards a posterior growth rotation of the mandible (Fig. 13.4a). In these cases, the vertical growth of the anterior intermaxillary height exceeds the growth potential of the alveolar processes and the open bite may extend to involve the buccal segments so that only the last molars are in occlusion.

Soft tissues

In Class III cases, the soft tissues do not generally play any part in the aetiology of the malocclusion. Indeed, they tend to encourage dentoalveolar compensation for skeletal malrelationships, both anteroposterior and transverse, so that the arch malrelationships are less severe than might have been expected from the skeletal pattern. Where there is a severe anterior open bite, the lips are usually incompetent and an anterior oral seal may be obtained between the tongue and upper lip or between tongue, alveolar mucosa and lower lip. The upper incisors are in a position of balance between the upper lip and the tongue, and the lower lip has little part to play. The lower lip may be rather full and pendulous (Fig. 13.4b) and in these cases, the lower incisors may even be proclined, exaggerating the reverse overjet. The different occlusal malrelationships that maybe found in Class III cases may necessitate a variety of adaptations in obtaining an anterior oral seal and in swallowing behaviour. These are of little importance in diagnosis and treatment planning because they will modify in response to orthodontic treatment. When surgical treatment is planned, however, it must be remembered that if the volume of the oral cavity is reduced, the tongue may have to be postured forward to avoid encroachment on the airway and so dental relapse may occur. In addition, orthognathic surgery will affect the balance of the circumoral musculature and, if presurgical decompensation has not been undertaken, this may happen spontaneously under the influence of the soft tissues, and the occlusion may relapse to some extent. This is discussed at greater length in Chapter 18.

Mandibular function

The occlusal malrelationships frequently lead to mandibular displacements (see Fig. 13.2). If this is left uncorrected, muscle dysfunction and pain may be experienced. Correction of the occlusal malrelationship, which is usually possible with orthodontic appliances in these cases, eliminates the displacement and relieves the pain and dysfunction.

Lateral mandibular displacements are often found where there is a unilateral crossbite. These are not associated with mandibular overclosure, but in the long run may well give rise to muscle dysfunction and pain. Even when the patient does not complain of discomfort, areas of muscle tenderness can frequently be found on palpation, and electromyographic records will demonstrate a disrupted pattern of muscle activity. Correction of a unilateral crossbite in a Class III case is not always simple. The upper teeth are often already inclined buccally and further upper arch expansion is neither very effective nor stable. In some of these cases, rapid maxillary expansion to separate the mid-palatal suture may be undertaken but this may have the undesirable side-effect of propping open the occlusion and reducing any overbite. In cases where the anteroposterior skeletal discrepancy is to be corrected surgically, this will at the same time lead to some improvement in the transverse arch relationship.

Occlusal function in Class III cases is often disturbed. Where there is a severe anterior open bite, for example, only the last standing molars may meet in occlusion. However, in the absence of mandibular displacements due to premature occlusal contacts, symptoms of pain and dysfunction are surprisingly uncommon (see also pp. 10–12).

Treatment objectives

Correction of the occlusal malrelationships with orthodontic appliances is possible only in the mild malocclusions, although these do form the greater proportion of all Class III cases. In severe cases, surgical intervention is required if the malocclusion is to be corrected (see Chapter 19). The greatest diagnostic problems arise in young patients who are already at the limits of orthodontic correction. Even if orthodontic treatment is reasonably successful at that age, further facial growth may produce a relapse and, if surgical treatment is then undertaken, the earlier orthodontic treatment may have been not only inappropriate but may prejudice the quality of the result. For example, if lower first premolars have been extracted to allow retraction of the lower labial segment, which later has to be proclined as part of the decompensation before surgery, the extraction spaces may then be very difficult to close.

It is therefore highly desirable to correct a Class III incisor relationship early in the mixed dentition whenever possible. Cooperation at this time will usually be excellent and tooth movement can be accomplished rapidly. Further, as this initial treatment does not require the removal of permanent teeth it preserves a number of later treatment options.

Treatment

Early mixed dentition

The patient can often obtain an edge-to-edge incisor occlusion but displaces forward to obtain occlusion of posterior teeth, thereby creating a reverse overjet. There is often some overclosure of the mandible, although this appears to be rather rarer than once supposed (Bryant, 1981). Provided that the upper incisors are not already proclined and that there is an adequate overbite, they are proclined with a removable appliance to correct the incisor malrelationship and eliminate the displacement as early as possible (see Fig. 13.2). This should take only a few weeks of treatment with a removable appliance. In the more severe cases or where there would be insufficient overbite to retain this simple form of incisor correction, a decision on treatment should be delayed until the early permanent dentition.

In many Class III cases, the upper arch is narrow and the lateral incisors are trapped palatally (see Fig. 13.3). They will then erupt into lingual occlusion, even when the central incisor position has been corrected. In addition, the upper permanent canines may lie labial to their roots, preventing labial movement until the canines have erupted and can be retracted. Where this problem is recognized before eruption of the lateral incisors, extraction of the upper deciduous canines may provide space for the lateral incisors to escape labially and erupt in alignment with the central incisors. This is not always successful but is worth attempting in suitable cases (see p. 20).

Even when the incisor relationship has been corrected in the early mixed dentition, relapse may occur later because of unfavourable facial growth. Where this happens it is generally an indication that the case is beyond correction by orthodontic means alone.

Late mixed/early permanent dentition

Where there is a positive overjet

The patient whose incisor malrelationship was successfully corrected earlier may still require treatment to relieve crowding and align the other teeth. The principles of treatment are the same as those for the Class I case with crowding. There may be problems with lateral incisor alignment if these teeth are still positioned palatally. Frequently they will be in crossbite and labial movement may require a fixed appliance; and even when they have been corrected, the overbite may not be sufficient to hold them there. If the overbite is tenuous, some extrusion of all the upper incisors may be attempted with a fixed appliance, but as the face continues to grow vertically, the overbite is liable to reduce again and upper incisors may slip back into reverse overjet. Patients and parents should be warned of this possibility.

Frequently the upper permanent canines erupt rather far forward where lateral incisors are positioned palatally, lacking the normal guidance from the lateral incisor roots. Occasionally an acceptable result can be obtained by extracting the lateral incisors themselves, rather than first premolars. However, as is the case where lateral incisors are absent developmentally, the appearance of the canine adjacent to the central incisor may not be ideal.

Where there is a reverse overjet

In deciding whether orthodontic treatment to correct the reverse overjet is advisable, the first step is to assess whether the facial appearance would be acceptable without surgical correction of the skeletal pattern. This evaluation must be undertaken with the mandible in the rest position so that a misleading impression is not given by an anterior displacement or overclosure.

Having decided that the facial appearance would be acceptable, the incisor relationship can be evaluated. If the patient cannot obtain an edge-to-edge occlusion of the incisors, or if there is an anterior open bite, orthodontic correction is probably not feasible. Finally, the incisor inclinations have to be taken into account. Only if the teeth can be tipped to obtain a normal overjet and a secure overbite, without the upper incisors being excessively proclined, is it reasonable to proceed with orthodontic correction of the incisor malrelationship.

Appliance techniques

Treatment of the Class III case with a removable appliance is possible only where a corrected incisor overjet can be achieved with an adequate overbite and without undue proclination of the incisors. The upper arch is often crowded and first premolars are the teeth of choice for extraction, assuming that all other permanent teeth are present, sound and satisfactorily positioned. Distal movement of the upper buccal segments to relieve even mild crowding is generally contraindicated because the molars are often rather distally inclined and because any possible restraint to forward growth of the maxilla and upper arch is to be avoided. Any crowding in the lower arch will usually be dealt with by the extraction of lower first premolars, even though this may leave residual spacing at the extraction site. This encourages the lower labial segment to drop back if there is a worsening of the skeletal pattern with

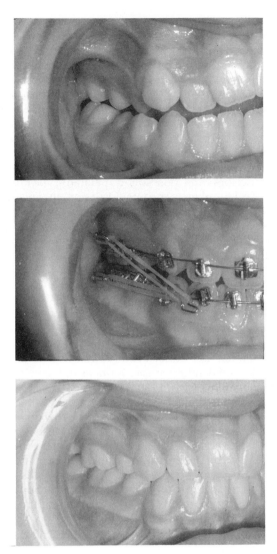

Figure 13.5 A patient with a moderately severe Class III incisor relationship that was successfully treated by means of fixed appliances incorporating intermaxillary traction.

growth, provided that there is an adequate overbite and that the lower incisors are not already very retroclined.

In the more severe case where the overjet cannot be corrected simply by proclining the upper incisors, or where the overbite is tenuous or where other teeth are positioned unfavourably, fixed appliance treatment will be indicated (Fig. 13.5). It is usually a good policy to aim to obtain as much improvement of the overjet as possible by retroclination of the lower incisors, because this does not reduce the overbite. This will usually necessitate the extraction of the lower first premolars, which will also provide space for the relief of any crowding. If the lower incisors are already retroclined, further retraction may not be possible, but this may well indicate that the case is at the limits of orthodontic treatment and surgical correction should at least be considered. Having decided how much retraction of the lower labial segment is feasible, it is clear how much labial movement of the upper incisors will be required.

Orthognathic surgery

Where it is decided that orthodontic correction is not practicable, or where earlier correction has relapsed due to unfavourable growth, either the arch malrelationship will have to be accepted and any orthodontic treatment directed towards alignment of the teeth, or surgical correction, possibly in conjunction with orthodontic treatment, will be required (Bell, Proffit and White, 1980) (see Chapter 19). This decision is usually best delayed until facial growth is nearly complete so that there is no uncertainty about later and possibly unfavourable growth changes.

References

Bell, W. H., Proffit, W. R. and White, R. P. (1980) *Surgical Correction of Dentofacial Deformities*, W. B. Saunders, Philadelphia

Bryant, P. M. F. (1981) Mandibular rotation and Class III malocclusion. *British Journal of Orthodontics*, **8**, 61–75

Chapter 14

Tooth movement

A tooth is suspended in its socket by the periodontal ligament, which, consisting of collagenous connective tissue, cells, blood vessels and tissue fluids, has viscoelastic properties. The periodontal ligament thus cushions the tooth and absorbs the forces of mastication and tooth contacts; it allows the tooth to erupt and to maintain its relation to the alveolar crest in the growing face; its sensory receptors are important in the control of masticatory activity; and it allows tooth movement to take place in response to muscular imbalance or orthodontic forces.

Periodontal ligament and alveolar bone remodelling do not occur in response to the transient imbalance in forces applied to the teeth produced by mastication, speech, swallowing or laughter, for example. Continuous and intermittent forces of sufficient duration and magnitude do prompt a cellular response and, if the loading is consistent in direction, alveolar bone remodelling and tooth movement occur.

The threshold in terms of pressure, duration or periodicity below which bone remodelling will not occur has not yet been quantified. Intermittent and interrupted forces are capable of producing tooth movement: for example, certain functional appliances generate intermittent forces and are worn only part time, yet are capable of producing extensive tooth movements. The force threshold required to produce tooth movement must be rather low; the slight muscular imbalance produced by labial movement of lower incisors, for example, is often followed by relapse. The question of what constitutes muscular balance is difficult to answer because recordings of the forces applied to the teeth when the orofacial musculature is at rest, and during function, indicate that it is rare for all the forces applied to a tooth at a particular moment to cancel one another out. It must be assumed that when the teeth are in a position of muscle balance, the force thresholds are not exceeded in some critical respect.

The nature of the initial tooth movement within the confines of the periodontal ligament depends on the forces applied to the crown and so determines the distribution of pressure changes within the ligament. The centre of resistance to movement lies at about 40 per cent of the root length from the apex and so, when a simple force is applied to the crown, it will tip about a fulcrum close to this point (Christiansen and Burstone, 1969; Yettram, Wright and Houston, 1977). Thus, the pressure within the periodontal ligament varies along the root length (Fig. 14.1),

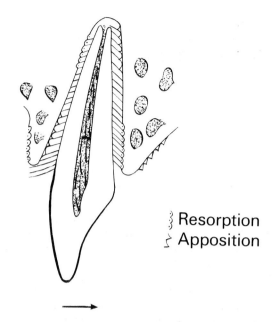

} Resorption
} Apposition

Figure 14.1 The distribution of bone remodelling changes on socket walls and alveolar process when a gentle force tips an upper central incisor palatally. The centre of rotation is at about 40 per cent of the root length from the apex.

the greatest pressure changes occurring close to the alveolar crest. When a tooth is moved bodily, the pressure distribution is more uniform along the root length but varies around its circumference.

Histological changes in areas of compression

The observed changes depend on whether or not capillary blood pressure is exceeded. Where this happens, the blood vessels are crushed, the cells die and the compressed connective tissue has a structureless glassy appearance when viewed in histological sections under the light microscope: this is called hyalinization (Rygh, 1974). This commonly occurs close to the alveolar crest in the area of maximum compression when teeth are tipped, even with quite light, continuous orthodontic forces. If excessive forces are used, hyalinization may be extensive. Areas of hyalinization are less common with true bodily tooth movements because of the more uniform pressure distribution along the root; but, of course, even with fixed appliances it may be difficult to avoid some tipping of the tooth and hyalinization is still liable to occur at any irregularities in the socket wall.

Areas of compression below capillary blood pressure

Within a few days, there is proliferation of fibroblasts and other cells of the periodontal ligament. Osteoclasts, which are believed to migrate to these areas from the blood vessels, appear along the socket wall and bone resorption commences. Soon the osteoclasts come to lie within shallow depressions known as Howship's lacunae. Osteoclasts are large, complex, multinucleated cells and the one osteoclast may be responsible for resorption at several different locations. Resorption does not take place over a large, continuous front and so while some of the fibres of the periodontal ligament become detached, others remain intact. After some bone has been resorbed, the osteoclasts migrate or are replaced and bone is resorbed at the previously passive sites. Meanwhile the detached periodontal fibres become reattached at the former resorption sites and so the integrity of the ligament is maintained (Kurihara and Enlow, 1980).

The factors mediating between the change in pressure and the cellular response are still a matter of speculation. They are probably the same as those that come into play when pressure is applied directly to the periosteum. Suggestions have been made that changes in electrical charge occur at the surface of the bone and that these promote the observed cellular response (Zengo, Paioluk and Bassett, 1973). Experimental work has shown that the application of a direct current to the alveolar process close to a tooth does accelerate its movement in response to orthodontic forces (Davidovitch et al., 1980). However, it is not at all clear whether this is a specific effect or whether it merely reflects a general perturbation of cellular activity.

There is some evidence that local hormones, known as prostaglandins, may also have a role (Sandy and Harris, 1984). These have been identified in pathological lesions associated with bone resorption; their inhibition reduces but does not prevent resorption in areas of compression of the periodontal ligament; and the injection of prostaglandins into the alveolar mucosa has been shown to accelerate orthodontic tooth movement (Yamasaki et al., 1984). However, although prostaglandins may be important, other chemical factors also have a role in the promotion of osteoclastic activity.

Areas of compression exceeding capillary blood pressure

As explained above, where the capillary vessels are crushed, the cells die and the compressed connective tissue appears structureless under the light microscope. If the pressure is reduced, these hyalinized areas rapidly become revascularized and colonized by new cells (Rygh, 1974). Bone resorption cannot take place on the surface of the socket wall beneath a hyalinized area. However, peripheral to the hyalinized area, the periodontal ligament is compressed slightly and direct surface resorption occurs. This peripheral resorption may completely remove the bone underlying a small area of hyalinization. However, more extensive areas of hyalinization are removed by undermining resorption within the cancellous spaces deep to the affected area; osteoclasts appear and the bone is removed from below (Rygh, 1974). If the appliance continues to exert an excessive force, a further zone of hyalinization will be produced. However, when the force is reduced by the tooth movement so that the area is compressed only gently, the hyalinized area will be revascularized and direct surface resorption can proceed.

Histological changes in areas of tension

The periodontal fibres are stretched, and with excessive forces, some may be torn and blood vessels may be ruptured. However, there is no fundamental difference in the nature of the tissue response to light and heavy forces, in contrast to areas of compression. Within a few days, cellular proliferation occurs among the fibroblasts of the periodontal ligament and the osteoblasts lining the socket wall. The extension of the principal fibres occurs throughout their length and not specifically at either end. Osteoid is laid down along the socket wall and this becomes calcified and reorganized as woven bone. The irregular and vascular woven bone is very susceptible to resorption but is progressively remodelled into mature bone.

The supra-alveolar connective tissues

The transseptal fibres, which pass between adjacent teeth, also adjust to tooth movement. If two teeth are being moved apart, the fibres stretch, but the residual tension is sufficient to promote tooth movement. Thus, for example, when a first premolar is being retracted, the canine will follow if it is free to do so, although some stretching of the fibres will occur and there will be a space between the teeth. It is good practice to avoid elongating the transseptal fibres because when teeth are approximated these fibres do not seem to shorten readily and so the interdental contacts may be less tight than would be desired.

The free gingival fibres pass from the neck of the tooth into the connective tissue system of the mucoperiosteum. When a tooth is moved orthodontically, it does not pass through the mucoperiosteum but carries it with it; and any adjustment occurs within the mucoperiosteum. This is of particular relevance when teeth are rotated because the free gingival fibres seem to stretch but not to remodel fully (Reitan, 1959). Residual tension within the supra-alveolar connective tissue system is probably an important reason why teeth that have been rotated mechanically are so liable to relapse (Edwards, 1968).

Remodelling of the alveolar process

The tissue changes associated with orthodontic tooth movement are not confined to the periodontal ligament and socket wall. Any labiolingual tooth movement is associated with remodelling of the alveolar process: subperiosteal apposition occurs on the bone surface towards which the root is moving, and resorption on the surface from which the tooth is moving. Thus the alveolar process 'drifts' with the tooth (see Fig. 14.1). Remodelling is most complete close to the alveolar crest but may be neglible at apical level. Thus it is possible to move the root apex through the alveolar plate where it is thin. This may provoke root resorption and clearly is undesirable (Ten Hoeve and Mulié, 1976). However, if the root is moved back again, the alveolar bone may reform (Thilander *et al.*, 1983).

Tissue changes during the retention period

If a tooth is released immediately after having been moved with an orthodontic appliance, it will spring back due to residual tension in the periodontal ligament and the force may even be enough to produce some resorption of bone on surfaces that were previously formative. Although this reversal is clearly limited in amount, it is desirable to retain the tooth until the periodontal ligament has adapted fully. More important is the fact that the recently formed bone is very readily resorbed and even slight forces that would not normally provoke a tissue response may initiate resorption. Thus it seems prudent in most cases to retain the tooth position until more mature bone has been formed (see Chapter 18). This takes between 3 and 6 months. During this period a new lamina dura forms on previously resorptive surfaces, and some adjustments may take place in the supra-alveolar connective tissue. However, adaptation of the supra-alveolar fibres seems to be very slow and may cause relapse of rotations even after quite long periods of retention.

Pathological changes associated with tooth movement

From some points of view it is surprising that there are not more complications of orthodontic tooth movement. Even after extensive hyalinization of the periodontal ligament, recovery is complete. This does not mean that large forces can be used with impunity: other side-effects described below are more liable to occur with excessive forces; and there can be problems of anchorage control and appliance management.

Crestal bone loss

A slight reduction in crestal bone height occurs with many types of fixed-appliance treatment. This may be a direct result of tooth move-ment, or it may be secondary to a deterioration in plaque control. However, when treatment is well managed this crestal loss should be less than 1 mm and is of limited clinical relevance (Zachrisson and Alnaes, 1974). However, with poor oral hygiene it may be more severe and can be a matter of concern. Severe crestal loss and periodontal recession can occur when a tooth is moved labially or buccally with heavy forces where the buccal plate is already very thin. If hyalinization of the periodontal ligament occurs at the alveolar crest, and the plate of bone is thin with few or no cancellous spaces, undermining and peripheral resorption can result in the loss of crestal height. If at the same time oral hygiene is less than ideal, gingival recession will also occur. Labial movement of lower incisors and buccal movement of upper and lower canines is particularly liable to be associated with periodontal recession of this type.

Labial or buccal movement of a root apex may result in fenestration of the alveolar plate. This is not such an immediately serious periodontal problem because bone may reform when the apex is moved lingually again, and it does not predispose to gingival recession in an otherwise healthy mouth.

Root resorption

Small areas of root resorption are universally found on teeth that are being moved orthodontically, owing to osteoclastic activity in areas of pressure (Linge and Linge, 1983). These may occur laterally or apically, and are usually small in amount; they are repaired by secondary cementum and are of no long-term importance. However, appreciable apical resorption with permanent shortening of the root can occur, particularly where extensive apical movements are undertaken as with fixed appliances. It has been suggested that 'round tripping' where the apex is moved first in one direction and then in another, is particularly liable to produce root resorption (Goldson and Henrikson, 1975); but this may merely reflect the total distance through which the root is moved. Heavy forces have also been implicated, but again there is no objective evidence that this is so.

The teeth most commonly involved are the upper incisors and the first permanent molars. One quarter of the root length or even more can be lost from previously healthy teeth and clearly this is a matter of serious concern. The teeth retain their vitality, they do not generally suffer further spontaneous resorption, and after the normal retention period do not demonstrate increased mobility; and so there are no immediate problems for the patient. However, should periodontal disease with alveolar bone loss become established subsequently, the prognosis for teeth with appreciably shortened roots is poor.

Some teeth are particularly susceptible to root resorption during orthodontic tooth movement and very extensive root loss can occur, even with simple tipping movements. These teeth almost always have signs of idiopathic resorption before orthodontic treatment is commenced and it is very important to examine on radiographs the root length of all teeth that are to be moved. If there are signs of blunting and shortening of the roots, then orthodontic movement of these teeth should be avoided if at all possible. Not only may rapid and extensive resorption occur, but because the centre of resistance to tooth movement is closer to the crown they tilt more than usual with removable appliances or other simple forces. If it is essential to move teeth that have been affected in this way, the patient (and parent if appropriate) must be warned of the dangers of serious root shortening reducing the life expectancy of the affected teeth, and only if they are prepared to accept the risks should treatment be commenced. It may be wise to confirm the warning and discussion in writing as a defence against subsequent litigation.

Light forces are mandatory and it is better to use fixed appliances with controlled tipping about the apex in order to minimize apical travel. Root length should be monitored and standardized periapical radiographs taken at 3-monthly intervals; if further root shortening is detected, the tooth should be stabilized with the appliances for a period of 3 months in order to allow as much repair as possible by secondary cementum (Rygh, 1977): resorption ceases when the force is removed. This procedure of stabilization should also be followed if root resorption is discovered in previously normal teeth during orthodontic treatment.

The final tooth position should be planned to be as free as possible from occlusal or other stress. It is surprising how firm a tooth that has lost even three-quarters of its root length can be, and it may be functional for many years providing that plaque control and gingival health are maintained scrupulously. However, such teeth are always at risk from even minor trauma and their long-term prognosis is invariably poor.

Damage to the dental pulp

When a tooth is moved by an appliance, the apical vessels are under some tension and a minor degree of pulpal hyperaemia commonly occurs (Stenvik and Mjör, 1970; Unsterseher et al., 1987; Kvinnsland, Heyeraas and Ofjord, 1989). This is normally reversible, with no symptoms or long-term damage. However, if the pulp is already fibrotic with a poor blood supply, for instance following a blow to the tooth, orthodontic movement may strangulate the vessels and finally devitalize the already moribund pulp. The tooth will frequently become discoloured and this will be attributed to the orthodontic treatment. The teeth most commonly affected are of course the upper incisors, particularly in Class II, division 1 cases in view of their susceptibility to trauma. The patient may volunteer no history of an accident and may not even remember it. This makes it very important to examine the upper incisors carefully at the time of diagnosis. Enamel fractures, cracks or discoloration all indicate that a vitality test should be performed, and the radiograph should be inspected with particular care for root fractures, failure of apical closure or periapical radiolucencies. If the tooth is non-vital, it must be satisfactorily root treated before tooth movement is commenced.

The decision is more difficult in the case of a diminished vitality response. The danger of moving such a tooth is that the pulp may die and the crown may well become discoloured. On the other hand, the patient will be reluctant to have root treatment for a symptomless tooth. Clearly the problem must be discussed with the patient and parent, and if the tooth's vitality response is appreciably diminished, root treatment should be advised.

Mechanisms of tooth movement

All movements can be described in terms of rotations and translations. We shall deal here only with the small initial tooth movements that occur within the periodontal space. Clearly the larger longer-term movements are the results of a succession of such minor movements, depending on the pattern of socket remodelling; and these too can be described in terms of rotation and translation. However, these may have been achieved by widely different pathways and so any bio-mechanical description may be more misleading than helpful.

Although, for the purposes of illustration, forces and moments are often discussed in quantitative terms, orthodontic appliances cannot be used with this degree of precision. Clinicians should be aware of the general range of forces that they apply to the teeth, and of the mechanical properties of their appliances. However, the effectiveness of a force delivery system is judged by its results: if a tooth is tipping too much as it is retracted with a fixed appliance, the couple will be increased or the force will be reduced at the next visit of the patient. A sound background knowledge is important so that the appliance can be designed and activated in an informed manner; and so that if the tooth movement is not as intended, an intelligent correction can be made to the force system.

When a simple force is applied to a single point on a tooth surface, it can be resolved into two components – one perpendicular to the surface at the point of contact and the other tangent to the surface. Unless care is taken in adjusting the spring correctly, unexpected and unwanted tooth movements may occur (see Fig. 15.2).

The centre of resistance to movement lies at about 40 per cent of the root length from the apex in a single-rooted tooth, and just apical to the furcation of most multirooted teeth. When the line of action of the force passes through the centre of resistance, the tooth will be translated in the direction of the force vector; but otherwise it will tip.

The further from the centre of resistance the force vector, the greater its tipping moment will be: the moment is calculated as the product of the force and its distance from the fulcrum. If we look at a tooth in cross-section, it is apparent that rotation can be induced when the force vector does not pass through the long axis. This is not an effective method of producing a controlled rotation but it is a common side-effect when, for example, a palatal canine retractor is adjusted incorrectly (see Fig. 15.2).

If translation of the tooth is required and the force vector does not pass through the centre of resistance, a mechanical couple has to be applied to the crown in order to counter the rotational effect of the moment. A controlled couple is very difficult to apply with a removable appliance, but is readily generated by a fixed appliance (see Fig. 10.1). It is evident intuitively and can be demonstrated mathematically that the ratio between the couple and the force determines the nature of the tooth movement. The forces generated by any orthodontic appliance must be in static equilibrium, otherwise it would not be stable. At the simplest level, for example when canines are retracted with a removable appliance, there is an equal and opposite forward force that is resisted by the anchorage. Within even a simple fixed appliance, the force system can be very complex indeed, and as the tooth moves, the forces change. It is neither possible nor is it necessary to analyse the forces within every fixed appliance in detail. However, it is essential to understand the general principles so that appliances can be designed and activated in a way that will produce the intended tooth movements without unexpected side-reactions. If treatment does not progress as planned, the reasons must be analysed and corrective action instituted. This can be done only by careful monitoring of tooth movements and with an appreciation of the biomechanical principles of fixed appliances. Horizontal and vertical forces are always balanced by equal and opposite forces of reaction; and couples can be resolved into horizontal and vertical components with corresponding forces of reaction.

Forces for the movement of teeth

It is generally agreed that 'light' forces should be used to move teeth. A light force is one which does not produce hyalinized areas in the periodontal ligament for that type of tooth movement. The division between light and heavy forces depends on many factors including the root length and shape, the characterstics of that periodontal ligament and the nature of the tooth movement. It is neither possible nor necessary to calculate the appropriate force to be applied from first principles. Empirical clinical and histological evidence suggest that a force of 30 g applied to the crown of a single-rooted tooth is appropriate for tipping movements, and that over 100 g can be used for bodily movements. Particularly with fixed appliances, it is difficult to estimate how much force is actually being transmitted to the periodontal ligament and how much is dissipated by friction between the brackets and archwire.

Although early tooth movement will be delayed by areas of hyalinization, the rapid movement subsequent to their removal may mean that progress is similar with both levels of force. Clinical experiments have shown that the rate of tooth movement is not consistently greater with light or heavy forces, even on the opposite sides of the same mouth (Andreasen and Zwanziger, 1980).

The importance of light forces rests not with the rate of tooth movement but with the undesirable side-effects of heavy forces:

1 Where large forces are used with intraoral appliances, anchorage control becomes difficult. It is possible to dissipate all the space required for correction of the malocclusion by unplanned movement of anchor teeth. For example, when a removable appliance is used to retract upper canines after extraction of first premolars, it is only too easy to lose all the space in this way. Where extraoral anchorage is used, this danger is reduced or eliminated.

2 Control of tooth movement becomes difficult because fixed-appliance archwires are not stiff enough to counter the tipping movement created

by large forces. For example, where teeth are moved along an arch-wire, excessive tipping and 'dumping' may occur, even with wide brackets, owing to flexion of the archwire. The mechanical properties of sectional archwires are particularly unsatisfactory when they are activated excessively.

3 Large forces make the teeth tender, and the risks of root resorption and damage to the pulpal vessels are increased.

4 When removable appliance components are activated excessively, the patient may have difficulty in inserting the appliance correctly. For example, canine retraction springs may be positioned distal to, rather than mesial to, the teeth.

Conclusion

The safe and effective use of orthodontic appliances depends on a detailed understanding of: the immediate change in tooth position in response to applied forces; the change in pressure distribution that this produces within the periodontal ligament; and the response of the supporting tissues to these pressure changes. The potentially damaging effects of orthodontic appliances can be controlled, providing they are understood and appropriate precautions are taken.

References

Andreasen, G. F. and Zwanziger, D. (1980) A clinical evaluation of the differential force concept as applied to the edgewise bracket. *American Journal of Orthodontics*, **78**, 25–40

Christiansen, R. L. and Burstone, C. J. (1969) Centers of rotation within the periodontal space. *American Journal of Orthodontics*, *55*, 353–369

Davidovitch, Z., Finkelson, M. D., Steigman, S., Shanfeld, J. L., Montgomery, P. C. and Korostoff, E. (1980) Electrical currents, bone remodelling and orthodontic tooth movement. I. The effect of electric currents on periodontal cyclic nucleotides. II. Increase in rate of tooth movement and periodontal cyclic neucleotide levels by combined force and electric current. *American Journal of Orthodontics*, **77**, I, 14–32; II, 33–47

Edwards, J. G. (1968) A study of the periodontium during orthodontic rotation of teeth. *American Journal of Orthodontics*, **54**, 441–461

Goldson, L. and Henrikson, C. O. (1975) Root resorption during Begg treatment: a longitudinal roentgenographic study. *American Journal of Orthodontics*, **68**, 55–66

Kurihara, S. and Enlow, D. H. (1980) An electron microscopic study of attachments between periodontal fibers and bone during alveolar remodelling. *American Journal of Orthodontics*, **77**, 516–531

Kvinnsland, S., Heyeraas, K. and Ofjord, E. S. (1989) Effect of experimental tooth movement on periodontal and pulpal blood flow. *European Journal of Orthodontics*, **11**, 200–205

Linge, B. O. and Linge, L. (1983) Apical root resorption in upper anterior teeth. *European Journal of Orthodontics*, **5**, 173–183

Reitan, K. (1959) Tissue rearrangement during retention of orthodontically rotated teeth. *Angle Orthodontist*, **29**, 105–113

Rygh, P. (1974) Elimination of hyalinised periodontal tissues associated with orthodontic tooth movement. *Scandinavian Journal of Dental Research*, **83**, 57–73

Rygh, P. (1977) Orthodontic root resorption studied by electron microscopy. *Angle Orthodontist*, **47**, 1–16

Sandy, J. R. and Harris, M. (1984) Prostaglandins and tooth movement. *European Journal of Orthodontics*, **6**, 175–182

Stenvik, A. and Mjör, I. A. (1970) Pulp and dentine reactions to experimental tooth intrusion. A histologic study of the initial changes. *American Journal of Orthodontics*, **57**, 370–382

Ten Hoeve, A. and Mulié, R. M. (1976) The effect of antero-posterior incisor repositioning on the palatal cortex as studied with laminagraphy. *Journal of Clinical Orthodontics*, **10**, 804–822

Thilander, B., Nyman, S., Karring, T. and Magnusson, I. (1983) Bone regeneration in alveolar bone dehiscences related to orthodontic tooth movement. *European Journal of Orthodontics*, **5**, 105–114

Unsterseher, R. E., Neigberg, L. G., Weimer, A. D. and Dyer, K. K. (1987) The response of human pulpal tissue after orthodontic force application. *American Journal of Orthodontics*, **92**, 220–224

Yamasaki, K., Shibata, Y., Tani, Y., Shibasaki, Y. and Fukuhara, T. (1984) Clinical application of prostaglandin E1 (PGE_1) upon orthodontic tooth movement. *American Journal of Orthodontics*, **85**, 506–518

Yettram, A. L., Wright, K. W. and Houston, W. J. B. (1977) Centre of rotation of a maxillary central incisor under orthodontic loading. *British Journal of Orthodontics*, **4**, 23–27

Zachrisson, B. U. and Alnaes, L. (1974) Periodontal condition in orthodontically treated and untreated individuals. II: Alveolar bone loss; radiographic findings. *Angle Orthodontist*, **44**, 48–55

Zengo, A. N., Pawluk, R. J. and Bassett, C. A. L. (1973) Stress-induced bioelectric potentials in the dentoalveolar complex. *American Journal of Orthodontics*, **64**, 17–27

Chapter 15

Removable appliances

Removable appliances are well suited to the treatment of simple malocclusions where teeth have to be tipped about a fulcrum close to the middle of the root. Good results can be obtained in suitable cases but experience and careful case selection are required if they are to be used to maximal advantage. They can be used by the general dental practitioner and they require little surgery time. However, they are not suitable for the treatment of complex cases requiring bodily movement of teeth, and they are not well tolerated in the lower arch, because they encroach on the tongue space. General practitioners should not become involved in treatment of cases that are beyond the scope of removable appliances, or of their expertise: it is only too easy to maltreat a case so that the malocclusion becomes more complex than before and the patient is even worse off.

Removable appliance design

In designing a removable appliance, four requirements should be considered in sequence: active, retentive, anchorage and baseplate. Some components may contribute to more than one function: for example, clasps may be used for both retention and anchorage. A very large number of removable appliance designs have been suggested, and the concern of the present text is to illustrate the general principles of design by reference to specific components that have proved to be reliable in clinical practice, while recognizing that alternative methods may be equally satisfactory.

Active components

These may be grouped broadly as springs and bows, screws and elastics. In general where there is a choice, palatal springs give the fewest problems; screws are used only in well-defined circumstances because of their expense and bulk; and elastics should be used only with headgear.

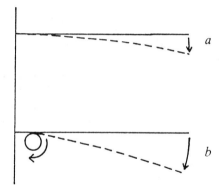

Figure 15.1 Cantilevered springs. (a) A simple cantilever. The deflection for a given load is proportional to the third power of the length of the spring and inversely to the fourth power of its diameter. (b) The incorporation of a coil increases the effective length of the spring. For maximum resilience the coil should be 'wound up' when the appliance is inserted and 'unwound' as the tooth moves.

Springs and bows

These are made from hard-drawn, stainless-steel wire. Removable appliance springs are generally variations of the cantilever spring (Fig. 15.1) modified according to local requirements. The force (F) delivered for a given deflection (d) depends upon the wire length (l) and radius (r) and elastic modulus (E) according to the formula:

$$F\alpha\ \frac{Er^4}{l^3}$$

From this it is apparent that small variations in the length and radius of the wire have a major effect upon its stiffness. Doubling the radius increases the stiffness by a factor of 16, while doubling its length reduces the stiffness by a factor of 8. In most circumstances, the force used to produce a simple tipping movement of a single rooted tooth should be in the region of 25–50 g (see Chapter 14).

It is convenient to have a spring deflection of 2–4 mm. This ensures that the typical spring will be able to self-activate as the appliance is inserted so that it is readily manageable by the patient. Further, the force does not drop off too rapidly as the tooth moves: too large a deflection makes it difficult to insert the appliance correctly, and a very small deflection of, for example, only 1 mm means that by the time the tooth has moved half of that distance, the force has declined by 50 per cent. The elastic modulus of wires generally used in removable orthodontic appliance varies little and spring length is constrained by the space available in the mouth.

The most important factor determining the characteristics of a particular design of spring is thus the diameter of the wire selected. In most circumstances, wire 0.5–0.7 mm in diameter will be used for the spring but it should be noted that the selection of 0.7 mm rather than 0.5 mm wire for a particular spring will increase its stiffness fourfold. In addition to its load/deflection characteristics the stability of the spring needs to be taken into account. If the spring is guarded by the baseplate or supported by a stiffer component, this may not be a serious problem, but where the spring has to be self-supporting, as in certain designs of buccal canine-retractor (see Fig. 15.5), there may have to be a compromise between stability and stiffness and so the properties of the spring are not entirely satisfactory in either respect: for optimal load/deflection characteristics the spring would be made in 0.5 mm diameter wire but it would then be so unstable vertically, that it would not function satisfactorily. Accordingly it is made from 0.7 mm wire, which improves the stability to a limited extent but makes the spring so stiff that for a buccal spring of average dimensions, a deflection of just 1 mm will generate a force of 75 g. This is not at all satisfactory.

Stability ratio

These problems highlight the necessity of taking account of spring stability when designing an appliance. The stability ratio is the stiffness in the direction of unwanted displacement divided by the stiffness in the intended direction of tooth movement (Houston and Waters, 1977; Waters, 1982). This ratio should be as high as possible, and at least 1. A simple cantilever spring is equally flexible in all directions of bending and so has a stability ratio of 1 when unsupported, but generally this will be increased by support from the baseplate. The typical unsupported buccal canine-retraction spring has a stability ratio of less than 1 and it is very liable to be displaced by lips or cheeks, or by its action on a sloping surface. This design is rather unsatisfactory and alternative patterns (see Fig. 15.5) will be found to be preferable in terms of both stiffness and stability ratio.

Coils

Most removable-appliance springs incorporate coils that increase their effective length and so reduce their stiffness. For the maximal effect, they should be made reasonably large (a diameter of at least 2.5 mm is required) and be placed close to the attachment point of the spring (Fig. 15.1). For small deflections, the direction in which the coil is loaded does not affect its stiffness but it is important in its resilience: a coil spring loaded in the direction of its formation (Fig. 15.1) has an enhanced resistance to permanent deformation.

Point of contact

When a tooth is contacted by a spring at a single point, it will move in the direction of the resultant force, which is perpendicular to the tangent at the point of contact with the tooth (Fig. 15.2). Thus great care must be taken to ensure that the spring is positioned and adjusted to move the tooth in the direction required. This should be considered at design stage. For example when a buccally positioned canine is to be moved distopalatally into the line of the arch, a palatal spring is not suitable and will tend to move the tooth further buccally and perhaps even to

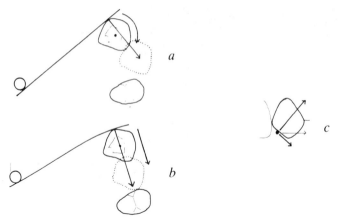

Figure 15.2 The design of a cantilever spring. The force applied to the tooth is perpendicular to the tangent at the point of contact. (a) It is a common mistake to have the contact of the spring on the tooth too far palatally. This means that the tooth will not move along the line of the arch but will be deflected buccally. Particularly with an upper canine, the force may also pass laterally to the centre of resistance of the tooth, setting up a mechanical couple, which will rotate the tooth. (b) The coil of the spring should be centred on the line through the midpoint of the tooth (i.e. its centre of resistance) and perpendicular to its intended path. Where necessary, the spring should be cranked so that the point of contact is positioned sufficiently buccally for this to be achieved. (c) If the spring acts on a sloping surface, an intrusive component may interfere with the eruption of the tooth; and the component along the tooth surface will make the spring unstable.

rotate it (Fig. 15.2). Even if the canine is in the line of the arch, it is very easy to produce unwanted tooth movements if the spring is designed or adjusted carelessly.

Spring design

Springs for mesial and distal tooth movements

Palatal springs. Where the tooth is in the line of the arch a palatal cantilever spring is indicated. Design principles are shown in Fig. 15.2. If the tooth is to be moved over an appreciable distance, the spring should be cranked to ensure the correct point of contact with the tooth. The coil is positioned so that it is 'wound up' when the appliance is inserted. The spring will usually be made from 0.5 mm diameter wire, giving a stiffness of about 15 g/mm for a spring 1.75 cm long. Stability of the spring is helped by boxing in by the baseplate (Fig. 15.3). The incorporation of a guard wire on the palatal aspect of the spring (Fig. 15.4) so that it acts in a slot between guard and baseplate enhances the stability further; but care must be taken to ensure that it can still move freely.

Adjustment. Detailed adjustment to ensure a correct contact between spring and tooth is undertaken first. The spring is then activated,

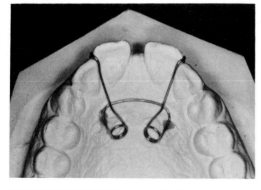

Figure 15.3 Springs to move central incisors mesially.

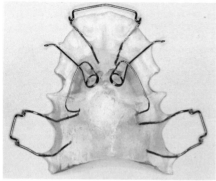

Figure 15.4 Palatal springs to retract upper canines. A guard wire lies between the spring and the palate. This helps to protect the spring from distortion when the appliance is inserted and removed. The boxing out by the baseplate and the guard wire both stabilize the spring. It is important that the spring moves freely between the baseplate and the guard wire.

typically by 2–3 mm. This is done in the free arm of the spring, not at its point of emergence from the baseplate nor in the coil where it is more liable to fracture from work hardening and stress concentration.

Buccal springs

These have to be used where a tooth is to be moved palatally as well as distally. They are often uncomfortable for the patient, their stability tends to be poor and they can be difficult to adjust. The classic design made from 0.7 mm wire (Fig. 15.5a) is unsatisfactory in all these respects. The supported design (Fig. 15.5b) is more stable, less stiff and is easier to adjust. All these designs are liable to be uncomfortable for the patient and to cause traumatic ulceration if they are extended too far into the buccal sulcus. The problem is that if they are not high enough, they are excessively stiff and have a very limited range of adjustment. However, other designs of buccal spring, of which there are many, tend to be even less satisfactory. It will be noted that in these springs, the coil is the wrong way round for maximal resilience. This is a minor disadvantage, but a coil made the 'correct' way round is more liable to be uncomfortable for the patient.

Adjustment. Self-supporting springs in 0.7 mm wire are very stiff and should be adjusted by only a small amount (about 1 mm). Supported

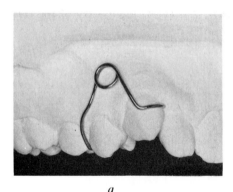 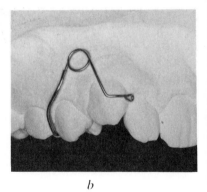

a   *b*

Figure 15.5 Buccal canine-retraction springs. (a) A self-supporting buccal spring in 0.7 mm wire. Note that this design controls the position of the tooth buccolingually as well as mesiodistally. However, this type of spring is very stiff and has a poor stability ratio (it is more flexible vertically than anteroposteriorly). (b) A buccal spring of 0.5 mm wire supported in stainless-steel tubing. This has a better stability ratio and at the same time is more flexible than the spring in (a).

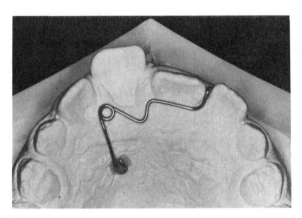

Figure 15.6 A cranked palatal finger spring. The crank keeps the spring clear of the correctly positioned central incisor. If the teeth were not spaced, the free end of the spring would be recurved palatally. Note the coil is positioned as far anteriorly as possible.

buccal springs are not so stiff and can be activated by 2–3 mm depending on the length of the free arm. Buccal springs are activated by inserting the round beak of a pair of spring-forming pliers into the coil and bending the anterior limb further round the beak. Palatal activation is in the anterior limb. Supported springs must not be adjusted where they emerge from the tubing, as they are most liable to fracture at this point.

Springs for moving teeth buccally

Incisors. Cranked (Fig. 15.6) or double cantilever springs (Fig. 15.7) are

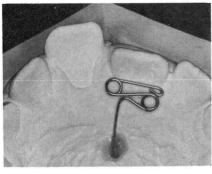
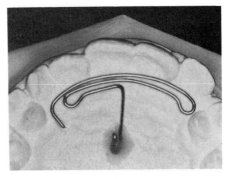

a   *b*

Figure 15.7 Double cantilever or Z-springs. (a) On a single tooth: on a narrower tooth such as a lateral incisor, the springs are stiff and have rather a poor stability ratio. (b) A double cantilever spring on four teeth. It is not necessary to incorporate coils as there is already a sufficient length of wire in the spring.

used most commonly. The spring is designed to be clear of other teeth throughout its action. Cranked springs have the point of attachment as far forward as possible so that they remain in contact with the tooth for the entire movement. Even when the tooth has moved away from the baseplate the spring is still supported by it and so stability is not a problem. The double cantilever spring is satisfactory if it can be made of sufficient width – as when two or more teeth are to be moved labially. When used on a single narrow tooth, it tends to be rather stiff and if the tooth has to be moved an appreciable distance from the baseplate, it tends to be unstable. For moving several incisor teeth labially, crossed cantilever springs (Fig. 15.8) can be useful.

Buccal teeth. A cantilever spring can be difficult for the patient to insert correctly and so, while a cranked finger spring can be used, a self-positioning T spring (Fig. 15.9) is usually more satisfactory. This works most effectively on a tooth such as a premolar or molar with a rather vertical palatal surface. The spring is constructed from 0.5 mm

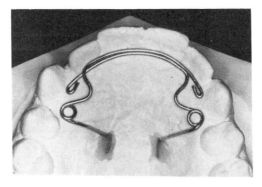

Figure 15.8 Crossed cantilever springs are an effective way of proclining all four upper incisor teeth.

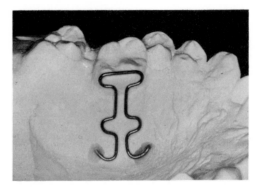

Figure 15.9 A T spring to move a molar buccally. These are also effective on premolars and canines. The adjustment loops allow the spring to be extended as the tooth moves. Note that the spring is constructed to lie well clear of the palatal mucosa.

wire and care should be taken that it stands clear of the palatal mucosa so that it does not dig in as the tooth moves. If appreciable tooth movement is required, adjustment loops should be incorporated to allow the spring to be lengthened (Fig. 15.9). It is activated by pulling it away from the baseplate, though not too far as it is difficult to bend it back again.

Where a canine needs to be extruded as well as moved buccally, as is often the case after surgical exposure, it be best to bond an attachment to the tooth, into which a removable appliance spring can fit.

Transverse expansion by springs

As an alternative to a screw plate (see below), a Coffin spring may be used (Fig. 15.10). This is constructed from 1.25 mm wire and has the advantage that differential expansion of the arch, anteriorly and posteriorly, is possible. These springs are cheaper and less bulky than screws but, unless they are well made and correctly adjusted, the appliance may be rather unstable.

Adjustment. Pits drilled into the baseplate allow the initial width of the appliance to be checked with calipers (Fig. 15.10). The spring is expanded anteriorly first, then posteriorly by pulling it apart, care being taken not to twist the appliance. This is easier and quicker than adjustment with pliers. An expansion of 2–3 mm will generally be appropriate.

Springs to move individual teeth palatally

The amount of movement is generally quite small and self-supporting buccal springs in 0.7 mm wire are satisfactory (Fig. 15.11).

Bows for incisor retraction

As with buccal canine springs, the problem is to design a retractor that

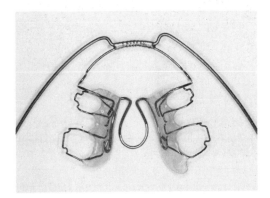

Figure 15.10 A Coffin spring in an 'en masse' appliance designed to retract the upper buccal segments. Small pits drilled in the acrylic allow the amount of expansion to be checked with dividers.

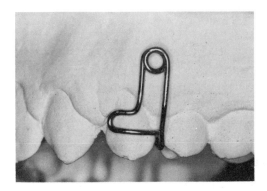

Figure 15.11 A self-supporting spring to move a tooth palatally.

will be flexible yet stable, and which will not be uncomfortable for the patient. Many bows in 0.7 mm wire have been devised but on the whole these have a poor stability ratio and are very stiff. They can be useful for minor adjustments to irregular teeth (Fig. 15.12) but are not really suitable for the reduction of large overjets. A 0.7 mm bow can be modified by splitting it (Bass and Robinson, 1969) (Fig. 15.13a) or by the addition of self-straightening wires (Fig. 15.13b). Both of these are light and flexible but it is very easy to flatten the labial segment too much and they have to be adjusted with care.

The supported incisor retraction bows are stable and flexible but are liable to break if they are adjusted incorrectly. The Roberts retractor made from 0.5 mm wire supported by tubing (Fig. 15.14) is an excellent retraction bow but is difficult to repair. However, provided care has been taken in its construction not to damage the wire, and provided that it is not adjusted where it emerges from the tubing support, fracture is not common. If the bow is made from Elgiloy wire (green grade) fracture is rare.

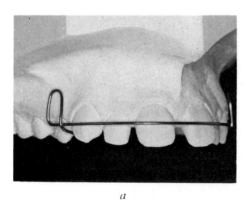
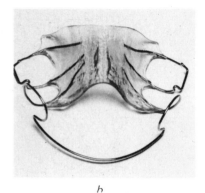

a   *b*

Figure 15.12 (a) A labial bow with reverse loops. It is too stiff for effective incisor retraction and the stability ratio is poor (it tends to slide up proclined incisors). It can be used for retaining tooth positions and for minor tooth movements. (b) A labial bow with large omega loops; this is more flexible but still has a poor stability ratio.

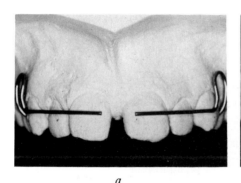
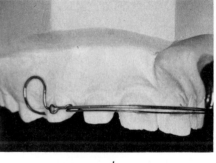

a   *b*

Figure 15.13 Modifications to a labial bow for incisor retraction. (a) Splitting the bow greatly reduces the stiffness. (b) A 0.4 mm wire attached to the bow as an auxillary spring. When in place it attempts to spring back to its passive straight form and so exerts a force on the teeth.

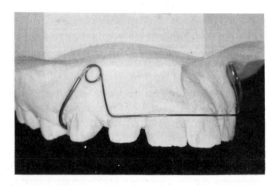

Figure 15.14 A Roberts retractor.

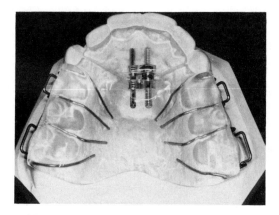

Figure 15.15 A screw plate to correct a Class III incisor relationship. This is less effective than an appliance employing palatal springs because there is no possibility of adjusting the direction of movement. Moreover, as with all screw appliances, their success depends on the ability of the patient to remember to turn the screw.

Screws

The orthodontic screw (Fig. 15.15) has its two ends threaded in opposite directions so that when it is turned, the metal end-plates move apart (or towards one another if a closing screw is to be used). Guide pins prevent the end-plates from rotating and enhance appliance stability.

Because the basic orthodontic screw is rigid it can be adjusted by only a small amount at any one time, otherwise the appliance cannot be inserted. The teeth are displaced within the limits of the periodontal ligaments and bone remodelling allows them to move. The screw can then be adjusted again. Typically, one-quarter of a turn of the screw will separate the parts of the baseplate by 0.2 mm and the patient will be instructed to turn the screw by one quarter turn each week. More frequent adjustment, up to a quarter of a turn every 3 days, is sometimes possible with children, but care must be taken not to adjust the appliance too frequently or it will not seat fully and will become progressively more ill fitting.

Many different designs of screw are available (Haynes and Jackson, 1962). Some are spring loaded, but it is questionable whether these are more effective than the conventional type. Others can hinge, allowing differential expansion anteriorly and posteriorly, which can be useful in the treatment of cleft palate (Haynes, 1964). Heavy-duty screws are used for rapid maxillary expansion (see pp. 220). Spring-pin screws are available for the labial movement of individual teeth. Although screw plates can be designed to undertake many of the tooth movements that can be achieved with springs, the latter are generally cheaper, less bulky and more adaptable. Screws are useful in anteroposterior (Fig. 15.15) and transverse arch expansion (Fig. 15.16a) and in contracting a wide maxillary arch (Fig. 15.16b) because they enhance appliance stability, but even for these purposes many orthodontists prefer to use springs of suitable design.

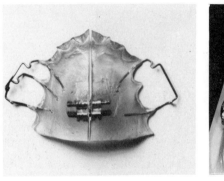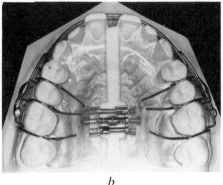

a *b*

Figure 15.16 (a) A screw plate to expand the upper arch. It is usually advisable to incorporate posterior bite planes to clear the occlusion so that the lower arch is not expanded at the same time. Note the different patterns of clasping that can be used to ensure adequate retention where the first molars alone do not provide this. It is important to avoid bringing two wires through an embrasure. (b) A screw plate to contract the upper arch. The appliance is made with the screw expanded. Buccal wires must contact the teeth to be moved palatally otherwise they will be left behind.

Elastics

Rubber or latex rings are used with extraoral traction (see Fig. 15.19); and to provide intra- and intermaxillary traction with fixed appliances (see Chapter 16). Ordinary 'rubber bands' obtainable from a stationery supplier are satisfactory for use with extraoral traction but latex elastics are preferred because they are more consistent in their quality. All elastics under tension exhibit some stress relaxation but this is not great enough to be a problem with orthodontic appliances.

Elastics are available in various sizes and one should be selected that gives an appropriate loading. The patient is instructed to renew the elastics every few days or sooner if they break. More frequent change is unnecessary. Elastics should not be used as the active components of removable appliance because of the risk of their slipping up the teeth and causing gingival damage. In particular, an elastic must never be placed directly around a tooth: it will tend to slip apically and gradually extract the tooth!

Retention

Adequate retention is essential because if the appliance is loose, the patient may have difficulty in wearing it. Adhesion between baseplate and oral mucosa contributes little to the retention of an orthodontic appliance, and this depends on clasps and bows. Retention is required anteriorly and posteriorly, and in general there should be three clasps distributed appropriately.

The most successful clasp for retention of removable appliances is the Adams clasp (Adams, 1950; 1953; 1954) (Fig. 15.17). The most useful

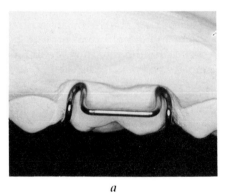
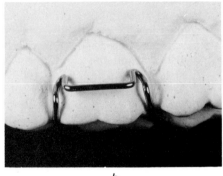

a   *b*

Figure 15.17 Location of undercuts utilized by the Adams clasp. (a) In a child the undercuts may be beneath the gingival margin and so the model must be trimmed carefully to expose them. (b) In an adult the undercuts may be quite deep and the arrowheads of the clasp must be located at the correct level if an appropriate degree of undercut is to be engaged.

undercuts for orthodontic appliance are at the mesiobuccal and disto-buccal aspects of the teeth. In children the gingival margin may still cover these and it is necessary to trim the model before making the clasp (Fig. 15.17a) so that it will slip into the gingival crevice and lie in the undercut when the appliance is fitted. In adults, the gingival margin may have receded so far that the undercut is excessively deep (Fig. 15.17b) (Seel, 1966). If the clasp is made to engage this fully, it will be too difficult for the patient to insert and remove the appliance, the clasp will have to be loosened and retention will then be poor. Thus the clasp must be designed to lie just far enough into the undercut to give adequate retention. The number of teeth clasped will depend on the factors tending to displace the appliance, and on the retention potential of the teeth. Where extraoral traction is used, particularly with a neckstrap that exerts a downward component of force on the appliance (see Fig. 15.20), retention has to be excellent and more teeth should be

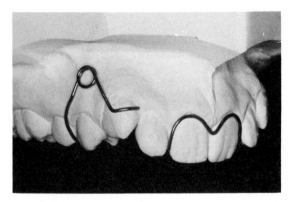

Figure 15.18 The Southend clasp: this is tightened by pushing it in at the interdental crest.

clasped than would otherwise be necessary. If the teeth are rather conical in shape with few undercuts, then more teeth may have to be used; excessive clasping should be avoided and the retention should be distributed sensibly. First permanent molars will usually be clasped and they alone will provide adequate posterior retention for many appliances.

An Adams clasp on the central incisors can be very effective in providing anterior retention but is less satisfactory when the teeth are proclined (Muir, 1971). The Southend clasp (Fig. 15.18) is preferred in most cases (Stephens, 1979). Stiff labial bows assist retention anteriorly, but unless they are also to serve another purpose, a Southend clasp will usually be found to be more effective and less obtrusive. Clasps should be adjusted only when necessary, not as a matter of routine at every visit. When the appliance is seated, the clasp should be passive, otherwise it can move the tooth palatally under the baseplate. This is most liable to occur when retention is poor due to lack of undercuts or poorly constructed clasps; and the retention potential of the tooth will be diminished still further as it is tipped palatally. If retention is inadequate, attempts should be made to improve it by adjusting the clasp to lie correctly within the undercut; and if this fails the appliance may have to be remade clasping other teeth. In some cases where no suitable undercuts are available, retention can be enhanced by fitting a band with buccal attachment to the tooth, or by directly bonding a buccal attachment, or even just a composite resin 'blob' on to the buccal surface of the tooth.

Retention problems may be caused by springs that tend to unseat the

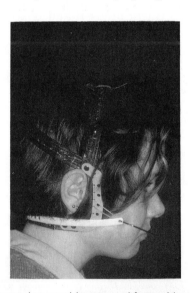

Figure 15.19 A headcap used to provide extraoral force either for anchorage or for traction – for example, to move upper buccal teeth distally. The direction of pull should always be slightly above the occlusal plane so that it does not tend to displace the appliance. This Interlandi design of headcap provides a choice of attachment points for the elastics. A safety mechanism – such as the Masel safety strap shown here – should always be fitted to reduce the chance of accidental injury.

appliance – for example, a spring acting on a sloping surface. Extraoral traction to a cervical strap (see Fig. 15.20) tends to displace an appliance and so it is wiser to use headgear with an upward force vector (see Fig. 15.19).

Anchorage

Anchorage is the source of resistance to the reaction from the active components. For example, if canines are to be retracted by springs, there is an equal and opposite force on the appliance, which has to be resisted by the anchorage. This will tend to move the anchorage teeth mesially by an amount that will depend on the forces used, the number of teeth incorporated in the anchorage and their resistance to movement.

In some circumstances, movement of anchorage teeth is desirable. For example, when the upper arch is to be expanded bilaterally to correct a crossbite, each side acts as anchorage for the other. This is called reciprocal anchorage. In other cases, limited movement of the anchor teeth is acceptable, as when extraction of premolars has provided excess space for retraction of canines and some forward movement of the posterior teeth is to be encouraged. Where space is at a premium, no movement of the anchor teeth is permissible. Clearly the greatest problems arise when little or no movement of the anchorage can be allowed. In these circumstances as many teeth as possible should be included in the anchorage and only a few teeth should be moved at any one time. The greater the root area of the anchor teeth relative to the teeth to be moved, the more secure the anchorage. If teeth can be prevented from tipping, their anchorage value is increased. This is a measure commonly used with fixed appliances but is difficult to obtain with removable appliances.

The forces applied to the teeth are very important. Light forces in the active components (30–50 g per single-rooted tooth) are sufficient but, when distributed over a larger number of anchor teeth, should fall below the threshold that appears to be necessary for rapid movement. Heavier forces generated by the active components will not move these teeth faster but, when distributed over the anchor teeth, may well be high enough to ensure their rapid movement (Crabb and Wilson, 1972). Where unacceptable movement of the anchorage teeth is occurring or where it is decided that it would be unwise to risk even a small amount of movement of the anchor teeth, reinforcement with extraoral traction is necessary.

Extraoral anchorage

Extraoral anchorage can be used either as the sole anchorage to retract buccal segments with an 'en masse' appliance (see Fig. 15.10), or to reinforce intraoral anchorage.

Where buccal segments are to be retracted, appreciable forces have to be used (250–500 g per side depending upon what the patient will tolerate) and it is desirable to use headgear with a slightly upward

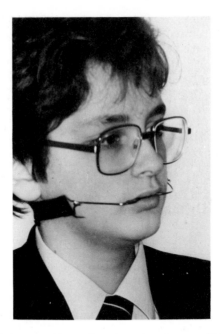

Figure 15.20 A neckstrap used to apply extraoral anchorage. Although this is less conspicuous than a headcap it usually delivers a downwards component of force, which tends to displace a removable appliance.

directed force (Fig. 15.19) rather than a neckstrap (Fig. 15.20), which tends to displace the appliance. The headgear and appliance should be worn for 12–14 h per 24-h day. It is helpful in monitoring the response to treatment, and it encourages motivation, if patients are asked to keep a record of wear and to produce it at each visit.

Where the extraoral anchorage is used to supplement intraoral anchorage, it should be adjusted to at least double the force generated by the active components and the headgear should be worn for 10 h in 24. If anchorage control is not achieved, patient cooperation is suspect: the need for conscientious wear should be emphasized and the amount of wear is increased to 14 h per day at least until control is re-established.

While headcaps can be made up from plastic or fabric tape, it is much more convenient to obtain them from an orthodontic supplier. They can be fitted in a few minutes, taking care to ensure that they are comfortable and do not rub on the ears. Many different designs are available and most are suitable for use with removable appliances. Select a type of headcap with a choice of attachment points for the elastics that will be connected to the face bow, so that the correct direction of traction can be assured (Fig. 15.19).

Extraoral traction can be connected to the appliance by a face bow, which will usually slide into tubes on the molar clasps (Fig. 15.21). J hooks, which are often used with fixed appliances, are best avoided with removable appliances because it is difficult to provide adequate

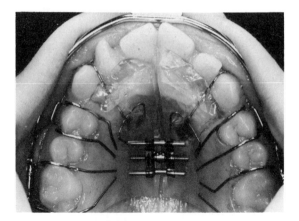

Figure 15.21 The face bow engages tubes either soldered to molar clasps, as shown here, or carried on the molar bands of fixed appliances.

safety precautions against their becoming displaced and lacerating the face or eyes. Face bows are adjusted so that the outer bow stands just clear of the cheeks when the elastics are fitted. The headcap may be elasticated so that the face bow can be attached to it directly, but better force control is possible with elastics. Elastics obtained from a stationery supplier are quite satisfactory for this purpose, or high-quality latex elastics may be obtained from an orthodontic supplier. The gap to be bridged by the elastic should be about 5 cm. Too small a gap means that a very small elastic with little extensibility has to be used, while a large gap may mean that the elastic rubs the patient's cheeks.

Hazards of headgear

Face bows are potentially dangerous to the patient or another child if they engage in horseplay, and it is important that they and their parents are warned of this, verbally and in a written instruction sheet (Postleth-waite, 1990). Another child may be injured by the extraoral hook and this danger can be minimized by finishing the hook neatly so that the end recurves. The face bow must never be removed from the mouth while still attached to the headgear, as there is a risk of its being released and lacerating the face or damaging the eyes. In order to minimize the risks to the patient of headgear, adequate precautions must be taken. The appliance must fit well and have adequate retention so that it does not tend to become displaced; and the headgear must have an upward component of force so that it does not tend to displace the appliance. For this reason, headgear and not a neckstrap should be used with removable appliances. The facebow must be robust enough to be stable when in position and, for this reason commercially manufactured facebows are preferred, except when the facebow is integral with the appliance, as in the 'en masse' appliance. A safety strap (Fig. 15.19b) should always be fitted so that the facebow cannot be removed when this is in position.

Safety headgear where the attachments break free if excessive force is applied reduces the risk of the facebow springing back against elastic traction, but does not eliminate the danger of the facebow coming out at night when the child could roll on it and damage an eye (Postlethwaite, 1989).

Finally, the appliance must be carefully finished and the patient and parents must receive careful but not alarmist instruction about correct use of the appliance.

The baseplate

The baseplate serves to hold together the other components of the appliance and may be built up into bite planes to clear the occlusal interferences or to help in overbite reduction. It contributes little to anchorage or retention in most appliances.

Scant attention is often paid to baseplate design but it is very important for patient comfort. A baseplate that is unduly bulky will be uncomfortable and may interfere with speech, while if it is incorrectly trimmed, it may allow food packing or hinder tooth movement. The baseplate is made from acrylic. Clear acrylic is usually preferred by the patient and has the advantage that any areas of undue pressure can be detected by observing blanching of the palatal mucosa when the appliance is in the mouth. Cold-cured acrylic is used most commonly because it is simpler for the technician and there is no risk of thermal distortion. However, heat-cured acrylic is appreciably stronger and its use is recommended for appliances with bite planes that will be loaded heavily, and for lower appliances, which are weak in the section behind the incisors.

Undercuts are rarely a problem in fitting upper removable appliances for children, but in adults and in lower appliances they may interfere with the insertion and removal of the appliances. It takes only a few moments to survey a model and to block out undercuts that might be a problem, and this should be done as a matter of routine in these cases. Thus it should never be necessary to trim the baseplate in order to allow the appliance to be inserted.

Bite planes

Bite planes are used to clear possible occlusal interference with tooth movement; and to reduce overbite.

Anterior bite planes (Fig. 15.22)

These are used for the purposes mentioned above. Overbite reduction is obtained by accelerated dentoalveolar development of the lower buccal segments; the upper buccal segments are restrained by the appliance and little intrusion of the lower incisors is produced (Cousins, Brown and Harkness, 1969). This is tolerated in children and subsequent

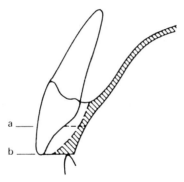

Figure 15.22 Bite plane design. Where overbite reduction is required the posterior teeth should be maintained at a 2–3 mm separation. It is customary to fit an appliance with the level at (a) to achieve this, and then add cold-curing acrylic resin during canine retraction. Full overbite reduction should be obtained in Class II, division 1 cases before incisor retraction is attempted. For this acrylic can be removed by 'undermining' the bite plane so that the lower incisors are still restrained from erupting.

facial growth will catch up so that the height of the intermaxillary space is not affected permanently. Attempts to reduce overbites in adults with anterior bite planes are not usually successful because the lower buccal segments may not grow vertically when the appliance is fitted. Even if this does happen, the overbite will often relapse: the orofacial muscula-ture may not adapt to the increased intermaxillary height and so the posterior teeth are intruded while the incisors slide past one another. Deep overbites in adults are difficult to reduce and fixed appliances are usually necessary.

The bite plane should be just deep enough to engage the lower incisors: there is no advantage in encroaching further on the oral space. For complete overbite reduction, the bite plane will have to be level with the upper incisor edges but few patients can cope with this height immediately. Initially a bite plane to the mid-height of the upper incisors should be tolerated and either this can be raised progressively by layers of cold-cure acrylic at subsequent visits, or the next appliance can be constructed with a full-height bite plane.

Posterior Bite Planes (see Fig. 15.15)

These are used to clear the occlusion where there is reverse overjet or where the overbite is tenuous and should not be reduced.

Fitting and adjusting removable appliances

As with all routine tasks, appliance fitting and adjustment is completed more quickly and more reliably if a standard procedure is followed. The procedures for fitting and for subsequent adjustment of appliances are similar to one another.

The baseplate

First ensure that there are no blebs of acrylic on the fitting surface. These should have been removed by the technician. The thickness of the baseplate is also checked and it is trimmed down if it is too bulky. This will not be necessary if the technician has received clear instructions. The well-constructed appliance should fit immediately. Difficulties in insertion are due to clasps carried too far into buccal undercuts, or failure to block out palatal or lingual undercuts on the model before the appliance was constructed. If the cause of the difficulty is not apparent immediately, bend the clasps back slightly in order to determine whether they are at fault. If there are undercuts on the baseplate, they are removed judiciously, taking particular care not to remove the edge of the acrylic at the polished surface where contact with the tooth must be maintained in order to avoid food packing and gingival hyperplasia. The clasps are now readapted.

Provided that the bite plane dimensions have been specified in the appliance prescription (Fig. 15.23), trimming will be minimal. Posterior bite planes are adjusted so that the patient occludes evenly on both sides with just enough clearance to allow the required tooth movements. The bite plane may be perforated over molar cusps but this does not matter. Anterior bite planes are trimmed so as not to extend further back than necessary and to a level that the patient can cope with. If the lower incisor edges are at different heights the bite plane is to be adjusted to allow at least three contacts and at subsequent visits it is flattened progressively by addition of acrylic.

Now the baseplate is trimmed to allow the teeth to move as intended.

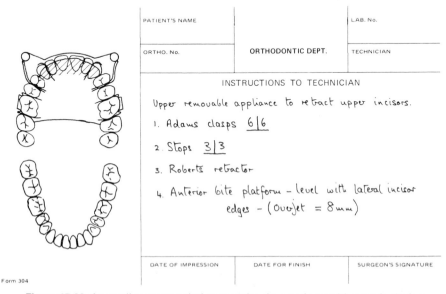

Figure 15.23 An appliance prescription must be clear and unambiguous in design specification.

Acrylic is cut back as generously as possible so that the teeth will be free to move throughout the period between visits. If the tooth is too close to the baseplate, not only will its movement be impeded, but the gingiva will tend to pile up between tooth and baseplate, and this can be uncomfortable for the patient. Sometimes, when one tooth is moved along the line of the arch, it is helpful to allow adjacent teeth to follow, and the baseplate should be trimmed to permit this.

Where incisors are to be retracted and there is an anterior bite plane, this will have to be cut back to allow the teeth to move, while maintaining contact with the lower incisors (see Fig. 15.22). This is not possible if the bite plane is too low and it may first have to be built up with cold-cure acrylic.

Retention

Retention components should be adjusted only if this is necessary. The correct method of adjusting Adams clasps is shown in Fig. 15.24. If retention is still poor after the clasps have been adjusted correctly, it may be necessary to construct a new appliance to an improved design, possibly with extra clasps. It is quite unreasonable to expect a patient to wear an appliance that is unstable.

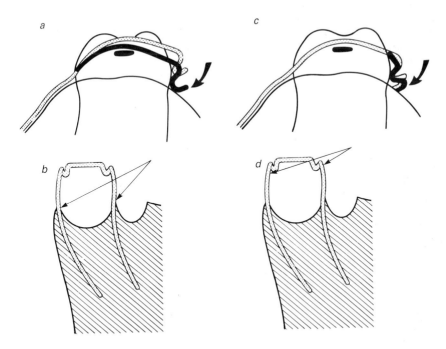

Figure 15.24 (a) Where the arrowhead lies occlusal to the buccal undercut, adjustment to the clasp should be made where the tag emerges from the baseplate as shown in (b). (c) Where the arrowhead is correctly placed but does not fully engage the undercut, adjustment should be made adjacent to the arrowhead as shown in (d).

Anchorage

Anchorage is planned at the stage of appliance design and nothing has to be done when the appliance is fitted, unless extraoral traction is to be used. The important points have already been mentioned and instructions to patients are discussed below.

Active components

At the first visit, these are adjusted only to a small extent. This is sufficient to initiate the tissue changes in the supporting structures and allows the patient to get used to the appliance. Full activation at the first visit may make the teeth tender and the patient may insert the appliance incorrectly (e.g. canine retraction springs may be incorrectly positioned distal not mesial to the teeth). Care should be taken to ensure that buccal springs and bows do not impinge on the gingiva or oral mucosa. The correct adjustment of the different springs has been described along with their construction (see pp. 280–285). Care should be taken not to damage the spring during the adjustment: if the wire is nicked with pliers, or if it is regularly adjusted at the same spot, subsequent fracture is more likely. This is also liable to happen if the spring is adjusted at the point of stress concentration where the wire emerges from the baseplate or from a supporting tube.

Instruction and motivation

The clarity and conviction with which instructions on appliance wear are given can greatly influence subsequent cooperation. It is unreasonable to expect a patient to remember instructions that are given casually and without reinforcement. It is preferable to restrict the number of new instructions given on each visit to two or three and so advice on oral hygiene and general information on the wear of appliances should be given on visits before the fitting of the appliance. Practical points, such as cleaning the teeth and appliance, and its insertion and removal should be demonstrated to the patient and then practised under supervision in the surgery. The most effective way of reinforcing instructions given to a child is to ascertain that they are understood and then ask the child to repeat or demonstrate them to the parent (having first checked that they can do so unaided). This approach emphasizes that the primary responsibility for appliance care and wear is the patient's, but provides the parent with the opportunity of asking for clarification of any points should they wish. Ideally, a leaflet containing the same instructions in writing should also be given to the parent.

The conviction and commitment of the dentist has an important effect on patient cooperation in appliance wear, particularly of headgear and functional appliances. Instructions given with confidence that the patient can and will wear the appliance as prescribed are much more effective than if the same information is given in a manner lacking conviction that the treatment is worthwhile or likely to be successful.

Particularly with children wearing headgear and functional appliances, which should be worn for as many hours as possible but not full time, it is effective to give the patient a target and ask them to keep a log-book or chart of wear. This record of treatment progress is readily appreciated by the patient and can boost their interest and cooperation. At each visit, progress should be compared with the account of wear, and praise or reproach given according to the results. Obviously, it is counterproductive to ask the patient to keep a record of wear but take no further interest in it; or to emphasize the need for full-time wear of the appliance but be unable to detect when this is not happening!

Follow-up visits

First of all chat to the patient, asking whether they have had any problems. Do not ask leading questions as to whether the appliance has been worn as instructed because almost inevitably the reply will be affirmative and it may then be difficult for them to retract this when clinical evidence suggests that the appliance has not, in fact, been worn correctly. Observe whether speech is affected by the appliance: most patients adapt to appliances within a few days, and if speech continues to be affected this may be a sign that the appliance is not worn full time.

A thorough inspection of the general oral condition, with the appliance removed, follows. Examine the oral mucosa for trauma or ulceration from the appliance and check the teeth for caries. The standard of oral hygiene is recorded and, if it is not satisfactory, a plaque or bleeding index is estimated and recorded. Any deficiency in general oral care is discussed with the patient. A persistently poor standard of oral hygiene may necessitate abandonment of orthodontic appliance treatment.

The orthodontic review begins with an assessment of the changes that have occurred since the previous occasion. Whenever possible, measurements are taken and noted so that an objective record of progress can be obtained. First check anchorage. Anchorage problems generally arise during retraction of teeth when the natural tendency to mesial drift of the anchor teeth is increased. Provided that no active lower appliance is being worn, the lower arch can be used as a reasonably reliable reference against which to check the upper anchorage. Care must be taken to ensure that the lower jaw is in true centric relation when this is done: if the upper buccal teeth are coming forward, the patient may posture the mandible, masking a change in occlusal relationships and giving a misleading impression that nothing has altered. Where the upper incisors are not being retracted but the appliance contacts them palatally, a measurement of the overjet provides a simple record of anchorage stability. Where active appliance treatment is being carried out in the lower arch, and particularly if the lower incisors are contacted by the appliance, it is not easy to monitor anchorage and, on occasions, it may be necessary to obtain a lateral skull radiograph to check it.

Clearly, if the anchorage is not stable, measures must be taken to control it. If the spring or bow has been activated too much, this is adjusted, but if the problem lies with the anchorage, then reinforcement with headgear (or increased wear if it is already fitted) is necessary. Only when the anchorage has been checked can a reliable record of the intended tooth movements be obtained. If it is known that the anchor teeth are stable, measurements from them can be used to record the tooth movements. The landmarks selected for the measurement must be readily identifiable: cusp tips and buccal fissures are good landmarks, and the margins of fillings may also be used. It is best to obtain the measurement with dividers and then record it directly on the patient's notes by punching holes through the page. A comparison with previous measurements gives an indication of whether or not the teeth are moving at the rate anticipated. If the teeth have moved less than expected, a series of points should be checked:

1 *Are the teeth free to move?* The baseplate, wirework or contact with opposing teeth may impede tooth movement.

2 *Is the spring correctly activated?* The spring (or bow) may be passive, or may be excessively active, and both faults may impede tooth movement.

3 *Is there any reason to expect a slow rate of movement?* Buccally placed teeth or 'necking' of the alveolar process may result in very slow movement because of the dense cortical bone surrounding the tooth. Provided that light forces are used, tooth movement will be progressive but slow.

4 *Is the appliance being worn as instructed?* The patient may position the spring incorrectly or the appliance may be left out. Even short periods of non-wear may greatly delay progress.

Appliance adjustment

Now it is time to adjust the appliance components, following the procedures outlined above.

References

Adams, C. P. (1950) The modified arrowhead clasp. *Dental Record*, **70**, 143–144

Adams, C. P. (1953) The modified arrowhead clasp – some further considerations. *Dental Record*, **73**, 332–333

Adams, C. P. (1954) Variations of the modified arrowhead clasp. *Transactions of the British Society for the Study of Orthodontics*, 71–75

Bass, T. P. and Robinson, S. I. M. (1969) Forces involved in incisor retraction. *Transactions of the British Society for the Study of Orthodontics*, 132–134

Cousins, A. J. P., Brown, W. A. B. and Harkness, E. M. (1969) An investigation into the effect of the maxillary bite plate on the height of the lower incisor teeth. *Transactions of the British Society for the Study of Orthodontics*, 105–110

Crabb, J. J. and Wilson, H. J. (1972) The relationship between orthodontic spring force and space closure. *Dental Practitioner*, **22**, 233–240

Haynes, S. (1964) A study of some conventional and unconventional orthodontic screws with some practical recommendations concerning their use. *Transactions of the British Society for the Study of Orthodontics*, 65–71

Haynes, S. and Jackson, D. (1962) A comparison of the mechanics and efficiency of 21 orthodontic expansion screws. *Dental Practitioner*, **13**, 125–133

Houston, W. J. B. and Waters, N. R. E. (1977) The design of buccal canine retraction springs for removable orthodontic appliances. *British Journal of Orthodontics*, **4**, 191–195

Muir, J. D. (1971) Anterior retention in the removable appliance. *Transactions of the British Society for the Study of Orthodontics*, 178–184

Postlethwaite, K. (1989) The range and effectiveness of safety headgear. *European Journal of Orthodontics*, **11**, 228–234

Postlethwaite, K. (1990) Safety headgear – dare we ignore it. *Dental Update*, **17**, 278–284

Seel, D. (1966) A rationalisation of some orthodontic clasping problems. *Transactions of the British Society for the Study of Orthodontics*, 112–118

Stephens, C. D. (1979) The Southend clasp. *British Journal of Orthodontics*, **6**, 183–185

Waters, N. E. (1982) The mechanics of buccal canine retraction springs for removable orthodontic appliances. *British Journal of Orthodontics*, **9**, 164–172

Further reading

Adams, C. P. (1984) *The Design and Construction of Removable Orthodontic Appliances*, 5th edn., Wright, Bristol

Houston, W. J. B. and Isaacson, K. G. (1982) *Orthodontic Treatment with Removable Appliances*, 2nd edn., Wright, Bristol

Chapter 16

Fixed appliances

Removable appliances can only tip teeth, while fixed appliances can produce any type of tooth movement. By applying a mechanical couple of forces to the tooth crown in conjunction with a simple force, apical and bodily movements, as well as rotations can be obtained (Fig. 16.1). Controlled intrusion and extrusion of teeth is also possible.

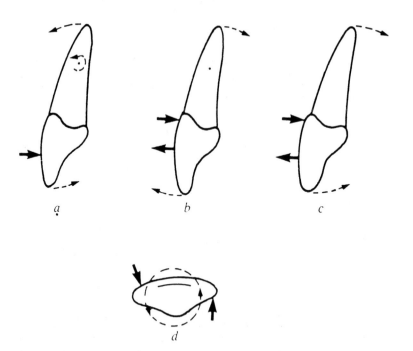

Figure 16.1 Force applied to teeth. (a) A simple force applied to the crown of a single-rooted tooth will tip it about a fulcrum within the root (see Chapter 14). (b) A pure mechanical couple of equal forces in opposite directions applied to the crown of a tooth will tip it about a fulcrum within the root. (c) An appropriate tooth without tipping. (d) Rotation of a tooth about its long axis will be produced by a pure couple applied in an appropriate manner to the crown.

Components

The principal components of fixed appliances are attachments, archwires and auxiliaries. It is not possible to separate the active and anchorage components in fixed appliances because both these functions are served by the archwires and auxiliaries. However, in planning and monitoring treatment, anchorage and active tooth movements must be evaluated separately.

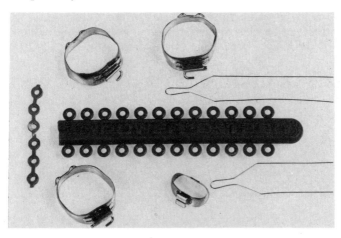

Figure 16.2 Bands and brackets used in the edgewise technique together with different methods of fixation: wire ligatures, polyurethane rings on a dispenser and a polyurethane chain. Whilst bonded brackets are now used routinely, anterior bands still have a place where the anterior teeth are hyoplastic or fractured

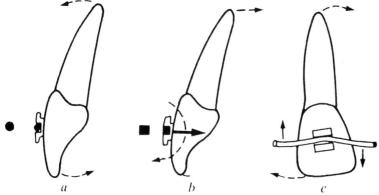

a   *b*   *c*

Figure 16.3 Force systems in the edgewise technique. (a) Retraction of an incisor with a round wire generates no mechanical couple and so the tooth is free to tip. (b) Retraction of an incisor with a rectangular wire: the fit of the wire in the bracket means that as the tooth tends to tip this is constrained by the fit of the wire in the bracket. A mechanical couple is generated and so the tooth undergoes a translational movement. Play between the wire and the bracket, or flexure in the archwire, may allow some tipping to take place. (c) If the bracket slot is not parallel to the archwire a mechanical couple will be generated, which tends to move the crown and root in opposite directions. If a force is applied to the crown so that it cannot move, only the root will move.

Attachments

The main attachments are brackets and tubes. Buttons and cleats may also be used in some situations (Fig. 16.2). The different fixed-appliance techniques are characterized by their attachments. For example, the brackets and tubes used in the edgewise technique and its variants have a rectangular channel, and the archwire is secured to the bracket by soft stainless-steel ligatures or by plastic rings (Fig. 16.2). Round archwires are used in the initial stages of treatment but labiolingual movement of the tooth apices is achieved by rectangular archwires (Fig. 16.3).

In contrast the bracket in the Begg technique is designed to allow free tipping of the teeth, both mesiodistally and labiolingually (Fig. 16.4).

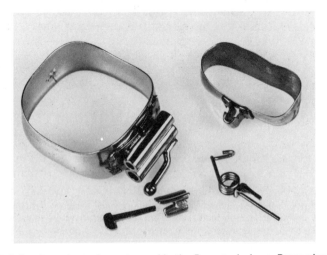

Figure 16.4 Bands and attachments used in the Begg technique. Brass pins secure the archwire in the bracket slot. These can be replaced by uprighting springs to produce root movement in Stage 3 (see Fig. 16.16c).

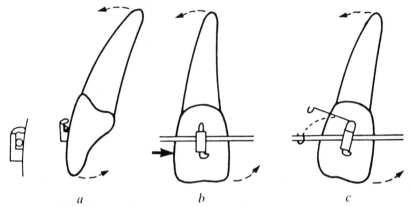

a   *b*   *c*

Figure 16.5 The force systems used in the Begg technique. (a, b) The round wire fits loosely in the bracket slot allowing the tooth to tip freely but not to rotate about its long axis. (c) Auxiliary springs are used to generate mechanical couples so that controlled root movement can be undertaken in Stage 3.

Round archwires are used and secured to the brackets by metal pins. Control of apical movement is obtained by auxiliary springs (Fig. 16.5) rather than by the fit of the archwire and bracket.

Bonds

Attachments may be fixed to the teeth directly with composite resins after acid etching of the enamel surface (see Figs. 16.16, 16.17). Chemically cured resins are generally used. The fitting surface of the bracket is designed to allow a mechanical locking with the composite resin because there is no chemical adhesion to stainless steel. The tooth surface is etched for about 15 s with phosphoric acid gel and is then washed and dried (Carstensen, 1986). The attachment is fixed to the tooth with a small amount of the composite resin. Special orthodontic resins are now available but conventional restorative filled resins may be modified for orthodontic use (Årtun and Zachrisson, 1982). It is very important that the attachment is positioned accurately and that excess resin is cleared away before it sets, otherwise it will encourage plaque accumulation and gingival irritation. This must be done with care, otherwise the set of material will be disturbed and the bond will fail later.

In ideal conditions, modern filled composite resins are strong enough to withstand all orthodontic forces, including those of headgear. However, bond strength is reduced greatly if the tooth surface is not dry when the attachment is placed. In areas where moisture control is difficult, in particular the lower buccal segments and upper molar regions, direct bonding may not be satisfactory (Carstensen, 1986). Most orthodontists prefer to use metal bands, to which the attachments are welded, in these areas.

Ceramic brackets are available for direct bonding and these have the great merit of being inconspicuous (see Fig. 10.8). However, at the present time they are brittle and are liable to fracture, particularly during their removal. They are also abrasive and so tend to wear teeth that occlude with them. For these reasons most orthodontists continue to use metal brackets, although ceramic brackets can be useful on the upper incisors in adults when only simple tooth movements are required. Various types of plastic bracket have also been produced but are not very satisfactory. Although they are inconspicuous when fitted, they tend to discolour, the wings are liable to fracture, and the brackets are not sufficiently rigid to apply torque effectively with rectangular archwires.

Bands

The original method of fixing attachments is by welding them to metal bands, which are then cemented to the teeth with zinc oxyphosphate or similar cement. This is still generally used for molar attachments. The cement not only holds the band in place but prevents the accumulation of plaque between band and enamel. It is very important that the integrity of the cement is checked regularly because, if it leaches out, plaque will accumulate and serious enamel demineralization can occur rapidly. All that is required is a firm pull upon each band from time to time, which will dislodge a partially cemented attachment. The risk of caries and demineralization under bands is reduced by application of fluoride to the tooth surface before the band is cemented (Dimitriadis, Sassouni and Draus, 1974; Adriaens, Dermaut and Verbeeck, 1990). This offers only temporary protection when cement is lost, and so does not absolve the practitioner from inspecting the bands at each visit. Some practitioners advocate the routine use of a fluoride mouth rinse but this is not usually necessary where good oral hygiene is maintained, using a fluoride toothpaste. More recently an increasing number of clinicians have adopted glass-ionomer cement for band cementation (Norris *et al.*, 1986). This material has the advantage that it releases fluoride and has a significantly lower failure rate in clinical use (Stirrups, 1991).

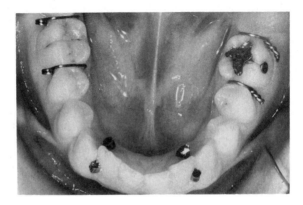

Figure 16.6 Different methods of separating the teeth; on the patient's left, brass separating wire has been twisted tightly around the contact areas of the molar. Separating springs have been placed mesially and distally to the right molar; a short arm of the spring passes under the contact area and applies a separating force to the teeth. Elastic separating strips have been placed mesially to the lower canines.

While bands can be made up from stainless-steel tape, preformed bands are much more convenient (see Fig. 16.4). These are usually supplied with brackets already welded in place. The band must fit the tooth well so that the bracket is at the correct height on the tooth crown and so that the gap that must be filled with cement is minimal. Molar bands and the lingual aspects of premolar bands should fit into the gingival crevice so that there is no unprotected enamel. Elsewhere the bands should be sufficiently clear of the gingival margin to allow plaque control. So that the bands can be placed accurately, the teeth have to be separated if the contacts are tight. This can be done by 0.5 mm brass ligature wire tightened around the contact area or by springs or elastics (Fig. 16.6), left in position for a few days. If it is necessary to use incisor bands, contacts can be separated by rubber strips cut from a broad elastic band and placed 1–2 h before the bands are placed (Fig. 16.6). The patient can insert these on the day of the appointment for banding.

Bonds and bands compared

Nowadays, directly bonded attachments are used almost universally on anterior teeth and premolars, while bands are generally used on molars.

Direct bonds have a number of advantages over bands. The attachments can be positioned more precisely and more quickly than when bands are used. Teeth of unusual shape or that have not erupted fully can be bonded readily, whereas banding may be very difficult. Frequently, teeth need to be separated before banding, which may entail an extra visit; and at the end of treatment band spaces have to be closed. Although the band material is not thick, the band space in each arch can amount to 3–4 mm and this is a disadvantage, particularly in cases where space is at a premium. Bands make the appliance more conspicuous. Thus the bonding of attachments is quicker, more precise and less stressful to the patient.

Bonding of attachments does, however, have some disadvantages. The most important of these is the need for excellent moisture control during bonding, which can sometimes be difficult. Removal of bonds and composite after treatment is tedious and more time consuming than for bands. If plaque control is less than excellent, the enamel is more liable to be demineralized with bonded attachments: the bands themselves protect the most vulnerable areas of enamel, provided that the cement is intact, while plaque gathering approximally and around bonded attachments results in rapid demineralization of the tooth surface (Zachrisson, 1974). The risk can be minimized by ensuring that there is no excess resin around the attachments to encourage plaque accumulation and by insisting on a high standard of oral hygiene, backed up by fluoride mouth rinses (Lundström, Hamp and Nyman, 1980).

Archwires

Originally archwires were made from gold alloys but these were very expensive and stainless-steel became the material of choice. Recently a number of titanium alloys have been introduced (Burstone and Goldberg, 1980; Miura, Mogi and Hamanaka, 1986). These 'super-elastic' wires have a lower modulus of elasticity and so are more flexible than a stainless-steel wire of the same dimensions (Kusy and Greenberg, 1982; Kusy and Stevens, 1987). This is useful in some situations. The elastic recovery is also superior to that of stainless-steel and while this makes the archwire more difficult to form, their resistance to permanent deformation in use is clearly advantageous. Braided, multiple-strand, stainless-steel archwires are also available (Kusy and Stevens, 1987). These have a much higher elastic recovery and a lower flexural rigidity than solid stainless-steel wires of the same nominal diameter, and are useful for the alignment of irregular teeth (Stephens, Houston and Waters, 1971). However, for most stages of orthondontic treatment, high-tensile stainless-steel wires are used.

Archwires have to satisfy many different requirements, some of which may be mutually contradictory. Non-toxicity; resistance to corrosion, fatigue and fracture; ease of formation and economy are all important considerations. Suitability for welding and soldering are advantages. Elastic recovery (spring-back) and flexural rigidity (stiffness) are two of the most important physical characteristics of an archwire.

A good elastic recovery is important, otherwise the arch is liable to become distorted in use, which at best will render it inactive but may result in unwanted tooth movements. Where the archwire is to be used to align irregular teeth, a low flexural rigidity is desirable so that the wire can be deflected through a reasonable distance without generating an excessive force (Waters, Houston and Stephens, 1981). With a stiff archwire, even a small deflection will produce a large force and either the teeth will be subjected to undue loads or the arch will have to be activated very frequently. While a low flexural rigidity is desirable for the alignment of irregular teeth, the archwires may also have to resist external forces such as those generated by elastics (Fig. 16.7). In this case, too flexible a wire may allow unwanted tooth movements. There are a number of other situations where a rather high flexural rigidity is desirable to maintain control – for example, when retracting a canine into a premolar extraction space, too flexible a wire will allow the tooth to tip. These conflicting demands may be met in

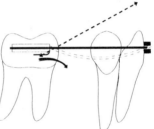

Figure 16.7 When elastic traction is applied to a lower molar, the unsupported span of the archwire tends to flex. If this happens to an appreciable extent, the tooth will tip. In order to prevent this, either the wire must be stiff enough to resist this effect or, where flexible wire is used, a 'tip-back' bend must be incorporated to counter the effect of the elastic.

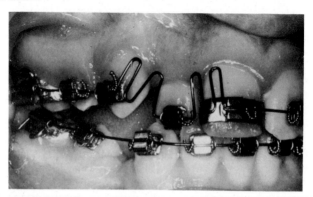

Figure 16.8 Vertical loops are incorporated in an archwire to increase its flexibility locally.

one of two ways. A relatively stiff wire (e. g. 0.016 inch diameter round wire) may be used, and its flexibility can be increased locally by the incorporation of loops (Waters, 1976) (Fig. 16.8). Alternatively, the initial alignment of irregular teeth can be achieved with a thin, flexible arch, and the use of elastics or other operations requiring a higher flexural rigidity can be delayed until stiffer arches are placed.

Active tooth movement with fixed appliances

In most appliance systems, the archwire itself is the major active component in the alignment of irregular teeth, both vertically and radially. Because the span between adjacent brackets is short, the archwire segments tend to be stiff and if a full-size archwire (e.g. 0.018 inches in diameter, or more) is used, a straight span would be almost rigid and quite unsuitable for tooth alignment. This problem can be circumvented by using very thin wires initially and then working up through progressively thicker wires until a full-size arch can be engaged (see Fig. 16.15); or by using thicker wires of low flexural rigidity, such as braided wires or one of the titanium alloys.

Alternatively, a relatively heavy stainless-steel wire (0.016 inch) can be used and its flexibility can be increased at irregular contacts by the incorporation of loops (Fig. 16.8) (Waters, 1976). Looped segments are very much more flexible radially to the arch than vertically, but this is generally advantageous because the major tooth irregularities are usually labiolingual. The force systems generated by looped arches are very complex and adverse side-reactions can occur, and so it is desirable to progress to a plain archwire at as early a stage as possible. There is a trend away from using looped arches for alignment and toward using plain arches of low flexural rigidity because they are simpler and take less chairside time.

Loops may also be used to retract incisors or to bring forward buccal segments to close spaces (Fig. 16.9). These are activated by pulling the

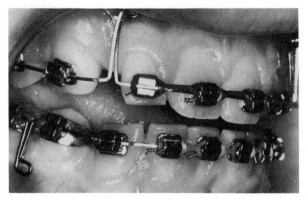

Figure 16.9 Loops incorporated in an upper archwire in order to retract the incisors and the lower archwire to close extraction spaces. The loops are activated by pulling the distal ends through the brackets and either tying them back or turning them down the distal part of the arch behind the molar tube.

archwire through the molar tubes by a small amount and holding it either by a ligature or by turning up the end.

Fabrication of archwires must be accurate because the teeth are generally drawn to the form of the archwire and any faults will be difficult to correct. Arch form and symmetry must be preserved.

Movements of teeth along the archwire may be accomplished by auxiliary coil springs, or elastics. Appreciable binding may occur between brackets and archwire but care has to be taken to avoid the use of excessive forces, otherwise the archwire may be deformed, allowing unwanted tooth movements and prejudicing the stability of the anchorage.

Adjustment of arch relationships is often achieved by the use of intermaxillary elastics (see Fig. 16.16b). Anchorage balance is very important here and the arch malrelationship must not be corrected at the expense of the stability. For example, in the correction of a Class II arch malrelationship with intermaxillary elastics, it is only too easy to

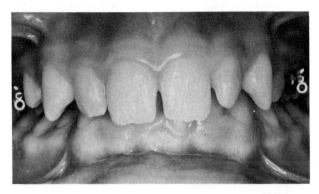

a

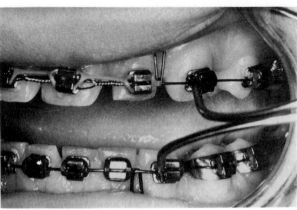

b

Figure 16.10 (a) Molar bands with double tubes. The more gingival, rectangular tube will carry an archwire while the lower tube will receive the face bow for extraoral traction. (b) J hooks being used to retract upper and lower canines along an archwire. The J hooks are attached to a headcap by extraoral elastics.

advance the lower incisors unintentionally, particularly when lower premolars have not been extracted.

Headgear is commonly used to reinforce anchorage or to achieve active tooth movement. Retraction of the upper buccal segments and of upper and lower canines are the tooth movements undertaken most commonly with extraoral traction (Fig. 16.10). High-pull headgear can be valuable in intruding the upper incisors in certain Class II cases (Fig. 16.11). In conjunction with a rectangular archwire, high-pull headgear is also very effective in achieving bodily retraction of the upper incisors.

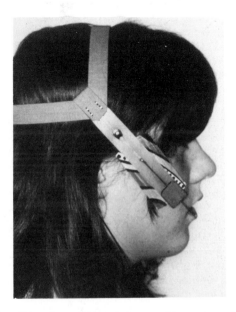

Figure 16.11 High-pull headgear. This is being used to apply a retrusive and retracting force to the incisor segment of the upper arch.

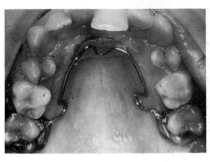 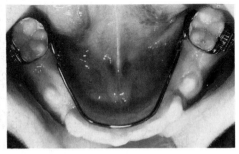

a   *b*

Figure 16.12 (a) An upper palatal arch attached to bands on the upper first permanent molars. This increases their anchorage value by preventing them from rotating or tipping. Note the button of acrylic anterior, which prevents the archwire from becoming buried in the palatal mucosa if the teeth do tend to tip, so reinforcing the anchorage. (b) A lower lingual arch to enhance anchorage of the lower molars.

Palatal and lingual arches (Fig. 16.12) may be used for anchorage reinforcement. They may also be used for arch expansion and, in some techniques, they may carry auxiliary springs that tip teeth.

Anchorage control with fixed appliances

As with removable appliances, anchorage control is fundamental to successful treatment. Loss of anchorage can mean that essential space is dissipated and this can be very difficult to regain.

The anchorage value of a tooth or group of teeth depends in part on root areas and in part on the type of movement that is allowed. With fixed appliances it is possible to prevent anchor teeth from tipping or rotating, and their anchorage value is increased greatly by ensuring that only bodily movement can occur. Equally this means that when a tooth does have to be moved bodily, substantial demands are made upon the anchorage.

Anchorage balance must be taken account of when treatment is planned. For example, if substantial space is required for the relief of incisor crowding and correction of a large overjet, and particularly if the tooth inclinations are unfavourable so that teeth cannot be tipped simply into the correct positions, the demands on anchorage will be considerable. It will usually be appropriate to extract first premolars so that the maximum number of teeth can be included in the anchorage (Fig. 16.13a) and to ensure that the maximum anchorage is obtained by preventing the tipping or rotation of anchor teeth, and by using headgear where appropriate.

On the other hand, if only a small amount of space is required for the correction of labial segment irregularities, the extraction of first premolars is undesirable because active closure of excess space can easily result in too much retraction of the labial segments (Fig. 16.13b). In these circumstances a better anchorage balance would be given by the extraction of second premolars, which encourages a greater amount of space closure by forward movement of the molars during correction of the labial segments. If, by the time the labial segment irregularity has been corrected, substantial space remains at the extraction site, the anchorage value of the anterior teeth should be maximized by ensuring that they are not allowed to tip.

One of the major benefits of fixed appliances compared with removable appliances is that excess space at extraction sites can be closed by forward movement of buccal teeth in a controlled manner, but if full advantage is to be taken of this, attention needs to be given to anchorage balance during planning and treatment.

Monitoring anchorage with fixed appliances

One of the major problems in evaluating treatment progress with fixed appliances is in monitoring anchorage. In fully banded appliances, there are no assured, stable reference points within the dentition. Cephalometric radiographs can be used to check the stability of the lower incisor

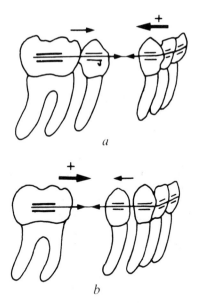

Figure 16.13 The concept of anchorage balance. (a) When the lower first premolars have been extracted and intermaxillary traction is applied to close the space, the labial segment tends to move more than the buccal teeth because of its smaller root area. The anchorage value can be enhanced by using an archwire, which prevents the labial teeth from tipping. (b) When second premolar teeth have been extracted, anchorage balance encourages closure of the space by forward movement of the molars.

position relative to the A-Pog line, for example, and then other tooth movements can be related to the lower incisors. However, cephalometric control of this sort can be used only very occasionally – not more than once or twice during a course of treatment. This means that anchorage management depends greatly on the clinician's acumen and ability to control the force systems that are used, with few opportunities to check objectively that unwanted anchorage loss is not occurring. This is one of the reasons why prolonged training in the use of fixed appliances is required.

Fixed-appliance techniques

A large number of different fixed-appliance techniques have been developed and there would be little value even in enumerating these. Many are variants of the edgewise technique, while others attempt to combine the best features of several different systems but rarely succeed in doing so. Continual development of materials and refinement of techniques has resulted in a number of powerful appliance systems that are capable of achieving good results for most malocclusions. For the orthodontic specialist, the limitations to what can be achieved should be biological rather than technical. The orthodontist will usually confine his or her practice to one or at the most two fixed-appliance techniques in the interests of practice efficiency. Although the proponents of each appliance system extol its virtues, the expert will be able to obtain

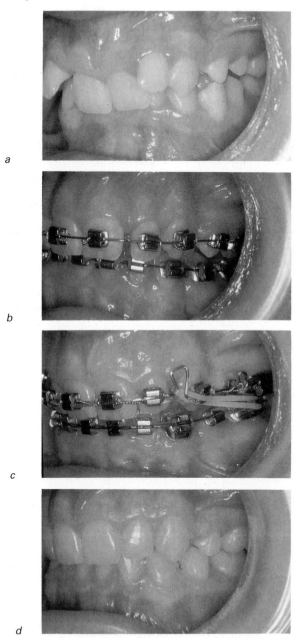

a

b

c

d

Figure 16.14 A case treated with edgewise technique: stages (a) initial irregularity; (b) alignment achieved by a nickel–titanium archwire now replaced by 0.016 and then 0.018 inch round wire; (c) retraction of the upper labial segment with a rectangular, 0.018 × 0.025 inch archwire; (d) on completion.

excellent results whatever system he or she uses. Advances in one appliance technique are soon matched by developments in its competitors.

Edgewise technique (Fig. 16.14)

This was introduced by Edward Angle (1928) but has evolved radically since that time. It is based on the use of brackets with a rectangular slot. In some versions of the technique the slot is 0.018 inches wide and in others it is 0.022 inches (Fig. 16.14). It is a very versatile system with many variants, only one of which will be outlined here.

The brackets are placed on the tooth surfaces so that when the teeth are in ideal positions, the bracket slots will be level. Initial bracket levelling and tooth alignment is obtained by first using a flexible archwire (Fig. 16.14a, b) (0.012 inch stainless-steel or 0.015 inch multiple-strand wire) and then progressively heavier arches (0.014 inch to 0.018 inch). The 0.018 inch archwire is suitable for achieving bodily movements of teeth around the arch and labiolingual tipping movements, as well as overbite control. Many simpler malocclusions can be treated completely with round archwires and can be finished with a 0.018 inch archwire. The heavier archwires (0.016 inch and 0.018 inch) should incorporate offsets to allow for the differing thickness of the teeth. These offsets are usually required mesial to the canines and first permanent molars. The upper and lower archwires must be coordinated in form so that the dental arch malrelationships are corrected in all dimensions.

Where buccolingual root movements are required, a rectangular arch is used after either an 0.016 or 0.018 inch round wire (Fig. 16.14c). By incorporating torque in the rectangular archwire, controlled buccolingual root movements and bodily tooth movements can be obtained. The rectangular arch must be formed very carefully so as not to produce unwanted torque and adverse buccolingual movements in teeth that were originally correct.

Techniques using pre-torqued brackets

Archwire fabrication is simplified if each bracket slot is inclined in such a way that, when the teeth are positioned ideally, the bracket slots lie on the one plane (Fig. 16.15b). Thus the final rectangular archwire would not require the incorporation of any torque. The bracket slot orientation for each tooth is different and thus separate bracket specifications are required. The base thickness of each bracket is designed to allow for the different thicknesses of the teeth and so the need for offsets in the archwires can be eliminated. The pre-torqued systems work well on teeth of 'average' form but, of course, in most patients at least some of the teeth vary from this and so some individualization of archwires is required.

Pre-torqued bracket systems do offer a number of advantages in ease of archwire fabrication over the conventional edgewise systems; but

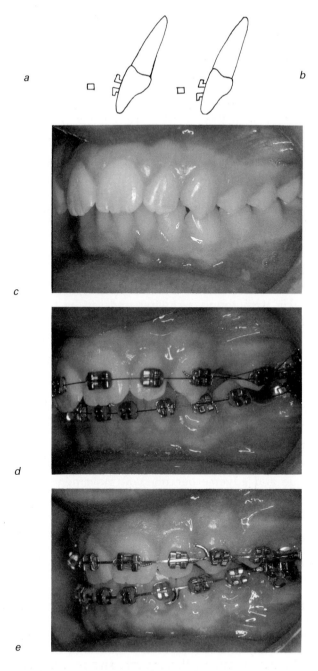

Figure 16.15 (a) With a conventional (standard) edgewise bracket the slot is not parallel to the occlusal plane when the tooth is in the correct position and so the archwire must be torqued. (b) This is not necessary in pre-torqued (straight-wire) brackets. (c–e) A case treated with pre-torqued brackets: (c) pretreatment; (d) initial alignment achieved with nickel–titanium round wires; (e) retraction of the upper labial segment and root alignment of all teeth achieved with flat rectangular arches.

with the variety of brackets, inventory control is more complex and they tend to be more expensive than conventional brackets.

The idea of pre-torquing brackets is an old one but the advantages could not be fully realized before direct bonding of brackets was developed, allowing them to be much more precisely positioned on the tooth surface. In addition, the introduction of low-modulus titanium alloy wires allows arches that nearly fill the slot from an early stage, so that the torque and tip incorporated in the bracket can be expressed fully. It must be emphasized, however, that although preadjusted brackets reduce the amount of wire bending required in the initial stages of treatment, finishing arches require to be adapted precisely to allow for variations from the average in tooth morphology, otherwise an optimal aesthetic and functional result will not be obtained.

The earliest commercial appliance system using preadjusted brackets was the straight-wire appliance introduced by Andrews in the 1970s (Andrews, 1979). This is still widely used. A number of other pre-adjusted systems were introduced subsequently and have minor differences in the orientation of their slots.

Begg techique (Fig. 16.16)

With edgewise appliance systems, very large forces can be generated when heavy arches are used. Begg, an Australian orthodontist, introduced a technique based upon tipping teeth with light forces, followed by root movements with auxiliary springs (Begg, 1954). The Begg technique has developed greatly since it was introduced in 1956 (Begg and Kesling, 1977), but although it has won widespread acceptance, it is now used by only a minority of orthodontists, in part because the archwires are complex to fabricate and manage.

The Begg bracket (see Fig. 16.4) is designed to allow free tipping of teeth in all directions. Treatment is divided into three stages (Fig. 16.16). The objectives of Stage 1 are to align the teeth and to correct the incisor and molar malrelationships. This is done using 0.016 inch round arches with vertical loops at interdental contact irregularities. Recently, more flexible wires have been used to align the teeth to avoid the problems of looped arches. Overjet and overbite are corrected with the aid of intermaxillary elastics. At the end of Stage 1, the teeth should be well aligned, and the incisors should meet edge to edge and the molars should have a Class I relationship.

In Stage 2, the extraction spaces are closed using plain 0.016 inch arches and intra- and intermaxillary elastics. The edge-to-edge incisor relationship is maintained while the incisors are tipped further back. At the end of Stage 2, the upper and lower incisors are often very retroclined (Fig. 16.16c).

In Stage 3, the inclination of the incisors and of teeth adjacent to extraction spaces is corrected by the use of auxiliary springs (Fig. 16.16c). The objectives at the end of Stage 3 are to have the teeth well aligned with correct axial inclinations but with arch relationships somewhat over corrected. Occlusal guidance will then carry the teeth into the correct relationships during the retention and settling-in phase. This

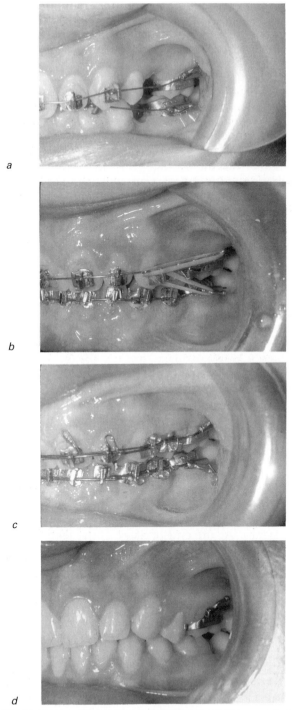

Figure 16.16 The stages of Begg treatment: (a) stage 1; (b) stage 2; (c) stage 3, showing torquing auxiliaries; (d) end of treatment.

may seem a little haphazard, but it is what happens during the normal development of the occlusion and excellent results can be obtained with the Begg technique.

Lingual techniques

This approach involves brackets and other attachments bonded to the lingual surfaces of the teeth (Fujita, 1979). The advantage is that the appliance does not show and this is more acceptable, particularly to adults who might otherwise be unwilling to undergo fixed-appliance treatment. However, this approach has a number of disadvantages and limitations. It is more exacting to attach brackets to the lingual surfaces of teeth because of their shortness and irregular surfaces; access is much more difficult for the orthodontist and complex archwire adjustments are very exacting and time consuming; the appliance systems cannot control tooth movements as effectively as conventional appliances. Thus treatment with these appliances is expensive and limited in scope.

Finishing procedures

At the completion of treatment, bands and bonded attachments have to be removed. This is a somewhat tedious task that is accomplished with special pliers. Band cement can be removed with scalers but residual composite resin from bonds has to be removed carefully with specially designed slow speed tungsten-carbide burs which ensure that the enamel is not damaged by these instruments.

Retainers are then fitted, as with cases treated by removable appliances (see Chapter 19).

Fixed–removable appliances

In some cases, treatment could be undertaken successfully with a removable appliance, apart from a specific malposition of one or two teeth. In these circumstances the best solution may be to use a removable appliance with fixed attachments only to the teeth in question. Rotations and traction to teeth (for example, of a palatally positioned canine that has been exposed surgically) are the operations most successfully undertaken with this approach. This treatment can be undertaken by the general practitioner who is skilled in the use of removable appliances. It is important to obtain brackets designed for direct bonding.

Derotation of teeth

An edgewise bracket is bonded to the labial surface of the tooth and a whip engages in a bow (Fig. 16.17). It is important that the whip is free to slide along the bow as the tooth derotates, and that it is constructed so that the patient can take out the removable appliance for oral hygiene.

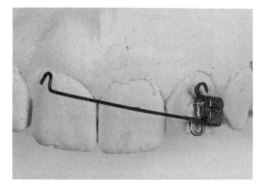

Figure 16.17 A whip spring and edgewise bracket can be used to derotate a tooth. A wire ligature between the loops in the whip spring holds the spring in place. The free end engages on the labial bow of a removable appliance.

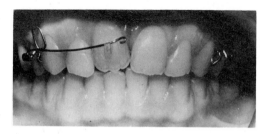

Figure 16.18 A removable appliance being used to extrude a tooth by the action of a buccal arm on a plastic edgewise bracket bonded to the crown .

Traction to unerupted teeth

Fixed–removable appliances are particularly useful for this purpose because, with a conventional fixed appliance, there is the danger of intruding and tipping adjacent teeth owing to reciprocal effects on the archwires. In some circumstances, composite material can be used to build up a ledge that can be engaged by a spring or buccal arm. More frequently a bracket is required. A Begg bracket lends itself particularly well to this purpose (Noble and Butcher, 1991) but an edgewise bracket can also be used (Fig. 16.18).

Indications for and disadvantages of fixed appliances

Fixed appliances are not suitable for use by practitioners without special training, and specialist treatment may not be available locally to patients in some communities.

The main advantage of fixed over removable appliances is in the possibility of precise control of all tooth movements. Thus they are indicated in malocclusions where rotations, bodily tooth movements and controlled root movements are required, and for controlled closure of extraction spaces.

The principal disadvantages are that they are unsightly, oral hygiene requires special care and treatment is expensive. With direct bonding and relatively narrow brackets, modern fixed appliances are less unsightly than when bands were used on incisors. Plastic brackets and lingual-appliance systems both have serious limitations despite their superior appearance. It is probable that future developments will improve the properties of ceramic brackets and that they will then be used routinely on at least the upper anterior teeth.

Provided that the patient maintains oral hygiene carefully, using a suitable toothbrush with disclosing tablets as necessary, and supplemented with fluoride mouth rinses, plaque control should be good and oral health should not deteriorate during appliance treatment. The adult patient with periodontal recession may need to use extra aids such as flossing, using a floss threader to feed the floss over the archwire, and plaque control can be difficult and time consuming.

References

Adriaens, M. L., Dermaut, L. R. and Verbeeck, R. M. H. (1990) The use of 'Fluor Protector', a fluoride varnish, as a caries prevention method under orthodontic molar bands. *European Journal of Orthodontics*, **12**, 316–319

Andreasen, G. F. and Quevedo, F. R. (1970) Evaluation of frictional forces on the 0.022 × 0.028 inch edgewise bracket. *Journal of Biomechanics*, **3**, 151–160

Andrews, F. (1979) The straight wire appliance. *British Journal of Orthodontics*, **6**, 125–143

Angle, E. (1928) The latest and best in orthodontic mechanisms. *Dental Cosmos*, **70**, 1143–1158

Årtun, J. and Zachrisson, B. (1982) Improving the handling properties of a composite resin for direct bonding. *American Journal of Orthodontics*, **81**, 269–276

Begg, P. R. (1954) Stone age man's dentition. *American Journal of Orthodontics*, **40**, 298–312; 373–383; 462–475; 517–531

Begg, P. R. and Kesling, P. C. (1977) *Begg Orthodontic Theory and Technique*, 3rd edn., W. B. Saunders, Philadelphia

Burstone, C. J. and Goldberg, A. J. (1980) Beta titanium: a new orthodontic alloy. *American Journal of Orthodontics*, **77**, 121–132

Carstensen, W. (1986) Clinical results after direct bonding of brackets using shorter etching times. *American Journal of Orthodontics*, **89**, 70–72

Dimitriadis, A. G., Sassouni, V. and Draus, F. J. (1974) The effects of topical fluoride applications underneath loose orthodontic bands. *Angle Orthodontist*, **44**, 94–99

Fujita, K. (1979) New orthodontic treatment with lingual bracket mushroom archwire appliance. *American Journal of Orthodontics*, **76**, 657–675

Kusy, R. P. and Greenberg, A. R. (1982) Comparison of nickel–titanium and beta titanium archwires. *American Journal of Orthodontics*, **82**, 199–208

Kusy, R. P. and Stevens, L. E. (1987) Triple stranded stainless steel wire – evaluation of mechanical properties and comparison with titanium alloy alternatives. *Angle Orthodontist*, **57**, 18–32

Lundström, F., Hamp, S-E. and Nyman, S. (1980) Systematic plaque control in children undergoing long term orthodontic treatment. *European Journal of Orthodontics*, **2**, 77–89

Miura, F., Mogi, M. and Hamanaka, H. (1986) The super elastic property of the Japanese NiTi alloy wire for use in orthodontics. *American Journal of Orthodontics, and Dentofacial Orthopedics,* **90**, 1–10

Noble, P. M. and Butcher, G. W. (1991) A removable appliance for the three dimensional movement of ectopic maxillary canines. *British Journal of Orthodontics,* **18**, 135–138

Norris, D. S., McInnes-Ledoux, P., Schwaninger, B. and Weinberg, R. (1986) Retention of orthodontic bands with new fluoride releasing cements. *American Journal of Orthodontics,* **89**, 206–211

Stephens, C. D., Houston, W. J. B. and Waters, N. E. (1971) Multiple-strand arches. *Transactions of the British Society for the Study of Orthodontics* 105–107

Stirrups, D. (1991) A comparative clinical trial of a glass ionomer and a zinc phosphate cement for securing orthodontic bands. *British Journal of Orthodontics,* **18**, 15–20

Waters, N. E. (1976) The mechanics of plain and looped arches. *British Journal of Orthodontics,* **3**, 75–78; 161–167

Waters, N. E., Houston, W. J. B. and Stephens, C. D. (1981) The characterisation of archwires for the initial alignment of irregular teeth. *American Journal of Orthodontics,* **79**, 373–389

Zachrisson, B. U. (1974) Oral hygiene for orthodontic patients – current concepts and practical advice. *American Journal of Orthodontics,* **66**, 487–497

Chapter 17

Functional appliances

Functional (myofunctional) appliances depend for their action upon the activity of the orofacial musculature.

The anterior bite plane

In its simplest form a functional appliance can be an anterior bite plane that produces a small amount of lower incisor intrusion through the direct action of the muscles of mastication. This is not generally thought of as a myofunctional appliance because the term is usually associated with the correction of anteroposterior arch relationships.

The oral screen

This is also a very simple functional appliance that takes the form of a curved shield of acrylic placed in the labial vestibule. It displaces the muscles of the lips, thereby generating a force on the appliance to reduce an excessive overjet. In the past the appliance has been used to discourage thumb sucking. It has also been advocated for 'lip training' in patients with incompetent lips.

The oral screen has no place in modern orthodontics: it is inefficient and limited in scope as an orthodontic appliance; and there is no evidence that its use as a lip training device is of any long-term benefit to the patient (Thüer and Ingervall, 1990).

Lip bumper (Fig. 17.1)

This is a functional component that has a use in conjunction with a lower fixed appliance either for traction or for anchorage (Salzmann, 1957). It has also been suggested that it can be incorporated into lower removable appliances (Bell, 1983).

Typically, a vestibular arch carrying an acrylic or silicone rubber pad engages tubes carried by lower molar bands (Fig. 17.1a). The arch is adjusted until the pad stands 2–3 mm clear of the attached gingiva at a level about 4 mm below the cervical margins of the lower incisors (Fig.

a

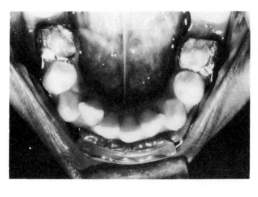

b

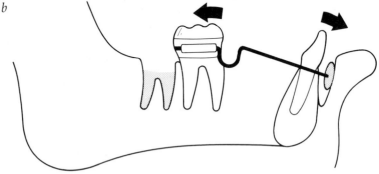

Figure 17.1 The lip bumper. (a) The appliance in the mouth. Note that the pad is 2–3 mm clear of the gingiva of the lower incisor teeth. (b) The greatest distal movement of lower molars is obtained where the second molars have been removed. The appliance has a tendency to procline the lower incisors but where this effect is undesirable it can be reduced by placing the pad as low as possible in the labial sulcus.

17.1b). The lower lip is thus held slightly forwards. The force of reaction from the lip can move the lower molars distally, and it also has a tendency to procline the lower incisors, which may or may not be desirable (Fig. 17.1b) (Osborn, Nanda and Currier, 1991). The lip bumper can also occasionally be useful in Class II, division 1 cases where there is strong lower lip contraction behind the upper incisors that may interfere with their retraction: by holding the lip clear, overjet reduction is expedited.

Origins of modern functional appliances

The first functional appliances were developed from the use of removable appliances incorporating bite planes. Catalan in Spain in the late nineteenth century used an inclined anterior bite plane with the intention of causing the mandible to be postured forward in the hope that this would cause a 'jumping of the bite' and stimulate growth of the mandible. Robin (1902) was the first to describe an appliance that was specifically designed to act on the maxillary and mandibular arches simultaneously, but it was the publication of the text on functional jaw orthopaedics by Andresen and Haupl in 1936 that popularized the concept of such appliances.

Categories of functional appliance

Various attempts have been made to categorize what is now a very large number of variants. Graber and Neumann (1984) have suggested that all functional appliances can be allocated to one of two groups, depending on the degree of displacement of the mandible: those that displace the mandible only to a moderate extent and are intended to stimulate muscle activity (myodynamic); and others that induce a more extreme displacement and rely on the elastic properties of the muscles and fascia for their action (myotonic). As functional appliances have become more complex and because such a classification is of no real help in indicating the quality of response an appliance will produce, others have proposed a classification based on the components that each appliance incorporates (Vig and Vig, 1986) These components are:

1 *Bite planes* – which produce differential eruption.
2 *Lip/cheek shields* – which alter the linguofacial muscle balance.
3 *The working bite* – which affects the mandibular posture as already described.

Proffit (1986) on the other hand proposes the following classification:

Tooth-borne passive
Tooth-borne active
Tissue-borne

More recently, Isaacson, Reed and Stephens (1990) have proposed dividing these appliances into those that are primarily rigid and made of acrylic (Andresen, Harvold, activator, bionator, etc.) and those that are more flexible (e.g. function regulator of Fränkel).

Despite such attempts there is no widely accepted classification and most functional appliances retain the name of their originator.

The use of functional appliances

Functional appliances are most effective in the correction of Class II arch malrelationships in children in the mixed dentition. They have limited application in the permanent dentition, particularly when facial growth is more or less complete. Many ingenious variations have been proposed to deal with individual tooth malpositions, but these are seldom very useful. Major dental irregularities are best dealt with either by a preliminary removable appliance or, if detailed tooth alignment is required, a course of fixed-appliance treatment following the functional appliance. Although crossbites, anterior open bites and Class III malocclusions can be treated with certain functional appliances, they are generally dealt with more effectively and more rapidly in other ways. For example, many of the cases of anterior open bite for which successful treatment is claimed could have been expected to resolve spontaneously had the appliance been withheld: some are the results of a digit-sucking habit and others are normally developing dentitions in which an overbite has not yet been established by full eruption of the incisors. The Class III cases that can be treated with a functional appliance are mild and these could often be corrected equally well with a simple upper removable appliance.

The main effect of a functional appliance is to apply traction between the arches (intermaxillary traction), which results in tooth movement by the usual processes of bone remodelling (see Chapter 14). Some appliances produce arch expansion by mechanical devices such as screws, by guidance of eruption of buccal teeth or, as in the Fränkel appliance, by holding the lips and cheeks away from the teeth so that their muscular balance is disturbed. As with any other orthodontic appliances, stability of expansion depends upon a permanent change in muscle balance. Claims have been made that this does occur, but they have not been substantiated by long-term controlled clinical trials or by other scientific evidence.

Proponents of functional appliances maintain that part of the correction in arch relationships is due to a change in jaw relationships produced by the appliance. Case reports have been published showing the improvement in facial pattern that can accompany functional-appliance treatment. However, these are usually specially selected, and there are few comparisons with matched control groups treated with other appliances. Many children with Class II malocclusions experience favourable growth changes whether or not they are receiving orthodontic treatment, and an objective evaluation of the studies that have been published has found little evidence of an effect on facial growth (Tulloch, Medland and Tuncay, 1990). Experimental work in monkeys has shown that the forward displacement of the mandible by splints, in a manner comparable to that of certain functional appliances, can promote growth of the condylar cartilage as well as remodelling of the glenoid fossa (McNamara and Carlson, 1979; McNamara and Bryan, 1987). It is interesting that the effect seems to be limited in duration and that further displacement of the mandible seems to be necessary to maintain the condylar response (McNamara, 1980).

On balance it seems probable that certain functional appliances may have a favourable effect on mandibular growth in some children; and they may also restrain maxillary growth to a small extent. However, these effects are limited in amount and most of the correction occurs by dentoalveolar change. Indeed it is very easy to procline lower incisors and to produce other tooth movements, which may not be stable. Claims of the correction of severe Class II malocclusions in a matter of weeks by 'jumping the bite' must be regarded with scepticism. This happens when the patient adopts a forward mandibular posture, which may be difficult to disclose but which will not be stable in the long term, and which cannot be regarded as an acceptable outcome of orthodontic treatment.

In a number of functional-appliance techniques, great emphasis is laid on retraining the orofacial musculature by means of the appliance and by exercises. It is certainly true that the activities of lips, cheeks and tongue may be atypical in the presence of a malocclusion but these are very frequently adaptations to the malocclusion (see Chapter 3) and improve spontaneously as the malocclusion is corrected, whatever type of appliance is used. Whilst it is possible to train lips to become stronger there is no evidence that this increases the forces applied to the teeth. Moreover, the effect of training is soon lost once exercises are discontinued (Thüer and Ingervall, 1990). There is little likelihood that training of the orofacial musculature by a functional appliance produces any extra modification that enhances occlusal stability or facial appearance.

Patient motivation is very important with functional appliances. They are bulky and inconvenient and the patient is tempted to wear them for less time than is necessary: treatment does not progress well and motivation deteriorates still further. A typical success rate with removable functional appliances is around 30 per cent (Cohen, 1981; Mills, 1983) and though this can sometimes be attributed to lack of favourable growth, the patient's failure to achieve sufficient wear is just as likely to be responsible (Sahm, Bartsch and Witt, 1990).

In addition to the usual techniques of motivation, it is particularly valuable to set the patient a target and to ask them to record truthfully their appliance wear each day. If the appliance has to be left out, for example for a social occasion, the time should be made up. Nevertheless, recent work that recorded electronically the number of hours for which bionators were worn (Sahm *et al*, 1990) showed that patients who were asked to wear their appliances for a mean of 15 h per day only achieved half this amount and this degree of compliance declined further to only 35 per cent after the first 6 months of treatment. Hence, if there has been no significant movement in the first 6 months there is usually little point in continuing with this form of treatment.

A considerable degree of expertise is required in the management of functional appliances, and they are not suitable for use in general practice, except perhaps for the treatment of rather mild, uncrowded Class II, division 1 malocclusions (which some would argue can usually be just as well and more simply treated by other means). In most other cases, a period of fixed-appliance treatment is required after correction of the arch relationships in order to obtain optimal alignment and tooth relationships.

The following discussion refers only to the treatment of Class II malocclusions, because it is in these cases that functional appliances are most successful. The reader who is interested in the treatment of other types of case is referred to the texts of Graber and Neumann (1984) or Isaacson, Reed and Stephens (1990).

Preliminary treatment

When a Class II malocclusion is to be corrected, the upper arch has to be expanded transversely to a minor extent in order to conform to the lower. Some authorities suggest that this expansion should be incorporated into the functional appliance, while others believe that it may be simpler to do this with an initial removable appliance. However, adjustment in posterior arch width can almost always be relied upon to occur spontaneously where the appliance is worn part time provided that there was no tendency to crossbite at the onset of treatment and the appliance does not constrain this (for example, by including upper molar clasps).

In a Class II division 2 case, the upper incisors can be proclined to somewhat more than average inclinations with an initial removable appliance. Having achieved this movement it is necessary to design the functional appliance so that this position can be maintained during sagittal correction of the arches. Where an initial appliance is to be used in this way it is wise to include an anterior bite plane to assist in reduction of the overbite where this is deep.

Registering the construction bite

Although functional appliances differ greatly in design, this important stage is similar for all of them. Variations in the amount of protrusion or opening are described with each appliance. The amounts of vertical and anterior displacement of the mandible are interrelated: the greater the anterior displacement, the less vertical opening can be achieved and vice versa.

The total amount of mandibular displacement depends on the type of appliance, the features of the malocclusion, the preferences of the operator and the compliance of the patient. For myodynamic appliances, the bite is opened within the normal working range of the muscles of mastication so that their activity is stimulated: while the opening is greater for myotonic appliances so that the muscles and other soft tissues are stretched. If only a small forward posture is required to correct the buccal segment relationship, a greater degree of bite opening will be required than if there is a more severe arch malrelationship.

The intended mandibular displacement is registered with a wax squash bite. It is helpful to get the patient to practise posturing the mandible by the required amount using a mirror, whilst receiving guidance from the clinician. For low construction bites (say up to 4 mm opening beyond the rest position) a suitable roll of softened wax is made up, formed to the shape of the lower arch, keeping it clear of the incisors. The wax is settled on the lower arch and the mandible is then guided forward by the required amount, taking care not to displace it laterally; and the patient is asked to close gently, maintaining the anterior displacement, until the required amount of opening at the incisors is obtained. The patient should be sitting upright when this is done.

It is important that the correct registration is obtained and that the occlusal surfaces of the teeth are clearly reproduced in the wax so that the models can be reliably articulated. Several attempts may be required to obtain the correct registration. The squash bite is then chilled and trimmed so that it does not extend beyond the last erupted molars or beyond the buccal cusps of the lower teeth. The chilled bite should be rechecked in the mouth to ensure that is has not warped and that the mandible is displaced as intended. The models are then mounted on an articulator, care being taken that the bite registration is not altered in any way.

Where wider opening is desired, it is easier to use a preformed, wedge-shaped wax bite. Before use the upper and lower surfaces are warmed to a depth of 2 mm using a spirit flame or gas burner. This method ensures that the bite remains resistant to distortion during efforts to remove it from the mouth and will also ensure that the larger vertical dimension is maintained by the hardened core.

The Andresen appliance (or activator)

The original Andresen appliance was designed as a passive retaining appliance to be worn during long summer vacations in Norway when fixed appliances were removed because they could not be adequately supervised. Andresen found that the malocclusion usually improved during the wearing of the retaining appliance and so this was developed to be used independently.

The appliance

In essence, the Andresen appliance consists of upper and lower base-plates sealed together. The acrylic caps the lower incisor edges to prevent them from overerupting and in an attempt to splint them to resist their proclination, although this may still occur. The acrylic is carried across the occlusal surfaces of the buccal teeth and there is an upper labial bow. If the upper incisors are spaced, this bow may be used to retract them, after clearing the palatal acrylic, but this makes the appliance more dificult for the patient to manage. Other springs can be incorporated but these are often troublesome and rather ineffective, and are not recommended.

The Andresen is a loosely fitted appliance, which is constructed to displace the mandible forward by a moderate amount with limited bite opening. It is thus a myodynamic appliance, designed to stimulate the muscles of mastication, although it has been found that this does not happen to any great extent during sleep.

The appliance is useful in the complete correction of mild to moder-ately severe Class II cases when there is no crowding in either arch. Preliminary treatment with a removable appliance to expand the upper arch to match the lower and to correct upper incisor inclination simplifies subsequent management, although the expert operator can obtain these changes with suitable adjustment of the functional appliance.

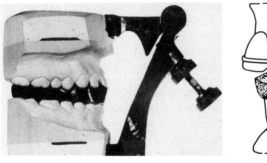
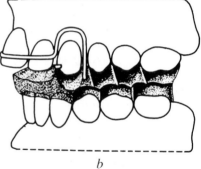

a b

Figure 17.2 An Andresen appliance. (a) Using the construction bite, the models are mounted on a plane-line articulator. (b) Channels are trimmed in the finished appliance to guide the eruption of the upper buccal teeth buccally and distally; and to guide the lower buccal teeth mesially. If the upper incisors are spaced the acrylic may be trimmed away from their palatal aspects to allow their retraction with the labial bow. The capping of the lower incisors must be left intact so that the overbite is controlled.

The construction bite

If it is possible to do so without undue strain, the construction bite is taken with the mandible displaced forward to obtain an edge-to-edge incisor relationship, with a vertical opening of 2–3 mm at the incisor edges to allow the lower incisors to be capped (Fig. 17.2). With large overjets, the advancement has to be done in two stages. It is possible to reactivate the first appliance by trimming it away from the lower teeth so that wax can be added to register the more advanced position of the mandible. The appliance can then be 'relined' with cold-cure acrylic. However, it is often more convenient to make a new appliance.

Clinical management

When the appliance is inserted initially, check that it fits well and that the mandible is displaced as intended. If the bite registration has been altered in the laboratory, the appliance will usually have to be discarded. In order to reduce a deep overbite, which will usually be present, channels are cut over the occlusal surfaces of the buccal teeth (Fig. 17.2). In the upper arch, these slope slightly distally and buccally, leaving interdental spurs to contact the mesiopalatal aspects of the teeth so that they are guided distally and buccally as they erupt. In the lower arch, the channels slope occlusally and the interdental spurs contact the distolingual tooth surfaces. Trimming is facilitated by marking on the appliance, with a wax pencil, the areas of acrylic that are to be left in contact with the teeth. If the upper incisors are to be retracted with the labial bow, the acrylic is trimmed away from their palatal aspects and the adjacent alveolar mucosa, but this is often better delayed until a subsquent visit because the appliance becomes rather unstable.

The patient is instructed to wear the appliance for 10–12 h in every 24. This will be at night, with 2–4 h wear in the evening. Evening wear is particularly important in the first few weeks when the patient is getting used to the appliance: it will often come out during the first few nights, but the patient should be reassured that this is normal and that they will soon cope with it easily.

The appliance requires little routine adjustment but the patient should be seen every 4–6 weeks. There should be definite progress at each visit. If there is no obvious change within 3 months, the appliance is not being worn as instructed and it may be best to discontinue treatment if full cooperation cannot be obtained. Unless treatment is monitored carefully, it may be allowed to run on for years with little improvement in the occlusion. This wastes everyone's time and undermines the possibility of future cooperation when treatment with a different type of appliance may be indicated.

A problem with the activator is that it is liable to procline the lower incisors while the lower buccal teeth are moved mesially. This may appear to be perfectly satisfactory while the appliance is being worn, but when it is discontinued lower incisors may drop back to their original position and become crowded. This is one advantage of the lower incisors being spaced in the first place.

The bionator

This appliance is derived from Andresen's activator but is greatly reduced in bulk (Fig. 17.3). Balters, who developed this appliance, emphasized the role of the tongue and respiration upon the development of malocclusion and based his treatment on theories that would not now be generally accepted. The appliance is effective in correcting mild Class II, division 1 occlusions, especially those that do not exhibit crowding (Eirew, 1981; Hunt and Ellisdon, 1985; Bolmgren and Moshiri, 1986). Its lack of bulk and its simplicity make it one of the easier functional appliances to use but until recently it has generally been neglected outside Germany. The effects of the appliance are primarily

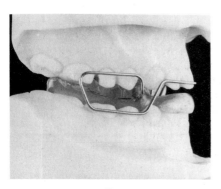
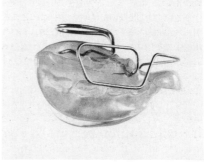

a   *b*

Figure 17.3 A bionator.

upon tooth position, with questionable influence upon skeletal growth and muscular patterns.

The appliance

The appliance consists of a lingual horseshoe of acrylic. In the lower arch, the acrylic base extends as far as the distal surface of the first permanent molars, contacting the mandibular teeth and the lingual alveolar mucosa. It does not extend far into the lingual sulcus. The base is clear of the upper incisors and extends over the occlusal surfaces of the premolars or deciduous molars, leaving the first permanent molars free to erupt. There are facets in the acrylic to accept the posterior teeth in both arches and these hold the mandible in the chosen postural relationship. The facets extend to cover approximately half the bucco-lingual width of the posterior teeth and are a relatively loose fit, which makes control of tooth position by eruptive guidance quite difficult.

The platform formed by the occlusal acrylic is ground flat so that the teeth contacting it are free to move buccally. The platform stabilizes the appliance and allows the molars to erupt so that the overbite is reduced. When this has been achieved, the platform can be removed, although this makes the appliance rather unstable.

A 0.9 mm labial bow almost contacts the incisors and extends distally to form a buccal archwire which is 2 mm clear of the buccal surfaces of the cheek teeth. Its function is to restrain the upper labial segment and at the same time to keep the cheeks away from the buccal teeth to allow some arch expansion. There is a midline palatal arch made in 1.2 mm wire. This is shaped like a reversed Coffin spring and extends distally over the palate, clearing the palatal mucosa by 1 mm. Variations of the basic bionator have been designed to deal with different malocclusions but usually there are simpler and more effective ways of treating them (Rutter and Witt, 1990).

Construction bite

In Class II cases, an edge-to-edge relationship of the incisors is aimed at, and the bite is opened just sufficiently to allow this. If the overjet is too large for an edge-to-edge incisor occlusion to be obtained readily, the mandible has to be advanced by stages and a corresponding number of appliances are required. (In these more severe cases it may be preferable to consider an alternative appliance).

When the mandible is displaced far enough to obtain an edge-to-edge incisor occlusion, the lower incisor edges are left free; but otherwise they are capped to prevent them from overerupting.

Harvold appliance

The Harvold appliance (Harvold activator) (Fig. 17.4) is derived from the activator of Andresen, but differs from it principally in the degrees of bite opening and in the trimming of the appliance (Harvold, 1974).

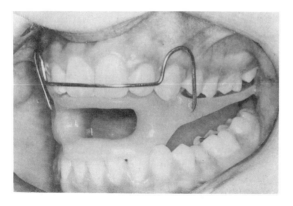

Figure 17.4 A Harvold appliance (Harvold activator).

This is a myotonic appliance that depends for its action on the elastic properties of stretched muscles and other soft tissues, rather than on muscular contraction.

Harvold stresses the importance of gaining anchorage from the lower lingual flanges, which should engage the full depth of the lingual sulcus. This combined with large working height also ensures that it is almost impossible for the patient to dislodge the appliance unintention- ally when asleep. The lower baseplate is also relieved around the lingual aspect of the lower incisors by plastering out the lower model in this region. This is believed to reduce the tendency of the lower incisors to procline during treatment.

The appliance

The upper labial bow (0.9 mm) contacts the upper incisors but it is not activated: it merely restrains the upper incisors and ensures that they are not left behind as the arch relationship is corrected. Palatal springs (0.9 mm) may be incorporated mesial to the upper permanent molars and are intended to unseat the appliance rather than to retract them,. They will be activated by about 1 mm. This means that the patient is constantly encouraged to bite into the appliance and this muscular activity complements the soft tissue stretch.

The baseplate extends deeply into the lingual sulci. The acrylic caps both the upper and lower incisors and passes between the occlusal surfaces of the buccal teeth to form a shelf that will contact the upper but not the lower teeth. To obviate very extensive trimming at the chairside, certain areas should be relieved before the baseplate is formed. These are plastered out if heat cured acrylic is to be used, but can be waxed out for cold-cure acrylic.

The acrylic should be well clear of the upper and lower incisors except incisally and labially. On the upper model, the palatal surfaces of the incisors and canines, and the anterior portion of the palate, are waxed out. This allows distal tipping of the incisors and alveolar bone remodelling as the upper arch is retracted. The displacing springs are also waxed out. The lower model is relieved over the lingual surface of the labial segment and immediately adjacent alveolar process. This means that the appliance should not exert any protrusive effect on the lower incisors and that the anterior displacement of the mandible is procured by contact with the lingual mucosa below the relieved area. The occlusal surfaces of the lower buccal teeth are covered with quite a thick layer of wax, which is carried over on to the lingual surfaces as a thin layer, leaving these teeth free to erupt and to aid overbite reduction. Depending on the degree of bite opening, 5–10 mm of clearance may be appropriate. The fitting surface of the lingual flange should not be relieved (Woodside, 1977). If the lingual undercuts are very deep they should be reduced on the model by the addition of wax, which should be applied to reduce the depth of the flange and not the degree of undercut itself. As the bite has been opened appreciably, a gap can be left in the incisor region, which allows the adept patient to speak with the appliance in place.

The construction bite

The typical bite has a horizontal registration that is 3.0 mm distal to the most protrusive position that the patient is able to achieve. Vertically the mandible is at 8–10 mm beyond the freeway space (Harvold and Vargevik, 1971). Others have advocated even more extreme degrees of opening (Woodside, 1977).

Clinical management

Provided that the models have been correctly waxed out as described above, trimming is minimal. However, it is important to ensure that the acrylic is checked to make sure it is adequately clear of the lingual surfaces of the incisors and of the occlusal surfaces of the lower buccal teeth.

A problem that may be experienced is how to insert the appliance! This is particularly true where there is any significant degree of lingual undercut. The clinician should insert the appliance first, preferably without a parent being present since the appearance can be very suprising. The lower teeth should be engaged first and to do this it may be necessary to carry the appliance distally so that the lingual flanges can be dropped down distal to the last standing tooth and the baseplate then slid into the lingual region using a mesial path of insertion. The patient should be warned that they will need to open very wide and not to panic if they get stuck with the occlusion propped on the lingual flanges. Just occasionally it will be found necessary to reduce the depth of the lingual flanges but on no account should the undercut be eliminated by reduction of the fit surface.

Once the lower arch has been engaged, the mandible can then be rotated up to engage the maxillary arch. When the appliance is fully seated, patients will find that they feel very stretched over the masseter area but this is quite normal.

The patient should be instructed to wear the appliance in the evenings and all through the night, aiming to eventually achieve at least 14 h per day. The appliance should be regarded as one that is worn full time except when in school or playing sports. Both these exceptions should be presented as concessions and every encouragement given to wearing the appliance as near full time as possible.

As with most functional appliances, claims are made that the growth of the mandibular condyle is stimulated, and that maxillary growth is restrained. The major effects are dentoalveolar. Harvold demonstrated that by manipulating the cant of the occlusal plane, a Class II buccal segment relationship could be corrected, and the appliance is effective in doing this. Bite opening occurs by eruption of the lower buccal teeth while the incisors are restrained, but where sagittal correction is very rapid the patient will be found to be propped on the incisors with a lateral open bite in the premolar region. This is nothing to be concerned about and the open bite will resolve during subsequent weeks as the posterior teeth erupt. The upper labial segment is tipped lingually, particularly when the appliance opens the bite to a major extent, but there is usually very little proclination of the lower incisors. There is therefore no reason for regarding patients who have proclined lower incisors as being unsuitable for activator treatment.

The Fränkel appliance

Named after its originator, Rolf Fränkel, this is one of the more recent functional appliances and it led to a resurgence in interest in functional appliance treatment (Fränkel, 1980). Fränkel termed it a function regulator (FR) because it is intended to correct functional anomalies in the circumoral musculature that he holds responsible for crowding and other aspects of malocclusion. The theoretical justification of the appliance may be questionable, but impressive occlusal changes can be obtained in suitable patients.

There are four variants of function regulator: FR 1 for Class I and mild Class II cases; FR 2 for Class II malocclusions of both divisions; FR 3 for Class III cases; and FR 4 for open bite and bimaxillary proclination.

The Fränkel appliance can be useful in the correction of Class II arch malrelationships but other malocclusions are generally treated more efficiently by other methods. The description here is confined to the FR 2 (Fig. 17.5) and is not intended to give more than a general idea of this complex series of appliances. Details of the other types can be found in the texts of Graber (see Further Reading), who has done much to popularize the appliance.

The appliance (FR2) (Fig. 17.5)

The *buccal shields* extend to the full depth of the buccal sulcus, and indeed the models are trimmed to allow this (see Fig. 17.7). Fränkel claims that this produces 'periosteal stretch' that promotes subperiosteal apposition of bone, but the validity of this is questionable. The buccal

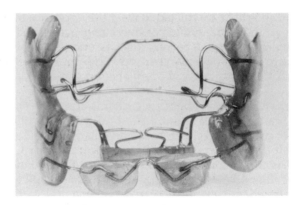

Figure 17.5 The Fränkel appliance.

shields lie clear of the teeth and so the arches are expanded: the teeth
are free of muscular pressures on the buccal but not on the lingual
surfaces. This expansion is undoubted, but adequately controlled long-
term studies of its stability are still awaited. The *lip pads* are also
intended to produce periosteal stretch and to control lower lip activity:
in conjunction with the forward posture of the mandible induced by the
appliance, the lip pads eliminate any trapping of the lower lip behind
the upper incisors.

The *lingual pad* contacts the alveolar mucosa on the lingual surface of
the mandibular alveolar process, but it is clear of the teeth. Thus a
forward mandibular posture is induced without any protrusive force on
the lower incisors. The labial and lingual pads both create stimuli that
result in a controlled forward posture of the mandible, and it is claimed
that this is more effective than the anterior displacement produced by
some other functional appliances.

The wire components are designed to connect the different parts and
to stabilize the appliance. The upper labial bow, upper palatal bow and
canine loops (in 0.9 mm wire), and the palatal arch (1.0 mm) with its
occlusal rests, stabilize the appliance against the upper arch. The palatal
arch passes interdentally, mesial to the first permanent molars: the
teeth should be substantially separated with elastic separators before
the impressions are taken, or the model can be trimmed so that the
teeth are separated as the appliance gradually settles into place.

The lower lingual arch (1.15 mm) supports the lingual pad; and this
in turn carries the lingual springs. These are designed to prevent
eruption of the lower incisors and so to control the overbite. They
should not be activated labially unless it is intended to procline the
lower incisors. All the wire components must be 2 or 3 mm clear of the
alveolar mucosa to avoid trauma or ulceration. The tags of all wire
components, except for the lingual springs, are embedded in the buccal
shields. The tags of the lower lingual and labial arches are disposed in a
way that allows reactivation of the appliance.

After the wire components have been fabricated, the models are mounted on a plane-line articulator using the construction bite. Wax relief is applied in the areas to be covered by buccal shields so that these will stand clear of the teeth and buccal mucosa. This clearance is greatest at the top of the shield (2–3 mm) and tapers to about 1 mm at the lower buccal sulcus.

Construction bite and impression technique

Unlike other appliances the Fränkel construction bite depends on several considerations including the type of appliance (FR1, FR2, etc.), the appearance of the facial profile and the avoidance of disturbing the muscle balance at the front of the mouth. Classically the bite registration is taken using a wax palate to which has been added lateral bite blocks.

The working impressions must extend to the full depth of the buccal and labial sulci, clearly reproducing muscle reflections. Even the well-taken impression will not generally reproduce the full sulcus depth, because the cheeks and lips are displaced outwards by the tray and impression material. To allow for this and to ensure some 'periosteal stretch', the sulcus should be deepened by carefully trimming the model.

Clinical management

Wear of the appliance is extended progressively. For the first 2 or 3 weeks it should be worn only in the evenings for about 2 h. When the patient is confident in its management, night-time wear is introduced and then as soon as possible the patient should wear it full time, except for meals and sports. The strongly motivated patient will cope with the appliance well. Fränkel lays great emphasis on obtaining habitual lip seal and recommends that the child should be reminded to do this whenever the parents observe the lips are parted. He also suggests that the child should practise holding a piece of paper between the lips when doing homework to focus attention on this!

If buccal shields have been over extended, ulcers may develop in the buccal sulcus and the shields will have to be trimmed very conservatively and polished. The lip pads may also cause trouble, but there is little scope for trimming them. These problems arise most commonly when the lip pads are not sufficiently upright, and so this needs attention during appliance construction.

Within 3 months of the commencement of treatment, progress should be obvious. If this is not the case, the appliance is probably not being worn as instructed. When there is initially good progress but this declines after 3–6 months, it is probably time to reactivate the appliance by advancing the lower labial and lingual pads.

Although lower incisor proclination should not happen unless the lingual springs have been activated intentionally, this is sometimes a problem. It is most liable to occur if the appliance is not adequately stabilized against the upper arch, or if the lower labial pads have been positioned incorrectly so that the lip is held away from the incisors.

The twin-block appliance

This ingenious appliance, first described by Clark (Clark, 1982; 1988), is becoming very popular in the UK. As yet there is no comprehensive study to evaluate fully the reason for its undoubted effectiveness. Unlike most other functional appliances it is made and worn as two independent parts. These carry inclined planes which meet and cause the mandible to be postured forward on closure (Fig. 17.6). Headgear is attached to the upper part of the appliance at night but the rest of the appliance is worn full time without difficulty and this may be the main reason for its effectiveness.

The twin-block appliance is excellent for the treatment of severe Class II, division 1 malocclusions, where progress is invariably good and occasionally spectacular. Class II, division 2 malocclusions can also be treated, provided the lower arch is well aligned and free of crowding. However, the appliance is not very effective in the treatment of a grossly increased overbite because eruption of the posterior teeth is impeded. A Class III version of the appliance is described, although this does not appear to have any clear advantage over conventional appliances and is not widely used.

The appliance can satisfactorily be used in the mixed or permanent dentition but is not able to perform individual tooth movements because of the close-fitting baseplates. However, this is of little consequence because the appliance works rapidly and a short course of twin-block treatment of the order of 3–6 months can precede conventional fixed-appliance treatment.

The appliance

The upper part of the appliance is similar to a conventional removable appliance with molar capping. The molar capping is limited to the posterior end of the arch with an inclined plane at the mesial end. This engages a similar incline on the lower appliance. A midline screw is incorporated to provide compensatory upper arch expansion as the anteroposterior jaw relationship is corrected. The modified arrowhead clasps are used to retain the appliance and span the second premolars and the first molars. A short coil is wound in the bridge of the Adams clasp and this enables a headgear face bow to be added to the appliance without the usual weakness associated with soldered tubes (Fig. 17.6), although many clinicians use a conventional attachment. There is a labial bow.

The lower appliance is retained posteriorly by Adams clasps. Anteriorly the retention should be designed to reduce proclination of the lower labial segment. This may be in the form of a labial bow, Southend clasp, or by acrylic incisal capping. Some recommend lingual extension of the appliance to distribute the mesially directed forces onto the mandibular alveolar process (Isaacson, Reed and Stephens, 1990). The lower part of the appliance carries capping in the premolar region only. The distal end of this is formed into an inclined plane which meets with that of the upper appliance and provides a vertical opening of about 7 mm.

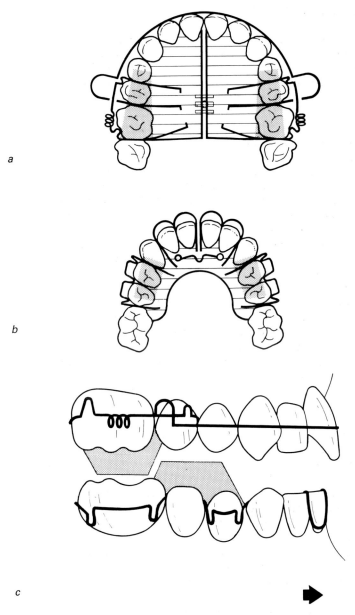

a

b

c

Figure 17.6 The twin block showing the two halves (a, b) of the appliance and (c) their relationship in the mouth. A variety of clasping can be used to suit the particular case.

In its original form, the lower appliance incorporated a hook connected by elastics to the extraoral face bow. The purpose of this was to encourage forward posture of the mandible. Many users omit this feature without any apparent detriment (Isaacson, Reed and Stephens, 1990).

Construction bite

The working bite is taken with enough opening to give 5–7 mm of molar separation with the mandible in comfortable protrusion. If there is any doubt about the ability of the patient to tolerate the chosen degree of opening it is sensible to use less, as resetting is quickly achieved by the addition of cold-curing acrylic resin at the chairside at a subsequent appointment.

Clinical management

Both parts of the appliance have to be fitted at the same time but otherwise the regimen is very much a matter of choice. Some authorities recommend a 2-week training period but this is not always required. Indeed, many young patients with a severe overjet prefer to wear the appliance full time from the start because of the immediate cosmetic improvement which they obtain. Eating with the appliance is difficult and should not be insisted upon, although many patients can manage this.

The headgear can be fitted at the same time as the rest of the appliance or may be delayed for 2 weeks. The amount of wear required depends on the severity of the case but 12–14 h a day would be typical. In mild cases, headgear may not be required at all.

Regular adjustment of the expansion screw should begin as soon as the headgear is fitted. This requires activation of about a quarter turn a month, and it is often sufficient for the operator to do this at routine visits. As soon as the patient can demonstrate the ability to posture the mandible forward from the working position reactivation should be undertaken by addition of cold cure acrylic to the inclined plane of the lower block.

During or after the correction of the anteroposterior relationship, the molar occlusion is re-established by progressive reduction of the blocks. If fixed appliances are to be used these can be fitted at this point. Headgear should normally be continued via conventional molar tubes.

The Herbst appliance (Fig. 17.7)

This appliance is a fixed functional appliance, the two halves of which are permanently connected by telescopic tubes that hold the mandible forwards (Pancherz, 1981). In many ways it is the fixed-appliance equivalent of the twin block. In its original form, the Herbst appliance consisted of two cast-metal skeleton splints, cemented to both upper and lower arches, which once placed by the operator could not be removed by the patient. In a more recent variation attachment to the teeth is by means of acrylic splints (McNamara and Howe, 1988).

Because of the enforced full-time wear the occlusal changes are very rapid. However, as the forces are applied directly to the teeth, there is an increased tendency for the lower incisors to become proclined during treatment (Pancherz and Anehus-Pancherz, 1982).

Headgear and functional appliances

In many Class II cases, some retraction of the upper arch is required and treatment will progress more rapidly if headgear is worn in conjunction with the appliance. Spurs to which J hooks can be attached are incorporated readily in a number of activators, but wherever possible headgear should be applied through tubes embedded into the acrylic or via molar bands, thereby reducing any risk of facial or ocular damage. Particularly where the extraoral traction is applied directly to the functional appliance, the pull should be directed slightly upward so that the appliance is not displaced, making it excessively difficult to wear.

Fixed appliance treatment in conjunction with functional appliances

In some cases, where the arches are initially well aligned, the results of functional appliance treatment will be entirely satisfactory and no further intervention is indicated. However, where there are dental irregularities or crowding necessitating extraction of teeth, a fixed appliance may be required for an optimal result. This should follow correction of the arch malrelationships with the functional appliance.

The transition from functional to fixed appliance is an area of controversy. Most clinicians agree that an interruption of treatment at this point is particularly valuable if the functional appliance has been used in the early mixed dentition. First, the patient may not be ready to proceed with fixed appliances for several years and it is an undue burden on their cooperation if the appliance has to be worn as a retainer during this period. Secondly, it is usually very desirable to allow a period of settling in without retention before the fixed appliance is fitted. This is especially desirable where untoward changes have taken

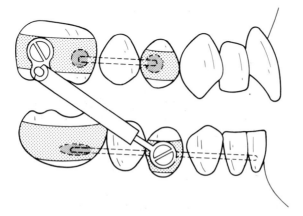

Figure 17.7 A diagrammatic representation of the Herbst appliance. The telescopic attachment permits opening to take place while maintaining the mandible in a forward position.

place, for example excessive arch expansion, or where the lower incisors have been proclined unintentionally and their stability is in question.

However, whilst a settling period of 12–18 months allows the orthodontist to commence fixed-appliance treatment in the knowledge that the teeth are in stable positions, it does extend the treatment time. For the patient who was rather late in starting the functional appliance phase of treament and who may now appear to be well into puberty, the benefit of such a delay must be weighed against the problems of

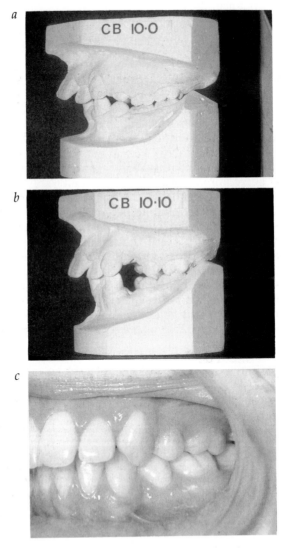

Figure 17.8 The use of an activator in the initial treatment of a severe Class II case: (a) before treatment; (b) after 10 months' treatment with a Harvold activator during which time all four first premolars were removed before the placing of a Begg fixed appliance; (c) after treatment.

loss of cooperation that may accompany such a prolongation of treatment. There is also the possibility that some relapse will occur once the functional appliance is discarded. It is believed by some that this is particularly likely to occur in the rapidly growing child with a treated Class II, division 1 incisor occlusion. In these circumstances it is probably best to fit an upper removable retainer, with a labial bow, a flat anterior biteplane and headgear support. This allows the lower arch to adopt a position of stability around which the later course of treatment can be based, while preventing maxillary relapse in the interim.

The role of functional appliances

Functional appliances can be useful in the treatment of mild, uncrowded Class II malocclusions with well-aligned teeth. In these circumstances an entirely satisfactory result may be obtained without any other appliances.

There is no advantage in using functional appliances for mild or moderate Class II malocclusions with crowding or dental irregularities. These can be treated more efficiently by using conventional removable or fixed appliances.

Functional appliances do have a place in the treatment of some more severe Class II malocclusions, particularly when these present in the mixed dentition. Advantage can be taken of facial growth in helping overbite reduction and correction of arch malrelationships (Fig. 17.8). If lower incisor advancement is planned, preliminary functional appliance treatment followed by a period without appliances is a good way of allowing its stability to be verified before definitive fixed appliance treatment is commenced (Pfeiffer and Grobéty, 1975). Although the effects of functional appliances on facial growth are still questionable, any changes that do occur can only be favourable. Scientific evidence and clinical anecdote does suggest that full time wear of functional appliances in the mixed dentition period may enhance facial growth in Class II cases, to at least a minor extent, and in the severe case all contributions to sagittal correction of the arch relationship are gratefully received by both patient and clinician.

References

Andresen, V. and Haupl, K. (1936) *Funktionskieferorthopädie. Die Grundlagendes 'norwegischen Systems'*, Herman Meusser Verlag, Leipzig

Bell, C. (1983) A modified lower removable appliance using lingual clasping and soft tissue anchorage. *British Journal of Orthodontics*, **10**, 162–163

Bolmgren, G. A. and Moshiri, F. (1986) Bionator treatment in Class II division 1. *American Journal of Orthodontics*, **56**, 255–262

Clark, W. J. (1982) The Twin Block traction technique. *European Journal of Orthodontics*, **4**, 129–138

Clark, W. J. (1988) The Twin Block technique. *American Journal of Orthodontics, and Dentofacial Orthopedics*, **93**, 1–18

Cohen, A. (1981) A study of Class II/I malocclusion treated by Andresen activator. *British Journal of Orthodontics*, **8**, 159–163

Eirew, H. L. (1981) The Bionator. *British Journal of Orthodontics*, **8**, 33–36

Fränkel, R. (1980) A functional approach to orofacial orthopaedics. *British Journal of Orthodontics*, **7**, 41–45

Graber, T. M. and Neumann, B. (1984) *Removable Orthodontic Appliances*, 2nd edn, W. B. Saunders, Philadelphia

Harvold, E. P. (1974) *The Activator in Interceptive Orthodontics*, C. V. Mosby, St. Louis

Harvold, E. P. and Vargevik, K. (1971) Morphogenetic response to activator treatment. *American Journal of Orthodontics*, **60**, 478–490

Hunt, N. and Ellisdon, P. (1985) The Bionator, its use and abuse. *Dental Update*, **12**, 51–61; 129–132

Isaacson, K. G., Reed, R. T. and Stephens, C. D. (1990) *Functional Orthodontic Appliances*, Blackwell Scientific, Oxford

McNamara, J. A. (1980) Functional determinants of craniofacial size and shape. *European Journal of Orthodontics*, **2**, 131–159

McNamara, J. A. (1988) Fabrication of the acrylic splint Herbst appliance. *American Journal of Orthodontics and Dentofacial Orthopedics*, **94**, 10–18

McNamara, J. A. and Bryan, F. A. (1987) Long term mandibular adaptations to protusive function – an experimental study in *Macaca mulatta*. *American Journal of Orthodontics, and Dentofacial Orthopedics*, **92**, 98–108

McNamara, J. A. and Carlson, D. S. (1979) Quantitative analysis of temporo-mandibular joint adaptions to protrusive function. *American Journal of Orthodontics*, **76**, 593–611

McNamara, J. A. and Howe, R. P. (1988) Clinical management of the acrylic splint Herbst appliance. *American Journal of Orthodontics and Dentofacial Orthopedics*, **94**, 142–149

Mills, J. R. E. (1983) Clinical control of craniofacial growth – a skeptics viewpoint. In *Clinical Alteration of the Growing Face* (ed. J. A. McNamara, K. A. Ribbens and R. P. Howe), *Monograph 14*, Center for Human Growth and Development, University of Michigan

Osborn, W. S. Nanda, R. S. and Currier, E.F. (1991) Mandibular arch perimeter change with lip bumper treatment. *American Journal of Orthodontics and Dentofacial Orthopedics*, **99**, 527–532

Owman-Moll, P. and Ingervall, B. (1984) Effects of oral screen treatment. *American Journal of Orthodontics*, **85**, 37–46

Pancherz, H. (1981) The effect of continuous bite jumping on the dentofacial complex: a follow-up study after Herbst treatment of Class II malocclusions. *European Journal of Orthodontics*, **3**, 49–60

Pancherz, H. and Anehus-Pancherz, M. (1982) The effect of continuous bite jumping with the Herbst appliance on the masticatory system: A functional analysis of treated Class II malocclusions. *European Journal of Orthodontics*, **4**, 37–44

Pfeiffer, J. P. and Grobéty, D. (1975) The Class II malocclusion: differential diagnosis and clinical application of actiovators extraoral traction and fixed appliances. *American Journal of Orthodontics*, **68**, 499–544

Proffit, W. R. (1986) *Contemporary Orthodontics*, C. V. Mosby, St. Louis, p.357

Robin, P. (1902) Observations sur un nouvel appareil de redressment. *Review of Stomatology*, **9**, 423

Rutter, R. R. and Witt, E. (1990) Correction of Class II division 2 malocclusions through the use of the Bionator appliance. *American Journal of Orthodontics and Dentofacial Orthopedics*, **97**, 106–112

Sahm, G., Bartsch, A. and Witt, E. (1990) Microelectronic monitoring of functional appliance wear. *European Journal of Orthodontics*, **12**, 297–301

Salzmann, J. A. (1957) *Orthodontics, Practice and Techniques*, Lippincott, Philadelphia, p.328

Thüer, U. and Ingervall, B. (1990) Effect of muscle exercise with an oral screen on lip function. *European Journal of Orthodontics*, **12**, 198–208

Tulloch, J. F. C., Medland, W. and Tuncay, O. C. (1990) Methods used to evaluate growth modification in Class II malocclusion. *American Journal of Orthodontics and Dentofacial Orthopedics*, **98**, 340–347

Vig, K. and Vig, P. (1986) Hybrid appliances: a component approach to dentofacial orthopedics. *American Journal of Orthodontics and Dentofacial Orthopedics*, **90**, 273–285

Woodside, D. G. (1977) The activator. In *Removable Orthodontic Appliances*, 2nd edn, (ed. T. M. Graber and B. Neumann) W. B. Saunders, Philadelphia

Further Reading

Isaacson, K. G., Reed, R. T. and Stephens, C. D. (1990) *Functional Orthodontic Appliances*, Blackwell Scientific, Oxford

Graber, T. M. and Neumann, B. (1984). *Removable Orthodontic Appliances*, 2nd edn, W. B. Saunders, Philadelphia

Chapter 18

Stability and retention

The position of teeth in the dental arch is dictated primarily by the shape and relationship of the jaws and by forces from the surrounding soft tissues (see Chapter 3). After a course of orthodontic treatment, the teeth should still be in a position of balance, but a period of retention is usually necessary to allow the supporting tissues to adapt (see p. 270). In some cases, permanent retention is required. A distinction should be made between relapse of orthodontic treatment, and changes that are a result of facial growth and occlusal maturation. For example, in a Class III case where upper incisors have been proclined but the overbite is inadequate to hold them, they will relapse (Fig. 18.1). Similar changes in incisor relationship can occur in the longer term, owing to unfavourable facial growth. Another situation where relapse can be mimicked by natural occlusal change is the development of lower incisor crowding: injudicious proclination of lower incisors may be followed by relapse and crowding; but similar lower incisor crowding may develop in the longer term, owing to late facial growth (see p. 39). For the patient, these changes are undesirable whatever the cause, but the clinician should recognize their different causes. Relapse should be anticipated and avoided wherever possible but the prediction of facial growth changes is much more uncertain. The clinician should be aware of the possibility of unfavourable occlusal change and should warn the patient accordingly (Wood, 1983).

The causes of relapse

Factors involved in stability are discussed under the following headings:

a soft tissue factors;
b occlusal factors;
c facial growth and occlusal development;
d supporting tissues.

Soft tissue factors

An occlusion before orthodontic treatment is in balance between occlusal and soft tissue forces; unless a new position of balance can be found,

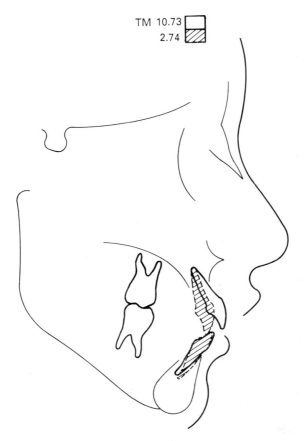

Figure 18.1 An incorrectly planned treatment of a Class III malocclusion where the overbite at the end of upper incisor proclination was insufficient to maintain stability.

changes will not be stable. As a general rule the size and form of the lower arch has to be accepted. Lower arch width is particularly difficult to alter with the assurance of stability and so this should not be done without good cause. Cases can be found where transverse lower arch expansion has been stable, but this is unpredictable and so is not a sound basis for treatment. Labiolingual movement of lower incisors is also liable to be unstable unless other factors are changed at the same time. For example, retraction of lower incisors may be stable in a Class III case if an adequate overbite is established. In a few Class II cases, the lower incisors have been restrained by contact with the palate or upper labial segment, or by a thumb-sucking habit, and so proclination to a position of true soft tissue balance will be stable (see p. 227). However, these changes in lower incisor position are problematical and have to be managed skilfully. Retraction of upper incisors in a Class II, division 1 case will be stable provided that their relationship to the lower lip is changed (Fig. 18.2) (see p. 227). Concomitant changes in the

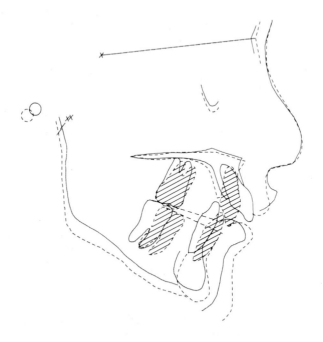

Figure 18.2 Successful reduction of an increased incisor overjet will usually require a change in the relationship between the upper incisors and the lower lip.

upper and lower arches have poorer prospects of stability because occlusal factors cannot help. Thus transverse expansion of both upper and lower arches to relieve incisor crowding is very liable to relapse and was discredited many years ago. It is still claimed that with some functional appliances, such as the Fränkel, the muscle balance can be changed so that tranverse expansion is stable (see p. 335) but this is a matter of controversy. Simultaneous proclination or retraction of both upper and lower labial segments is equally problematical. Proclination of upper and lower incisors in cases of bimaxillary retroclination would provide a simple solution to the deep overbite, but would not be stable. In many cases of bimaxillary proclination, retraction of upper and lower incisors would be advantageous, but this will be stable only if the soft tissue balance can be changed (see p. 212). Cases can be demonstrated that seem to disprove these general guidelines, but they are exceptions. The experienced orthodontist may be able to recognize these unusual cases where the general rules can be broken, but this is always at the risk of long-term relapse. Stability should not be claimed for such cases until all retention appliances have been abandoned for at least 2 or preferably 5 years.

Occlusal factors

Teeth that are retained by the occluᵤion will be stable without retention appliances. For example, instanding upper incisors that have been moved over the bite will be stable, provided that the overbite is adequate. Similarly, a unilateral crossbite corrected by upper arch expansion should be stable if there is a good intercuspation of the teeth. The occlusion is also important in maintaining a corrected anteroposterior arch relationship – for example, after retraction of upper buccal segments in a Class II case. Stability of overbite reduction depends on a change in the interincisor relationship; the edge–centroid relationship must be secure (see p. 239).

Facial growth and occlusal development

Dentoalveolar adaptation tends to maintain occlusal relationships even when skeletal relationships change with growth. However, if the intercuspation of the teeth is poor or if dentoalveolar compensation is already at its limits, occlusal changes can occur, particularly where skeletal growth changes are marked. For example, a Class III occlusion will often deteriorate if the underlying Class III skeletal relationship becomes more severe; and a skeletal open bite often becomes worse with growth in lower face height. Although the arch relationships remain stable in most cases, increase in labial segment crowding is often associated with dentoalveolar adaptation (see p. 263). Mesial drift of buccal teeth contributes to the development of labial segment crowding. Many causes of mesial drift have been postulated, including the anterior component of force, tensions in the supra-alveolar connective tissues and impaction of third molars. It is possible that all these factors can play a part but the evidence is not clear-cut, and certainly the early removal of third molars cannot be justified on these grounds alone.

Supporting tissues

In normal circumstances, transient variation in occlusal and muscular forces will not result in tooth movement. However, when a tooth has been moved by an orthodontic appliance, the recently deposited bone is particularly susceptible to resorption. Thus relapse can occur from minor imbalances that would normally have no effect. For this reason it is prudent to retain most tooth movements for a period of months until the supporting tissues have adapted fully. The supporting bone and principal fibres of the periodontal ligament will be reorganized within 3–6 months, but the supra-alveolar connective tissue takes very much longer (Reitan, 1959; Edwards, 1968). This can produce partial relapse of rotations; and of labial movement of instanding lateral incisor teeth unless they are held by an overbite. Pericision of the free gingival and transseptal fibres after the rotation (Fig. 18.3) helps to stabilize the correction, although it does not eliminate the risk of relapse (Edwards, 1970; 1988; Pinson and Strahan, 1974). Overcorrection and prolonged retention (see p. 270) also help to deal with this problem, although there

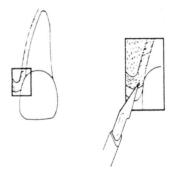

Figure 18.3 Pericision. A fine pointed scalpel blade is inserted through the gingival crevice as far as the alveolar crest and the incision carried circumferentially around the tooth. Care must be taken in this procedure to ensure that all the free gingival and transseptal fibres are severed.

are no precise quantitative guidelines because individual response varies so much.

In the adult patient with periodontal disease, appreciable drifting of teeth, particularly the upper incisors, may occur. This is in part due to pocket formation producing an imbalance in periodontal support, but to a large extent can be attributed to disruption of the transseptal and other supra-alveolar connective tissue fibres, which undoubtedly have an important role in stabilizing tooth positions against minor imbalance in occlusal and soft tissue forces. Particularly where the control of upper incisors by the lower lip is marginal, they may drift labially and space, while the lower incisors overerupt. Stabilization of these teeth after orthodontic treatment can be very difficult. Control of the periodontal condition is mandatory, and if there has been appreciable loss of periodontal support, some form of permanent retention will be required.

Retention

After orthodontic treatment, the occlusion may be self-retentive as when an upper incisor is moved over the bite, and so no retention appliance is required. Unless there is positive occlusal retention of the treatment result, it is usual to fit a retainer at least until the supporting tissues have reorganized fully. Retention can be: (a) short term, (b) medium term, or (c) permanent (see Reitan, 1969).

Short-term retention

This extends from 3 to 6 months while the supporting tissues reorganize. A removable appliance is most useful because it can be worn only part time towards the end of the retention period. A typical regimen would be full-time wear for the first 3 months, followed by night-only wear for a similar period. Some operators then ask the patient to wear it only on alternate nights to taper off the retention gradually. The advantage of concluding retention with part-time wear is that if the teeth become more mobile or if the appliance is difficult to insert after it has been left out, it indicates that the tooth positions may not be stable. There is little merit in then extending the retention period in the hope that things will improve. A decision has to be made whether to proceed with further orthodontic treatment; or to leave out the appliance to find out how much relapse will occur; or to institute permanent retention according to the features of the case and the wishes of the patient.

Where active treatment has been completed with a removable appliance, this may be rendered passive and used as a retainer. On some occasions it is better to make a new retainer. This is generally required after fixed-appliance treatment in the upper arch for the following reasons: to allow controlled occlusal settling; and to permit a period of part-time retention so that stability can be assessed; and because patients are invariably anxious to be rid of their fixed appliance as soon as possible. For most purposes, a Hawley type of retainer is adequate in the upper arch. A similar appliance can be used in the lower arch but is not advised because the patient may find it difficult to manage upper and lower retaining appliances (Fig. 18.4). It is often better to remove attachments of a lower fixed appliance progressively, so that the fixed appliance can be used as a retainer. Premolar attachments are removed first, and then molar bands and an anterior sectional arch used to retain the labial segment. Later this can be replaced with a bonded lingual retainer if necessary (see below).

Some orthodontists like to retain their cases with a positioner (Kesling, 1945). This is a flexible splint (Fig. 18.5) made from synthetic rubber or plastic material into which the patient bites. It is intended to adjust any minor dental irregularities (Vorhies 1960; Wells, 1970) although this should have been done with the active appliance. Preformed positioners are available but these have the serious limitations that unless one can be found that fits the occlusion precisely they may be ineffective as retainers and may even introduce unwanted tooth

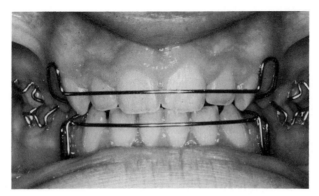

Figure 18.4 The simultaneous use of upper and lower removable appliances is not to be recommended.

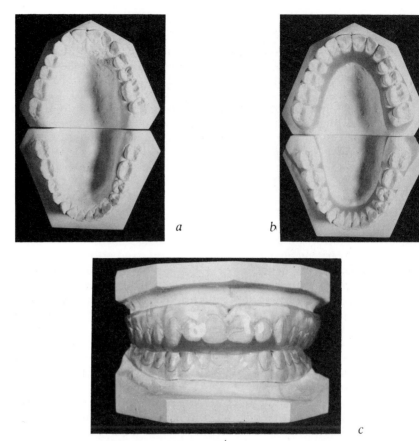

Figure 18.5 An individually prepared positioner. (a) At the completion of treatment, minor irregularities remain. (b) These teeth are removed from the model and repositioned to correct any minor irregularities. The adjustments to the tooth position are small and the arch size and form cannot be changed. (c) The positioner is made on the adjusted models from a plastic or rubber material.

movements. Individually prepared positioners are made on models that have been adjusted to correct any minor irregularities (Fig. 18.5).

Medium-term retention

This is appropriate where the supporting tissues will take longer to adapt, or where it is decided to stabilize the occlusion during the later stages of facial growth so that dentoalveolar adaptation does not result in adverse occlusal changes, and in particular lower incisor crowding. Medium-term retention may extend between 1 and 5 years. A fixed retainer will generally be used, and although some orthodontists use positioners in this capacity, this is of questionable benefit. Medium-term retention should be used only where there are clear indications that it will be beneficial and not merely to postpone the inevitable relapse of an unstable treatment result.

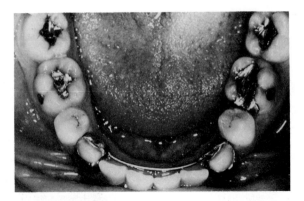

Figure 18.6 A lower lingual retainer attached to bands on lower canine teeth.

Bonded flexible retainers

Where a rotated tooth is to be retained for an extended period, a multiple-strand wire can be bonded to the lingual surfaces of the tooth in question and its neighbours (Zachrisson, 1977). The retaining wire may be applied directly to the teeth or prepared on a model and attached using an indirect bonding technique (Ferguson, 1988). With multiple rotations in the labial segment, for example, the retainer may extend from canine to canine (Fig. 18.6). The retainer must be clear of the occlusion. The flexibility of the wire allows a small amount of individual tooth movement in response to occlusal forces (attempts to bond together adjacent teeth directly usually fail because of these minor tooth movements). Retainers of this type will generally be used for 1 year to 18 months but, provided an excellent standard of oral hygiene is maintained, there is no reason why they should not remain in place for longer (see below).

Lower lingual retainers

These are particularly useful where the lower incisors were crowded or where the lower labial segment has been proclined and it is considered that relapse could be produced by late facial growth and associated dentoalveolar adaptation. A retainer of this type ensures that dento-alveolar adaptation has to occur in other ways, for example by some proclination of the upper incisor teeth; and mesial drift of the lower buccal segments is prevented from encroaching on the labial segment. This does not ensure, of course, that adverse occlusal changes will not occur after the eventual removal of the retainer.

In the past such retainers have usually been made from 0.7 mm wire attached to bands or gauze that will be bonded to the supporting teeth (Fig. 18.6). The retainer may be attached to the canines or premolars. In the lower arch, this form of retention, whilst it prevents a reduction in the intercanine distance that might produce crowding, does nothing to prevent relapse of actively aligned lower incisor teeth. For this reason, and because the lower intercanine distance tends to decrease with time,

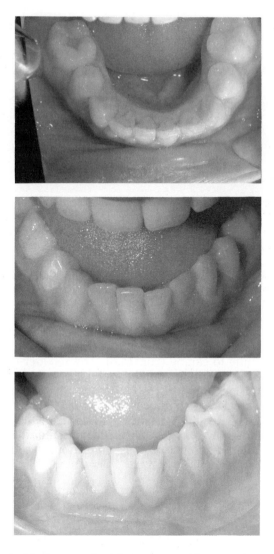

Figure 18.7 Views of the lower arch of the case treated by extraction of four second premolars and the use of fixed appliances shown in Fig. 16.16, showing how a slow return of lower incisor crowding is almost inevitable in many cases: (a) immediately after treatment; (b) 1 year out of retention; (c) 3 years out of retention.

many clinicians now prefer to use a bonded lingual retainer attached to the lower incisors only.

In many situations the retainer will be in place for 12–18 months. However, if they are to be effective in controlling dentoalveolar adaptation, lower lingual retainers have to be worn until growth is nearly complete. This may mean that the retainer must be left in place until 16–19 years of age in boys, and until 14–17 years of age in girls. It is now recognized that dentoalveolar growth changes continue slowly throughout life and a recurrence of lower incisor crowding is almost inevitable, even in cases where treatment has been carried out to the highest standards (Fig. 18.7) (Little, Wallen and Reidel, 1981; Little, Riedel and Årtun, 1988).

Prolonged retention to overcome this should not be embarked upon lightly. Regular inspection is essential to ensure that the appliance is satisfactory, and careful oral hygiene is necessary to prevent plaque accumulation.

Permanent retention

The general practitioner should not contemplate undertaking orthodontic treatment where permanent retention might be required. However, the orthodontic specialist may decide to use permanent retention in selected cases: for example in the patient with a cleft of the lip and palate where a prosthesis can act as retainer, and in adult patients with periodontal problems where there is no alternative but to stabilize the teeth permanently (Williams et al., 1982).

References

Edwards, J. G. (1968) A study of the periodontium during orthodontic rotation of teeth. *American Journal of Orthodontics*, **54**, 441–461

Edwards, J. G. (1970) A surgical procedure to eliminate rotational relapse. *American Journal of Orthodontics*, **57**, 35–46

Edwards, J. G. (1988) A long term prospective evaluation of the circumferential supracrestal fibrotomy. *American Journal of Orthodontics and Dentofacial Orthopedics*. **93**, 380–387

Ferguson, J. W. (1988) Multistrand wire retainers: an indirect technique. *British Journal of Orthodontics*, **15**, 51–54

Kesling, H. D. (1945) The philosophy of the tooth positioning appliance. *American Journal of Orthodontics and Oral Surgery*, **31**, 297–304

Little, R. M. Riedel, R.A. and Årtun, J. (1988) An evaluation of changes in mandibular anterior alignment from 10 to 20 years postretention. *American Journal of Orthodontics and Dentofacial Orthopedics*, **93**, 423–428.

Little, R. M., Wallen, T. R. And Riedel, R.A. (1981) Stability and relapse of mandibular anterior alignment – first premolar extraction cases treated by traditional edgewise orthodontics. *American Journal of Orthodontics*, **80**, 349–365

Pinson, P. R. and Strahan, J. D. (1974) The effect on the relapse of orthodontically rotated teeth of surgical division of the gingival fibres–pericision. *British Journal of Orthodontics*, **1**, 87–91

Reitan, K. (1959) Tissue rearrangement during retention of orthodontically rotated teeth. *Angle Orthodontist*, **29**, 105–113

Reitan, K. (1969) Principles of retention in avoidance of post-treatment relapse. *Journal of Orthodontics*, **55**, 776–790

Vorhies, J. M. (1960) Short intensive use of tooth positioners and an appraisal of the results. *Angle Orthodontist*, **30**, 248–254

Wells, N. E. (1970) Application of the positioner appliance in orthodontic treatment. *American Journal of Orthodontics*, **58**, 351–366

Williams, S., Melsen, B., Agerbaek, N. and Asboe, V. (1982) The orthodontic treatment of malocclusion in patients with previous periodontal disease. *British Journal of Orthodontics*, **9**, 178–184

Wood, C. M. (1983) The effect of retention on the relapse of Class II division 1 cases. *British Journal of Orthodontics*, **10**, 198–202

Zachrisson, B. U. (1977) Clinical experience with direct-bonded orthodontic retainers. *American Journal of Orthodontics*, **71**, 440–448

Chapter 19

Oral surgery for orthodontic patients

David Poswillo and Murray Foster

Craniomaxillofacial surgery

Techniques developed in Europe in the early 1950s, particularly those of Obwegeser and Trauner (1957), provided the basis for surgical movements of the jaws that would alter, in a stable fashion, the alveolar and basal bones. These techniques now provide the opportunity for orthodontist and oral surgeon to treat, in collaboration, severe orofacial disproportion that was not previously amenable to orthodontic therapy alone. In this chapter the guidelines for the planning and execution of orthognathic surgery of the maxilla and mandible will be discussed, with special emphasis on the aspects with which the orthodontist should be familiar.

Case assessment

Early in treatment planning the consultant responsible for overall case control should discuss, with the patient, the principal complaint and the motives for seeking treatment. At this interview, possible treatment options should be outlined and good written records begun. If it appears likely that the patient will proceed with treatment, or wish for further information, additional records such as photographs, study models and radiographs should be obtained. The initial radiographic views required are a lateral cephalogram, plus panoral and appropriate intraoral films. A facebow recording may assist with accurate mounting of the study models.

Early in the assessment phase, attention should be given to psychological and behavioural matters, career prospects, educational commitments, marriage plans and other personal matters. Family attitudes to facial appearance should be evaluated, signs of personal embarrassment should be sought (for example, covering the mouth with the hand while conversing) and the expectations of treatment should be compared with the likely results of surgery. An early meeting with parents, spouses or other important members of the family will help to provide a picture of home support and attitudes to treatment. These preliminary observations are essential if the true measure of the patient's concern with facial or dental appearance is to be appreciated.

At an appropriate stage of assessment the patient should be informed of all realistic treatment options, including the masking of deformity by less demanding camouflage or compromise procedures. The advantages, disadvantages and likely complications of the various options should be explained. Special attention should be given to obtaining an accurate history of the general medical status of the patient and the presence or absence of genetic disease in the immediate family. While eliciting all this essential detail the clinician can assemble information related to the specific facial problem. It should be remembered that many factors that affect assessment and the outcome of treatment are outside surgical control: factors such as skin quality, general health, hair, and the shape, size and position of the ears can rarely be changed. Ethnic factors should be considered when planning the 'ideal' facial form: cultural attitudes may not coincide with those that motivate the surgeon.

If treatment is to proceed, it must satisfy the patient's concern with respect to the presenting problem. There is an overriding need, at this stage, to define this area from the point of view of both surgeon and patient. Where the aspirations of the patient can be matched by the technical skills of the surgeon, there exists a realistic basis for a successful outcome.

Clinical inspection

When examining, first inspect critically and then gently palpate to confirm your findings. Note if the face and occlusion are symmetrical, for the ensuing discourse assumes this. If asymmetry exists, define the main area affected, think hard about which side is at fault and calculate which sites need to be corrected. Is the asymmetry limited to the lower face or are the orbits and temporomandibular joints included? Assuming it is lower facial, does the maxillary plane require lateral levelling and, if so, would it be best to raise one side or lower the other? Generally the former is felt to be more stable but the decision clearly depends on lip/incisor relationships, the need to alter the anteroposterior occlusal plane angle, existing nasal-airway patency and what mandibular procedure is anticipated.

The initial emphasis should be on general impressions, the balance, then proportions, of the face, both in profile and full face. Look at the chin, nose and lip balance, both vertical and anteroposterior. Use the labiomental/nasolabial angles for this, and supplement them with the frontonasal and chin–neck angles. Is the nasal profile alone a likely source of complaint by the patient (the size, width, symmetry, shape, humping), are the nostrils flared or pinched, is the columella particularly noticeable? Note the relative facial prominence of the zygomata, orbital rims and orbital globes in relation to the jaws and chin. A higher facial convexity is generally more acceptable in Caucasian females than males. Look at the vertical proportions of the face: are they within an acceptable range, or are the upper and lower face too long or short, or is the fault a combination of both? As a general rule the distance from glabella to subnasale and from subnasale to the base of chin should be about equal.

When viewing the patient's profile, remember that the patient himself cannot see this. Try to determine clinically whether any anteroposterior discrepancy between the jaws is mainly maxillary or mandibular in origin, or both. Relate this to the earlier assessment of upper and lower facial heights, and palpate the nasolabial areas to determine the underlying bony level. Likewise, palpate the infraorbital rims and glabella, and check the masseteric muscle bulk during clenching, and the symmetry of mandibular opening.

Circumoral assessment must include the relative prominence of the lips and the ratio of the upper/lower vermilion exposure. The degree of lip competence and lip tone is worth noting. What relationship has the upper lip to the upper incisors at rest? Usually 1–4 mm shows in adults. Note this, especially when the patient is smiling, and whether there is excessive or deficient upper gingival exposure. How are the lateral facial proportions in the full-face view? It is most common to see the inner canthus line up with the lateral alar margins, and the pupils with the oral commissures. Does the intercanthal distance look right (men 34 mm; women 33 mm)? Normal values of soft tissue proportion in the full-face view have been published, as have those of soft tissue profile proportion in the predominant ethnic groups (Bell, Proffit and White, 1980).

Radiological examination

The assessment can now move on to a more exact value analysis (but no more or less important) of the hard tissues, best done with radiographs in the light of clinical findings. In the UK it is unusual to analyse posteroanterior cephalograms for anything other than the site and broad degrees of asymmetry. Most emphasis is put on the proportional and absolute linear, vertical and anteroposterior measurements, in addition to angular assessments. The importance of having standardized lateral cephalograms cannot be overemphasized when comparing patient data.

When inspecting such a film, ensure that appropriate soft tissue outlines can be seen easily and that there is good quality and exposure, including nose, chin and hyoid, and that it is appropriately labelled with the patient's name, date and hospital of origin. Any of the currently accepted methods of cephalometric analysis may be used (see Chapter 6). The importance is that the clinical impression and diagnosis of the main source of skeletal and occlusal defects is sharpened or adjusted, and that possible solutions to the basic defect(s) or, alternatively, less complex masking procedures are generated during the analysis. Nowadays, this is most conveniently done with a computerized system, which allows the digitized image of the patient's cephalogram to be rapidly manipulated and displayed (Harradine and Birnie, 1985)

Special tests

At the conclusion of the clinical and radiographic analysis a clear impression should exist in the clinician's mind as to the sites of the main anteroposterior, vertical and transverse discrepancies. In addition, an assessment should be made of the compensations that have taken place naturally, and those corrections which it may be reasonable to offer, bearing in mind the patient's complaints and aspirations.

The principles of orthodontic assessment have already been covered in Chapter 7. The differences specific to surgical assessment include the following additional examinations: it is important to have periapical films of the teeth adjacent to a planned osteotomy within the dental arch, and vitality test results must be recorded where teeth are at risk during segmental surgery.

It is a good plan to retake preoperative radiographs after the completion of orthodontic treatment to reassess root and apical positions and any changes that may have followed appliance therapy. While with modern orthodontic techniques of arch levelling, many feel that the place for segmental surgery is receding, there are still instances where the patient and problem merit this type of solution to adjust the occlusal plane or level and achieve better occlusion, e.g. in open bites, both anterior and lateral. The most likely category will be where the patient's age or commitments or dental condition preclude protracted, visible appliance therapy and a surgical alternative can be offered. It is, of course, possible to create space orthodontically to enable easier and safer segmental osteotomy to be performed. Surgical correction of deep overbite and anterior open bite may still be preferred when long-term orthodontic stability is uncertain.

Extra study models should be requested and, if necessary, mounted on an articulator, but remember that the patient's own jaw provides the best guide to articulation. Using a fine plaster-cutting jigsaw blade, segmental surgery can be tried out by sectioning the model at the sites that would appear most suitable for arch expansion, realignment of anterior segments, or their vertical or anteroposterior repositioning, usually in the canine–premolar region. Beware of removing approximal tooth substance with a saw: and if small cuspal interferences arise, consider cusp grinding. If a stable final occlusion will result, mark where this has been done, recalling that excessive grinding will produce dentine sensitivity needing treatment. Remove segments of base plaster and keep them as a guide to the necessary bone removal, and make a note of what has been planned.

The mobilized segment may be held in the neutral position initially with soft pink carding wax, and later by sticky yellow wax or by dual pins in each segment joined by elastics. Test the new occlusion in protrusive and lateral excursive movements. Depending on the method of fixation to be used, a new occlusal impression may be needed to construct a wafer to tie the mobilized segments together.

Templates

On the few occasions when body or segmental osteotomies are to be carried out, templates are used by some surgeons. These must be prepared with great care. The template must locate firmly into position in such a way that it relates positively to the teeth, otherwise inadequate or excessive quantities of bone may be removed and require bone grafting or prejudice the stability of the result.

Mock up surgery

This is wise for certain complex osteotomies, in particular for facial asymmetry. It is desirable to make up full-scale models to facilitate mock surgery and pre-empt operative difficulties and unforeseen rotations. This may also be applicable to osteotomies of the body and anterior mandible, and certain midfacial procedures.

Final treatment planning

This is best undertaken at a joint orthodontic and oral surgery clinic, with the patient present and after each clinician has had an opportunity to see the patient or study the records. Having reached an agreed diagnosis and assessed the patient's needs and suitabilities, and thought out varying treatment options, these can be discussed with the patient, their merits compared and a plan of action evolved. Most treatment planning will be performed in this fashion. The emphasis is commonly towards predominantly orthodontic or predominantly surgical solutions and a variety of aids to the processes are used. These include the dental-model and jaw-model mock surgery, discussed already.

In instances where facial morphology will alter, it has become accepted practice for a number of clinicians to profile plan the changes. Some clinicians point to the value of conducting this process in the presence of the patient, as the planning exercise forms a method of communication with the patient, whose comprehension of the likely change can only be enhanced by seeing the predicted profile and a suitable explanation of its meaning and accuracy. In addition, the method can be used as a valuable teaching and thought-provoking procedure.

While the 'eye-balling' system that comes from experience is the more popular tool, profile planning should be outlined at this point. The method described by Henderson and Poswillo (1985) requires a transparent (celluloid) lateral facial photograph to be enlarged to a precise profile fit with the most recent lateral cephalogram. The points S, N, A, B, menton, gnathion, gonion, pogonion, ANS, PNS, are pricked through both the lateral cephalogram and the superimposed profile photograph and the incisor and first molar of each jaw are traced on to the photograph. This is then separated from the cephalogram and checked. The photograph is sectioned and repositioned to simulate the planned osteotomy movements. The soft tissue profile consequences are then calculated and the chin, nose and lip repositioned accordingly. Overlaps and defects are eliminated and the result represent a reasonable guide to the likely profile alterations; and it may also serve to reveal unfavourable effects of certain osteotomy plans (Fig. 19.1).

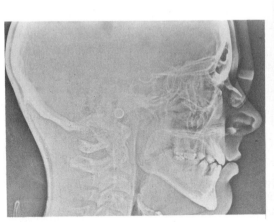
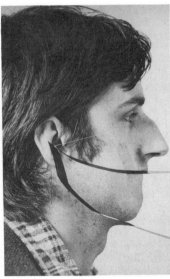

a   b

Figure 19.1 (a) Soft tissue profile with underlying skeleton and teeth shown on xeroradiograph before profile planning. (b) Paste up of profile segments on planning photographic print. (From David, D. J., Poswillo, D. and Simpson, D. (1983) *The Craniosynostoses*, Springer–Verlag, Berlin.)

Mandibular prognathism and retrognathism

Osteotomy techniques

In recent years there has been a proliferation of procedures used for the correction of dentofacial anomalies in which the collaboration of the orthodontist and the oral surgeon is paramount. The very fact that diverse techniques exist for the correction of almost every type of orthognathic problem means that no specific operative method is universally applicable to a given type of jaw deformity. Surgeons may prefer to operate by the intraoral route or by other approaches from the skin surface; and the choice between maxillary, mandibular, intraoral, extraoral, segmental and interradicular techniques allows the surgeon numerous options. Every effort should be made to avoid obviously inappropriate procedures, and generally, when the guiding principles of assessment and case planning are applied, an optimal solution is available for each individual problem of orofacial deformity. Clearly the plethora of technical modifications cannot be encompassed in a single chapter. Opportunity will be taken in this section to describe in broad outline those basic technical procedures that are frequently used in one modified form or another for the correction of most orthodontic/ orthognathic problems.

Body ostectomy

This method is valuable for closure of gaps in the dental arch, reduction of the abnormally long body of the mandible and the restoration of symmetry (Fig. 19.2). It can be used to close an anterior open bite, in conjunction with a reduction in lower facial height. The area of bone contact achieved is often less than adequate, however, and union is not always achieved in the expected time.

This method requires meticulous model planning on a plaster or acrylic mandible. Templates showing the precise amount of bone to be

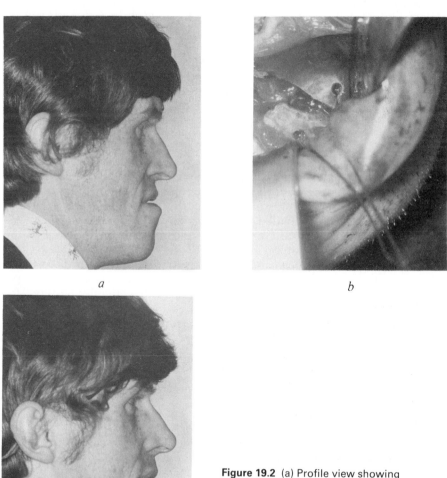

a

b

c

Figure 19.2 (a) Profile view showing prognathism with abnormally long body of mandible. (b) Gap in premolar region of body of mandible after body ostectomy and before tightening of fixation wires: mental nerve is protected in 'bone cave' at superior aspect of cut. (c) Profile after bilateral intraoral body ostectomy.

removed are constructed, due consideration being paid to the sites of teeth and roots adjacent to the bone cuts. The surgical approach is generally intraoral and bone grafts are useful additions to promote early union. While intermaxillary fixation is not always essential, great care must be taken with the method of splinting, especially where the crowns of the teeth are malposed or small.

The principal disadvantages of this procedure are those connected with the necessity to avoid injury to the mental nerve and the difficulty in fixing a small, anterior, semilunar segment on widely flared, posterior bone cuts. Union is impaired in these circumstances, even when grafting with iliac crest bone mush is employed. When large movements are undertaken, relapse is prone to occur, vertical steps may remain on the lower border of the mandible and excessive submental soft tissue may produce an unacceptable 'double chin' appearance. The procedure does nothing to overcome the poor aesthetics of an obtuse mandibular angle in cases of mandibular prognathism.

C and L osteotomies

These geometrically designed, ramal bone-cut procedures permit repositioning of the body and tooth-bearing segment of the mandible in relation to the rami within the pterygomasseteric sling. While the range of movement of the resected parts is somewhat limited, there is some advantage from the minimal positional disturbances of the muscles of mastication. The methods are particularly favoured for the closure of anterior open bite, provided that pure rotation is avoided, for this leads to instability. Bone grafts are usually incorporated in the area of the resection to promote union and stability (Fig. 19.3).

The surgical approach can be intra or extraoral. Care must be taken to match arches and attention should be given to good final cuspal interdigitation. If used intermaxillary fixation is generally required for 6–8 weeks postoperatively. These procedures have the advantage of interfering only minimally with the coronoid process and temporal muscle. The chief limitation is that of relapse: when considerable mandibular advancement is attempted, relapse may be dramatic. While paraesthesia of the lips is usually avoided, trismus may persist for a

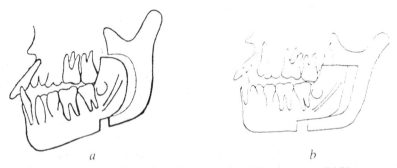

a   *b*

Figure 19.3 (a) Diagram of bone cuts in conventional C osteotomy. (b) Diagrammatic view of modified Trauner L osteotomy in mandible.

long period. The use of iliac bone grafts may leave an unacceptable external scar at the donor site.

Mandibular ramus osteotomies

The aim of these procedures is to reposition the entire body of the mandible in relation to the maxillary teeth, while operating within the pterygomasseteric sling, which envelops the site of surgery. While the procedures usually permit great flexibility in the repositioning of segments, there are limits to the degree of retrusion and/or advancement that can be achieved without loss of stability. Attempts to reduce or elongate much beyond 1 cm are often compromised by relapse.

In choosing these procedures, attention should be given to the adequacy of the final occlusion and arch fit; spot grinding and occlusal wafers may be needed at operation to facilitate these aims. The use of orthodontic archwires for intermaxillary fixation is essential if occlusal adjustment is to be carried out. It should be ensured that the condyles are correctly repositioned in the fossa before establishing intermaxillary fixation. These procedures usually produce large areas of cancellous bone for optimum healing of the fixed segments. Relapse is minimized by periods of fixation extending to 9 weeks. Rigid internal fixation with screws is a contemporary alternative.

In experienced hands there are usually few complications from these procedures. Postoperative swelling can be greatly reduced by the use of steroids, peri- and postoperatively; bleeding is usually slight, especially when local anaesthetic infiltration is employed and incisions are made with a cutting diathermy. Adequate drainage of the wound prevents haematoma formation. Often there is some alteration in sensation of the lips and tongue for variable periods after operation. Rarely, prolonged paraesthesia may occur. Relapse, in well-planned cases, is seldom severe and the patient acceptance of these procedures is uniformly high.

Sagittal split techniques

The original Obwegeser (1964) method, in the ramus, has great merit for push-back procedures. It is sparing of damage to the inferior dental nerve and is a particularly versatile procedure, allowing the correction of asymmetry and crossbite (Fig. 19.4).

The Dal Pont (1961) modification of Obwegeser's technique is widely used for mandibular advancement: it provides a large area of bony contact, but has the disadvantage of greater inferior dental nerve morbidity. It is probably the most widely used method of correction of prognathism and mandibular retrusion in the UK and Europe. Rare instances of severe haemorrhage and postoperative VIIth nerve paresis have been reported. The absence of facial scars and the relative stability of the procedure have enhanced the reputation of the sagittal split method as the operation of first choice whenever case assessment indicates the possibility of this approach to treatment.

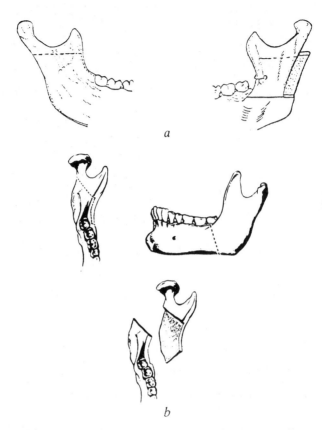

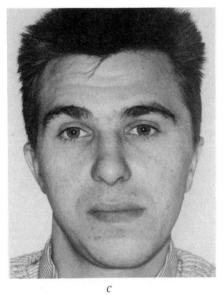

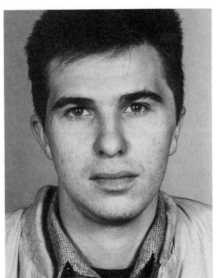

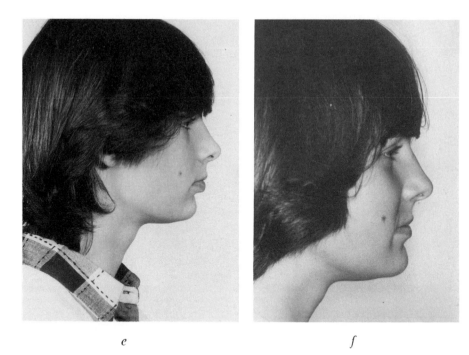

e   *f*

Figure 19.4 (a) High Obwegeser osteotomy cuts for classic sagittal split technique. (b) Dal Pont modification of Obwegeser sagittal split. (c, d) Pre- and postoperative views of asymmetrical prognathism with asymmetry corrected by Obwegeser 'high' sagittal split bilaterally with push-back and rotation. (e, f) Pre- and postoperative profile where orthodontic treatment combined with Dal Pont modification sagittal splits was used to advance the body of the mandible.

Vertical subsigmoid osteotomy

This technique is usually performed intraorally. It is very popular in the USA because of the low incidence of paraesthesia of the inferior dental nerves when the method is used to correct prognathism. The technique also produces an aesthetic improvement to the previously obtuse mandible, though care should be taken not to run the risk of a square facial pattern.

The procedure is not suitable for mandibular advancement and the degree of mandibular retrusion achieved may be constrained by the width of the ramus posteriorly or the impaction of the coronoid process on the temporal aspect of the zygomatic arch. Coronoidectomy may be necessary in some instances, but is associated with trismus. The procedure is performed very rapidly, with little postoperative swelling, especially in the pharynx. Although necrosis of the tip of the distal segment has been reported, this is not a common problem and the incidence of complications is extremely low.

The surgical approach to the ramus, in the intraoral technique,

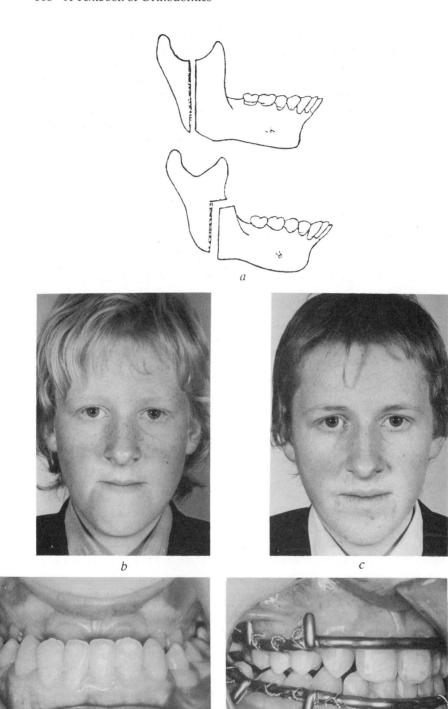

a

b   *c*

d   *e*

involves exposure of the lateral aspect of the ramus only. Retractors in the sigmoid notch above, and under the angle below, provide adequate access and visibility for sectioning of the ramus vertically, behind the antilingula, by means of an oscillating saw. Once the mandible has been sectioned by an oblique cut from the notch above to the lower border, the posterior fragment is overlaid on the lateral aspect of the ramus and the wound is closed. In the hands of the experienced operator the whole procedure takes less than 1 h and the patient is usually discharged from hospital the following day. Intermaxillary fixation may be needed for 4 weeks (Fig. 19.5).

Postcondylar cartilage grafts

Trauner (1954) and, later, Poswillo (1968) described these procedures for the correction of distocclusion in the adolescent who could posture forwards into an acceptable incisal relationship. Using bilateral preauricular incisions, blocks of autogenous or lyophilized cartilage are anchored to the root of the zygoma above, extra-articularly, between the posterior aspect of the head of the condyle and the bony auditory meatus. These blocks hold the whole mandible forwards in the anticipated position of intercuspation (Fig. 19.6). Although postoperative fixation with functional appliances has been used, it is not mandatory. Viability of the cartilage is maintained by tissue fluid perfusion. Forward movement by this technique is usually limited to the width of one premolar tooth. Long-term follow-up reveals that remodelling in the condyle and fossa produce permanent changes in the relationship of the mandible to the base of the skull. The function of the temporomandibular joint is not impaired and the correction of distocclusion and the associated retrognathism are not compromised by relapse. The procedure has been favoured by some authors because of the lack of interference with the periosteum of the ramus of the mandible. Where the choice of advancement lies between sagittal split procedures or postcondylar grafts, and the extent of the advance is not more than one premolar unit, the latter procedure may be preferred for the patient in the late mixed dentition. Early surgical correction of retrognathism by this method permits further functional catch-up growth of the retruded mandible.

Correction of micrognathia and retrognathia

While both micrognathia and retrognathia are often loosely used to describe anterior mandibular deficiency, these terms are not synony-

Figure 19.5 (a) Diagrams showing classic and L-modification vertical subsigmoid bone cuts used for correction of prognathism. (b, c, d, e) Pre- and postoperative views of mandibular prognathism treated by classic intraoral vertical subsigmoid procedure. The archbar fixation provides good visual repositioning of occlusal surfaces with reasonable aesthetics and minimum inconvenience to the patient although fixed orthodontic appliance archwires are just as good.

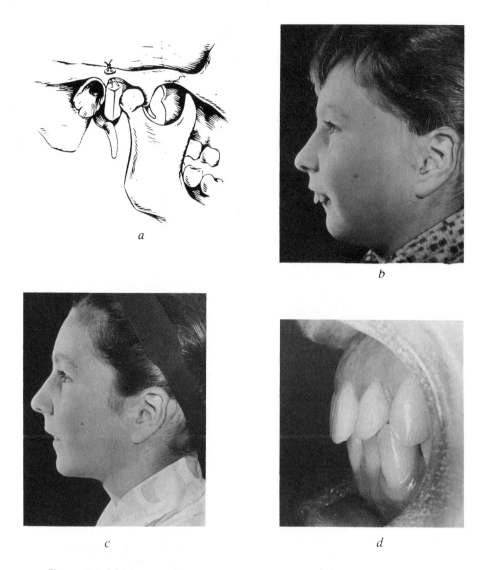

Figure 19.6 (a) Diagram of postcondylar cartilage graft technique. (b, c) Pre- and 1-year postoperative views of corrected distocclusion after this procedure. (d) Lateral view of anterior occlusion of the same patient 15 years after postcondylar cartilage grafts for mandibular advancement.

mous. Micrognathia refers to abnormal smallness of the jaw; a localized form of this is microgenia, where the chin is deficient. Retrognathia implies a retruded position of the mandible without diminution in size.

In surgical terms, correction of micrognathia is more difficult than the correction of prognathism for two principal reasons. First, it is more difficult to augment the mandible than to reduce it; and secondly, when

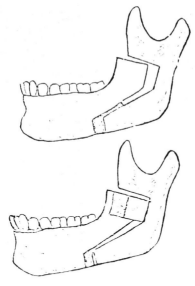

Figure 19.7 Hayes modified L sagittal split used to advance mandibular body. The onlay bone bridge is obtained from the split margin of mandibular bone, thus eliminating an additional operation to 'harvest' bone.

the mandible is small the investing soft tissues are correspondingly reduced. Expansion of the soft tissue envelope by elongation of the jaw may fall short of that which is adequate or desirable.

Ideally, surgical techniques for correction of micrognathia should provide an adequate Class I occlusion, overall aesthetic improvement, including restoration of the chin prominence, a satisfactory gonial angle and minimal disruption to the contents of the mandibular canal or lingual nerve. Innumerable operations have been described, many of which, while technically feasible, have fallen from regular use because of problems associated with relapse. The C osteotomy and the sliding L osteotomy previously referred to have been used with a degree of success, as have modifications of the sagittal split procedure. A combination of the L technique with sagittal splitting of the body portion of the mandible described by Hayes (1973), has probably been the most successful procedure for elongation of the micrognathic mandible (Fig. 19.7). The method appears to satisfy all the criteria mentioned above, with few, if any, of the disadvantages of the L osteotomy or sagittal split procedures when used alone. It would appear that plating has reduced relapse in most osteotomy types and where overlap occurs transfixation screws can also be used in the mandible.

Microgenia and genioplasty techniques

While osteotomy procedures and postcondylar grafts are frequently used to extend the body of the mandible forwards into a more acceptable occlusal and aesthetic position, compromise procedures may occasionally produce equally acceptable results with less morbidity.

When the occlusion is acceptable and all that is required is improvement in the appearance of the chin or in lip position or control relating to incisors, augmentation genioplasty may be the procedure of choice. The simplest method of augmentation is the implantation of a contoured wedge of Proplast into a pocket of periosteum over the chin point. Adjustments to the shape of the alloplastic material permit the correction of small degrees of asymmetry of the chin.

The major disadvantages of alloplastic augmentation of the chin, in the past, have been the degree of bone resorption that subsequently occurs beneath the implant and the migration of the onlays from the position in which they were originally placed. These problems have been most obvious when cartilage or Silastic have been used. It is anticipated, on the basis of short-term experience, that these difficulties may not arise when Proplast or Interpore is used; nevertheless most alloplastic augmentation techniques have their limitations.

The procedure that has best stood the test of time in the field of enlargement of the chin has been the anterior lower-border osteotomy procedure suggested by Obwegeser (1961). This is a modification of Hofer's (1942a) original method; by an intraoral approach, the anterior mandible is degloved and single- or even double-section horizontal sliding osteotomy cuts are made. The bone sections are pulled forwards, rotated and contoured, as occasion demands, and the forwards-sliding grafts are then fixed by transosseous wires plates or transfixation screws.

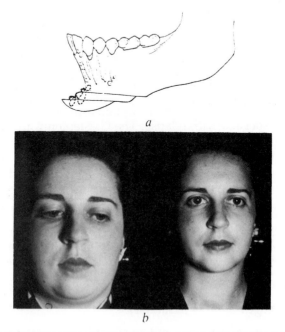

a

b

Figure 19.8 (a) Diagram of two-layer chin advancement by genioplasty. (b) Pre- and postoperative views showing chin contour enhanced by sliding genioplasty.

Slight overcorrection may be used; but lateral portions of the osteotomy segment that project slightly in the mental region are not usually contoured at the time of initial surgery in order to prevent undue rounding of the chin as remodelling proceeds (Fig. 19.8).

A similar technical procedure has been used to reduce chin prominence, often in association with upward movement of the lower border of the mandible in the long-face syndrome. Instead of advancing the upper sliding section in a two-section genioplasty, it is removed, thus reducing the depth of the chin and allowing aesthetic repositioning of the lip chin point and lower border. This flexible technique of genioplasty has been found to provide long-term stability when used both for chin augmentation and reduction. It is infinitely superior to onlay techniques in which autogenous bone grafts are used.

Condylar hyperplasia and mandibular hypertrophy

Developmental hyperplasia of the mandibular condyle usually appears about the time of the adolescent growth spurt. The result is excessive growth of the ramus and condyle on the affected side, leading to asymmetrical prognathism.

The most rapidly effective surgical treatment is excision of the condyle through the condylar neck on the affected side. This technique, timed as soon as opportunity arises after the condition is diagnosed, rapidly restores symmetry of growth and form to the affected side. Within 6–12 months of condylar excision a new condyle has regenerated. The phenomenon of excessive elongation of the condylar head and neck has not been observed in the condyle that appears *de novo*; this long-term stability is achieved by an uncomplicated surgical procedure in a condition which, if untreated, results in severe lateral open bite, or crossbite, with marked facial asymmetry (Fig. 19.9). Occasionally, orthodontic assistance is required to align the arches on the affected side after condylectomy, and to facilitate the closure of a lateral open bite.

If the developmental deformity is not observed until after the cessation of growth, and lateral shift of the mandible has resulted in severe crossbite and prognathism, a sagittal split osteotomy on the affected side, with or without condylotomy on the contralateral side (depending on the degree of rotation of the jaw likely to be required for the correction of acquired crossbite) is the procedure of choice (Poswillo, 1964).

In mandibular hemihypertrophy there may be a lowering of the occlusal plane on the affected side, with aesthetically unacceptable downgrowth of the lower border of the mandible. This produces a form of asymmetry that is difficult to mask without removal of excess basal bone from the lower border of the affected side of the mandible (Fig. 19.10), and where necessary simultaneous levelling of the maxillary occlusal plane.

The presence of the mandibular canal and its contents further complicates surgical approaches to lower-border reduction. The optimal pro-

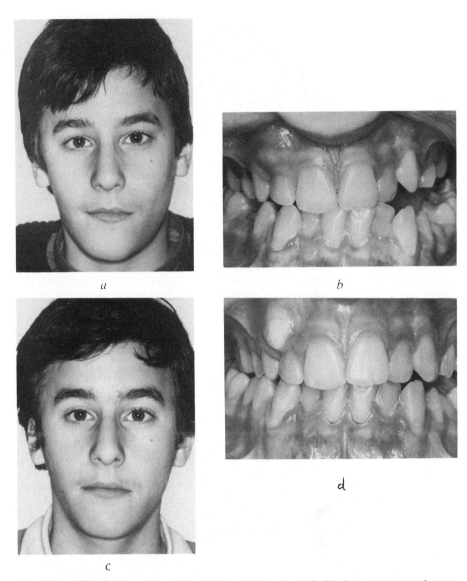

Figure 19.9 full face (a) and dental view (b) showing left-sided asymmetry and open bite associated with left condylar hyperplasia. Full face (c) and dentition (d) before definitive orthodontic treatment, 1 year after left total condylectomy.

cedure, which allows some shortening of the ramus, reduction of open bite (if it exists) and trimming of excess basal bone, is a sagittal split operation extending from above the lingula on the lingual side to the mental foramen labially. Once the mandible is split and the contents of the mandibular canal are dissected free, lower-border reduction can be done to the appropriate level on both labial and lingual plates; the ramus may be shortened, and finally, the nerve placed in the soft

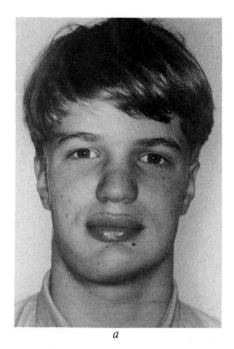

a

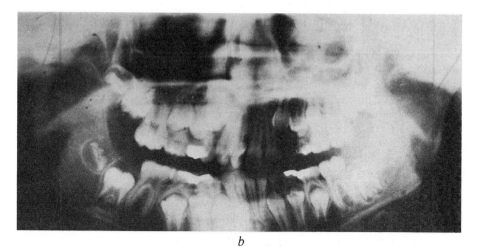

b

Figure 19.10 (a) Full face in right hemihypertrophy of mandible, before orthognathic correction. (b) Orthopantomogram showing increased size of mandible and permanent cheek teeth on affected side.

tissues below the resected border of the mandible before wound closure and skeletal fixation.

Collaboration with the orthodontist in the planning stages, when model surgery on a plaster or acrylic mandible is undertaken, can be of invaluable assistance to the surgeon when planning definitive treatment of these complicated, asymmetrical cases. It is generally unwise to proceed to surgical correction of this condition until adolescent growth is complete. In males this may mean deferring final assessment until the late teens, by which time the third molars will also be in place and their future status may be considered before completion of the treatment plan.

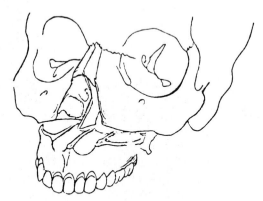

Figure 19.11 Diagram showing principle of 'down-fracture' for Le Fort I maxillary osteotomy.

Maxillary osteotomy procedures

Repositioning of the entire maxillary alveolar process has advanced dramatically in recent years. More than any other orthognathic operation the 'down-fracturing' modification of the earlier Le Fort I osteotomy has permitted access and visibility in areas of the maxilla that were previously unknown territory in the field of orthognathic surgery (Fig. 19.11). Access to the superior surface of the maxillary fragment has permitted a wide range of variations in the original one-piece repositioning procedure. Bell (1975) and others have made numerous important contributions to technique and it is not uncommon for the maxilla to be surgically segmented into numerous parts, which allow optimal positioning of tooth-bearing segments. With adequate illumination, good haemostasis and a substantial palatal pedicle to provide viability to the segments, the range of adjustments to the tooth-bearing maxilla is almost unlimited (Fig. 19.12).

Maxillary surgery has permitted greater attention to discrepancies in facial height (e.g. in the long-face and short-face syndromes and vertical maxillary excess), rotational anomalies (e.g. open bite), and antero-posterior deficiencies, especially maxillary hypoplasia. One of the outstanding advantages of this flexible approach has been the ease with which palatal expansion, elevation or lowering may be achieved. By improving the space available for the tongue, incisor stability is enhanced. These new maxillary techniques have involved, more than ever before, the collaboration of the orthodontist in the preparation of cases for orthognathic surgery.

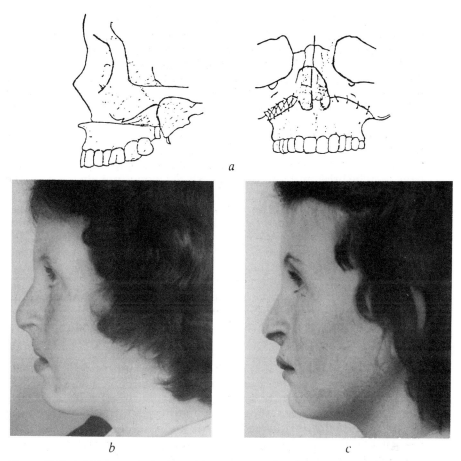

Figure 19.12 (a) Diagrammatic view of anterior repositioning of maxilla in Le Fort I osteotomy and asymmetrical adjustment of vertical facial height. The right side shows a stabilizing onlay rib-graft technique and the left, direct wire fixation. (b, c) Pre- and postoperative profile photographs of Le Fort I maxillary advancement in the secondary surgical correction of a cleft lip and palate defect.

All cases should be planned with an eye to excellent arch matching before surgery: such preparation greatly reduces the need for surgical arch levelling and reangulation of individual small segments. Sectional orthodontic arches are sometimes used to facilitate the definitive correction of occlusal irregularities by multiple sectioning of the maxilla; requiring less orthodontic correction preoperatively and possibly less relapse postoperatively.

The technique of maxillary down-fracture involves a vestibular incision, preferably with a cutting diathermy, from one malar buttress to the other. This is followed by osteotomy cuts above the apices of the teeth. The nasal septum, lateral nasal walls and pterygoid plates are separated with appropriate chisels and osteotomes. The maxilla is mobilized, appropriate bone cuts are made in the maxilla proper or in the attached bones above, in order to realign the tooth-bearing segments or move the maxilla upwards, forwards or even slightly backwards. Bone grafts, while not mandatory, are frequently used to stabilize the segments and promote union. Various methods of fixation, by external rods, internal wires or increasingly plates, may be used to support the maxilla in the correct relationship to the mandible below and the cranial base above.

While this short description of technique would suggest that the procedure is usually simple and uncomplicated, it is not always so. Occasionally, maxillae tethered by scar tissue are exceedingly difficult to mobilize. This is especially true of the post-traumatic injury. Haemorrhage may be brisk and tedious to arrest. Fixation is not always a simple procedure. When orthodontic collaboration has been provided preoperatively, it is prudent to use the bands and fixed, sturdy archwires (to which cleats for wires or elastics have been attached) for definitive intermaxillary fixation. A thin, acrylic wafer may be placed in the desired position of intercuspation to augment fixation and ensure ideal cuspal interdigitation and stability.

After removal of the intermaxillary wires, attention should be paid by the orthodontist to occlusal irregularities before fixed or orthodontic appliances are removed. These finishing touches are of the greatest assistance to the oral surgeon in the pursuit of excellence in orthognathic surgery.

It may be observed, in cases where multiple small segments of maxilla have been repositioned, that teeth do not respond to clinical vitality tests for long periods after operation. While teeth on smaller segments may be compromised to a greater or lesser degree by postoperative ischaemia, studies have shown that pulp viability, as distinct from vitality, is usually maintained. In the fullness of time, ingrowth of sensory nerves from the adjacent periodontal tissues provides a degree of recovery of traditional pulpal vitality (Poswillo, 1972).

Bimaxillary orthognathic surgery

Some cases of dentofacial deformity are sufficiently severe to warrant surgical repositioning of both maxillary and mandibular tooth-bearing segments. Where anteroposterior movements of greater than 1 cm are needed, or where, for example, the maxilla must be elevated and the mandible advanced, it is necessary to carry out simultaneous procedures on both jaws.

The bimaxillary approach has the considerable advantage of permitting the surgeon to reposition the total maxilla–mandible complex with respect to the cranial base. The jaws may be advanced, raised, lowered, rotated or asymmetrically moved in order to achieve the planned position. Maxillary osteotomies, while usually carried out at the Le Fort I level, may be at any other level, and in general, the entire dental arches of both maxilla and mandible are mobilized and repositioned (Fig. 19.13).

Technically, the basic procedures of mandibular and maxillary osteo-

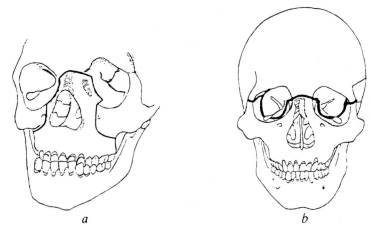

Figure 19.13 (a) Surgical bone cut lines used for Fort II osteotomy. (b) Bone cuts in Tessier I, Le Fort III osteotomy.

tomies (previously described) are carried out sequentially: the surgeon will decide which jaw is to be repositioned first. Stable internal fixation with plates is usually applied after bimaxillary procedures and it is now much less common to use external rods attached to cranial fixation even in conjunction with fixed orthodontic appliances (Ferguson, 1985). The complexities of the fixation and the degree of acceptability of each alternative method should be discussed with the patient before completion of the treatment plan.

The lengthy surgical procedure involved in bimaxillary correction produces additional burdens on patient and surgeon: blood transfusions (including autologous) may be required; bone grafts (with the added potential morbidity of a donor site) may be necessary; the risk of injury to peripheral sensory nerves is greater; and the chances of incorrect surgical repositioning are increased. All these matters should be discussed with the candidate for bimaxillary surgery when informed consent to the procedure is sought.

The versatility of combined maxillary and mandibular procedures makes possible the correction of almost any conceivable deformity that may present to the orthodontist and oral surgeon. The results will depend less on the imagination of the experts than on the degree of care taken with the case assessment and preoperative planning, and the ability with which the essential technical procedures are carried out.

Surgical correction of open bite

There are numerous ways to close anterior or posterior open bite. The choice of procedure is determined by the results of clinical and cephalometric analysis. Attention should be paid to the pattern of rotational development of the face, the relationship between the skeletal bases, anteriorly and posteriorly, the angles of the maxillary and mandibular occlusal planes, and the anterior and posterior facial heights. Measurements should be made of the relationship between the nasolabial angle, the upper lip and the upper incisors. The aim of the procedure is to produce lip competence and incisor control, an aesthetic nasal tip and lip/incisor relationships, pleasing nasolabial and labiomental curves. The orthodontist provides invaluable preoperative assistance by flattening the dental arches and realigning the incisors in such a way that an ideal interincisal angle may be achieved after surgery.

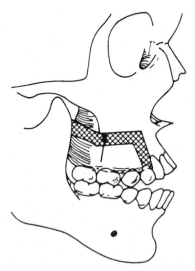

Figure 19.14 Schuchardt upper buccal segment repositioning procedure. Cross-hatched area represents excised bone.

While there are many technical options, including upper and lower segmental procedures, Le Fort I maxillary repositioning and antero-mandibuloplasty (Foster and Henderson, 1981), the choice will ultimately be made on the results of case analysis. Simple rotation of the mandible seldom produces a stable result. Similarly, intrusion of the upper buccal segments by a Schuchardt (1961) procedure is seldom successful unless it is combined with a mandibular sagittal osteotomy (Fig. 19.14). While the Schuchardt technique may be suitable when there is a convenient step in the maxillary arch, it may have to be varied considerably when the maxillary dental arch is well aligned. In general, the upper buccal segment is intruded more than the anterior segment, by any suitable maxillary procedure, and the mandible is then rotated forwards and upwards. If chin retrusion remains a problem, it may be corrected by a combined advancement and reduction genioplasty.

Finally, the role of the tongue in the maintenance of open bite is very much a matter for consideration during the planning of procedures to close, permanently, an anterior open bite. When abnormal tongue function cannot be controlled, a surgically closed anterior open bite almost invariably relapses. Lip competence and optimal interincisal angulation do much to reduce this problem, but it cannot always be eliminated. Anticipation is the best method of avoiding this form of relapse.

Segmental osteotomies

As early as 1849, Hullihen described the first anterior mandibular segmental osteotomy. In 1942 Hofer (1942a) used a similar intraoral approach to accomplish a forward movement of the anterior maxillary segment. Since these early descriptions, a plethora of small osteotomy procedures, carried out by an intraoral approach, have been described for the correction of severe malposition of the teeth, all on the same segment, when the basal bone is in a relatively satisfactory position. These techniques have the advantage over conventional orthodontic alignment in that the teeth can be moved a considerable distance, upwards, downwards, laterally or obliquely, by a one-stage surgical repositioning, with little likelihood of significant relapse. The anterior maxillary and mandibular segmental osteotomies rapidly produce the refinements of lip contour and anterior occlusion that orthodontic treatment might be hoped to provide, but with less likelihood of idiopathic root resorption, especially in adults.

The anterior maxillary osteotomy of Wassmund (1935) is a one-stage procedure to alter, to a more acceptable aesthetic and functional position, the premaxillary segment that is protruded (Fig. 19.15). The segment to be treated may include the premolar teeth bilaterally and all the anterior teeth on any of the various segments within these limits. The midline of the premaxilla may also be split to move the two halves independently and close a diastema between the incisors. The anterior maxillary arch may be recontoured, moved superiorly or inferiorly, rotated or even advanced (utilizing an interpositional graft) by this well-established technique.

Originally, the method involved vertical incisions in the midline and premolar regions that enabled, by a tunnelling approach, bone cuts to be made in predetermined sites so that the premaxilla could be separated from the maxilla without depriving it of essential blood supplies. On the palatal aspect, gingival margin and midline incisions enabled tunnels to be created, giving access to burs and chisels with which adequate bone was removed to effect the desired new position of the segment. After detachment from the nasal septum the premaxillary segment was moved to the new position and fixed with an archbar constructed on the surgically corrected models.

Numerous variations of the technique permit the surgery to be carried out from a palatal approach (Wunderer, 1965) or by a down-fracture of the anterior maxilla (Cupar, 1954). The principal advantage of the premaxillary osteotomies is that they can reduce maxillary excess in the adult who has a reasonable nose and mandible in circumstances where orthodontic treatment may not be acceptable. Occasionally the procedure is valuable in the realignment of upper incisors that are suffering severe gingival stripping on the palatal aspect. Rarely, anterior open bite may be corrected by this technique.

One serious disadvantage of the anterior maxillary osteotomy by the classic Wassmund or the down-fracture approach is the loss of the anterior nasal spine during sectioning of the anterior nasal rim. When this happens a flat, ugly lip, with obliquity of nasolabial angle, develops. This so-called Wassmund lip is seldom observed by the patient, but it mars the appearance in profile of the patient, who otherwise may be considered to have a satisfactory result. This complication can be avoided by careful dissection of the nasal rim, permitting bone cuts that free the anterior maxilla without detachment of the nasal spine. Attempts to restore the lost nasal spine by small bone grafts are doomed to failure through rapid resorption of the onlay.

Following the Wassmund-type procedure, the teeth on the premaxillary segment may remain unresponsive to sensory stimuli for periods of a year or more. Careful radiological review of such teeth is essential, for the incidence of pulp death, followed by periapical infection, is higher in this procedure than in many other orthognathic operations.

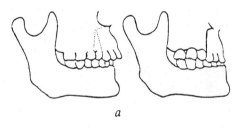

a

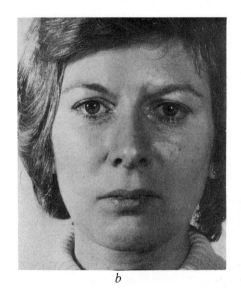

b

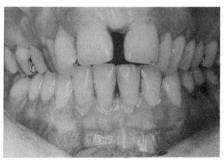

c

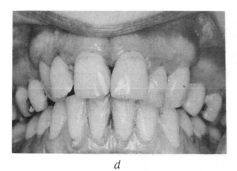

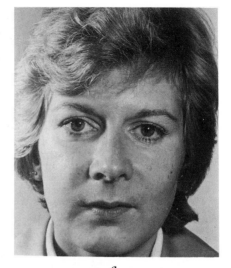

d

e

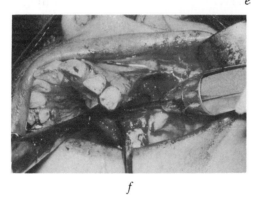

f

Figure 19.15 (a) Posterior repositioning of maxillary anterior segment by Wassmund technique. (b, c, d, e) Pre- and postoperative views of face and teeth where orthodontic treatment with removable appliances in adolescence had not been successfully completed. The residual aesthetic and occlusal problems were corrected by a compromise procedure of Wassmund repositioning with sagittal splitting of the premaxilla to close the diastema. Preservation of the anterior nasal spine has maintained columella prominence. (f) Surgical tunnelling to divide palatal bone before splitting the premaxilla.

The posterior maxillary osteotomy of Schuchardt is used for the treatment of posterior maxillary excess, the long-face syndrome and, occasionally, anterior open bite. By intruding the buccal segments upwards into the space provided by the maxillary sinus, the occlusal plane can be levelled both anteroposteriorly and laterally, and the anterior face can be shortened. Where much of the beneficial effect results from autorotation of the mandible, as mentioned in the discussion of open bite, results are disappointing because of the frequent tendency to early relapse.

The surgical technique usually involves a one-stage procedure in which a buccal approach is made to the lateral and palatal walls of the posterior osseous segment. Removal of the precise amount of bone from the lateral wall with an oscillating saw allows access to the alveolar and palatal bone on the deep aspect. Sectioning is completed by the use of a curved osteotome or bur, and the maxillary segment is finally separated from the pterygoid plates with a fine, curved osteotome. The freed segment is positioned exactly and fitted into a prefabricated wafer or archbar. Additional fixation is provided by a circumzygomatic wire. If mandibular surgery has been carried out at the same time, the circumzygomatic wire may be attached to the mandibular arch.

The complications from this procedure are few. As with all alveolar osteotomies in the maxilla, union of the fine bones may be slow. Rarely, an oroantral fistula may appear. The principal reason for the waning popularity of this technique is the unpredictable nature of the relapse and its declining applicability.

The lower labial-segment repositioning procedure of Köle (1959) is frequently used to reduce excessive anterior mandibular height, improve the labiomental curve and correct the occlusal plane with a reverse curve of Spee. Occasionally it is used to correct anterior open bite or realign proclined mandibular incisors.

Technically, the procedure is relatively simple. The reflection of the labial tissues allows a direct approach to the bone cuts. The vascular pedicle of the genial muscles nourishes the segment from the lingual side. Before surgery begins the operation must be planned to the last millimetre by model surgery. Critical attention must be given to the intercanine width and the feasibility of fitting the repositioned lower arch into an appropriate relationship within the curve of the upper arch. Changes in lower facial height must be calculated with care. Avoiding damage to the roots of teeth can often be a difficult exercise. The sulcus tissues must be closed in layers with great care to avoid seepage of fluid and subsequent infection.

This procedure, when performed with meticulous attention to detail, alone or in combination with other orthognathic procedures, can be of the greatest value to the oral surgeon and orthodontist. Under optimal circumstances the complications of numbness of the lip and denervation of the teeth are only transitory problems. Rarely, infarction and loss of the whole segment has occurred. This is a very high price to pay for what is, in the final analysis, aesthetic dentofacial surgery.

The Sowray-Haskell (1968) technique incorporates the lower labial segmental osteotomy with a step-excision of basal bone at the lower border (Fig. 19.16). If a block of basal bone is excised in the midline and the margins are pulled together, lateral crossbite and mild prognathism can be reduced. Removal of bone sections unilaterally permits correction of asymmetry. As with the Köle procedure, great care must be taken to obtain precise measurements of anticipated movements of segments at the model planning stage. The method is occasionally used to advantage in correcting mandibular discrepancies in the cleft palate patient. The principal advantage of this technique, and of other anteromandibulo-plasties, over the Köle procedure, is that there is a greater opportunity

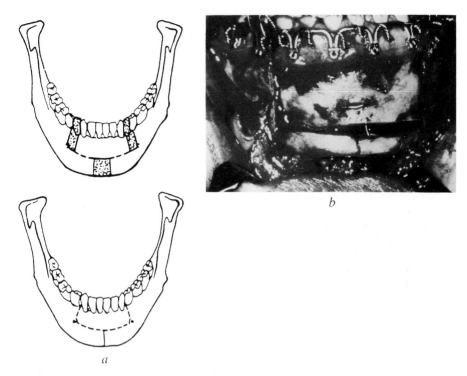

Figure 19.16 (a) Technical stages in Sowray-Haskell anterior mandibuloplasty. (b) Intraoral operative view after removal of central section of lower border of mandible, retrusion and intrusion of lower labial segment and stabilization by direct interosseous fixation.

to control chin prominence and minor asymmetry while varying the height and inclination of the lower labial segment.

The complications associated with these procedures are those previously described for lower labial-segment repositioning. Most difficulties can be prevented by careful model surgery and good preoperative radiological assessment of the position of the roots of the teeth and the location of the mental nerves.

Guidelines for orthodontic and oral surgical collaboration

Joint procedures between orthodontists and oral surgeons are more successful when there is early agreement on the likelihood of surgical intervention. Appropriate arrangements can then be made for clinical and radiological examinations and joint consultations throughout the preoperative treatment period. Decisions can be taken, during combined clinics, on such important factors as the amount of arch expansion for decompensation, the optimal interincisal angulation and the ultimate lip levels required to achieve competence and aesthetics.

Collaboration at the stage of profile planning permits the development of an ideal orthodontic prescription. Decisions can be made on the method and extent of surgery. If bimaxillary surgery appears likely, the associated orthodontic constraints, if any, can be determined.

Regular reviews of the progress of orthodontic treatment by both surgeon and orthodontist enable final technical details to be decided. Arrangements can be made concerning the type of fixation to be used, modifications needed in the fixed appliances can be discussed and arranged, and the patient can be advised of all likely events, orthodontic and surgical, that may arise during the postoperative period.

The attendance of the orthodontist during the final stages of the orthognathic surgical procedure is of great assistance to the surgical team. Definitive decisions can then be made jointly on such matters as the suitability of the position of the dentoalveolar segments and the load imposed on the orthodontic appliances by the surgical fixation; agreement can be reached on individual responsibilities for continuing care of the patient during the recovery period. Finally, mutual understanding between orthodontist and surgeon creates a climate for innovation and research, which is essential for the development of the art and science of craniomaxillofacial reconstruction. The pioneers of surgical orthodontics would agree that Blair's (1909) classic comment that the mandible 'is a hoop of bone capable of almost any kind of adjustment' is more relevant and realistic now than ever before. One suspects that his comment today to the orthodontists and their surgical collaborators would be to ask: 'Are there any restrictions on the timing or technique of orthognathic surgery; and if so, what are you doing to overcome them?'

References

Bell, W. H. (1975) Le Fort I osteotomy for correction of maxillary deformities. *Journal of Oral Surgery*, **33**, 412–426

Bell, W.H., Proffit, W. R. and White, R. P. (1980) *Surgical Correction of Dentofacial Deformities*, W. B. Saunders, Philadelphia

Blair, V. P. (1909) Underdeveloped lower jaw with limited excursion. *Journal of the American Medical Association*, **53**, 178–183

Byrne, R. P. and Hinds, E. C. (1974) The ramus 'C' osteotomy with body sagittal split. *Journal of Oral Surgery*, **32**, 259–263

Cupar, I. (1954) Die chirurgische Behandlung der Form-und Stellungsveranderungen des Oberkiefers *Oesterreichische Zeitschrift fur Stomatologie*, **51**, 565–581.

Dal Pont, G. (1961) Retromolar osteotomy for the correction of prognathism. *Journal of Oral Surgery, Anesthesia and Hospital Dental Service*, **19**, 42–47

Ferguson, J., Lewis, D. and Foster, M. E. (1985) Improved craniomaxillary fixation using orthodontic appliances. *British Journal of Orthodontics*, **12**, 46–48

Foster, M. E. and Henderson, D. (1981) Anterior mandibuloplasty. *British Journal of Oral Surgery*, **19**, 258–264

Harradine, N. W. T. and Birnie, D. (1985) Computer prediction of the result of orthognathic surgery. *Journal of Maxillofacial Surgery*, **13**, 245–249

Hayes, P. A. (1973) Correction of retrognathia by modified 'C' osteotomy of the ramus and sagittal osteotomy of the mandibular body. *Journal of Oral Surgery*, **31**, 682–686

Henderson, D. and Poswillo, D. (1985) *A Colour Atlas of Orthognathic Surgery*, Wolfe, London

Hofer, O. (1942a) Die vertikale osteotomie zur verlangerung des einseitig verkurtzen aufsteigenden unterkieferastes. *Oesterreichische Zeitschrift fur Stomatologie (Wein)*, **34**, 286–289

Hofer, O. (1942b) Operation der prognathie und microgenie. *Deutsche Zeitschrift fur Mun Kiefer und Gesichts Chirurgie (Munchen)*, **9**, 121–127

Hullihen, S. P. (1849) Case of elongation of the underjaw and distortion of the face and neck. Zurich, Swiss Society of Plastic and Reconstructive Surgeons, 1965.

Köle, H. (1959) Surgical operations on the alveolar ridge to correct occlusal abnormalities. *Oral Surgery, Oral Medicine, Oral Pathology*, **12**, 515–524

Obwegeser, H. (1961) Vorteile und moglichkeiten des intraoralen vorgehens bei der korrektur von unterkieferanomaliess. *Fortschritte der Kiefer und Gesichts Chirurgie (Stuttgart)*, **7**, 159–164

Obwegeser, H. (1964). The indications for surgical correction of mandibular deformity by the sagittal splitting technique. *British Journal of Oral Surgery*, **1**, 157–171

Obwegeser, H. and Trauner, R. (1957) The surgical correction of mandibular prognathism and retrognathism with consideration of genioplasty: Part I. *Oral Surgery, Oral Medicine, Oral Pathology*, **10**, 677–689

Poswillo, D. (1964) The surgery of orofacial deformity. *Australian Dental Journal*, **9**, 345–353

Poswillo, D. (1968) The aetiology and surgery of cleft palate with micrognathia. *Annals of the Royal College of Surgeons of England*, **43**, 61–88

Poswillo, D. (1972) Early pulp changes following reduction of open bite by segmental surgery. *International Journal of Oral Surgery*, **1**, 87–97

Schuchardt, K. (1961) Experiences with the surgical treatment of some deformities of the jaws: prognathia, micrognathia, and open bite. In *Transactions of the 2nd Congress of the International Society of Plastic Surgeons* (London, 1959) (ed. A. G. Wallace) Livingstone, Edinburgh, p. 73

Sowray, J. H. and Haskell, R. (1968) Osteotomy at the mandibular symphysis. *British Journal of Oral Surgery*, **6**, 97–102

Trauner, R. (1954) Die retrokondylare implantation eine operationsmethode zum vorbringen des unterkiefer beim distalbiss. *Deutsche Zahn-, Mund- und Keiferheilkunde mit Zentralblatt fur die Gesamte Zahn- Mund- und Keiferheilkunde (Leipzig)*, **21**, 391

Wassmund, M. (1935) *Lehrbuch der Praktischen Chirurgie des Mundes und der Kiefer*, Vol. 1, Barth, Leipzig

Wunderer, S. (1965) Surgical correction of the profile by operation on the maxilla. In *Proceedings of the 2nd Meeting of the Swiss Society of Plastic and Reconstructive Surgeons* (Zurich, November 1965) Swiss Society of Plastic and Reconstructive Surgeons, Zurich

Chapter 20

Clefts of the lip and palate

Michael Mars

Cleft lip and palate is the most common malformation in the craniofacial region and the reported incidence is 1 in 700 live births (i.e. 1000 new cases per year in the UK). The incidence varies according to the type of cleft, racial group and sex: cleft lip with or without cleft palate (CL(P)) ranges from about 3.6 per 1000 births for Indians to 0.5 per 1000 for negroes with an incidence of about 1 per 700 for Caucasians (Gorlin, Cervenka and Pruzansky, 1971). However, the reported frequency varies even within racial groups. Some of these differences may be due to variations in methods and efficiency of recording facial deformity. In Caucasians at least, CL(P) is more common in males (about 60 per cent) and unilateral clefts occur more often on the left side. Isolated cleft palate is less common, occurring about once in 2000 births, and more often in females.

The aetiology of clefts of the lip and palate is still a matter of debate. Certain types of cleft have a family history and so there is sometimes a genetic predisposition to clefting, which may be triggered by environmental factors. This hypothesis is supported by the results of studies in animals. Some strains of mice, for example, are particularly susceptible to clefting of the palate, which occurs spontaneously in a proportion of the offspring, but the frequency can be increased greatly by a variety of drugs and other environmental insults at critical periods in development (Loevy, 1962). However, the role of such teratogenic influences is not clearly established in man. Specifically, dilantin sodium when taken by epileptic women in pregnancy has been shown to significantly increase the incidence of cleft lip and palate.

Classification

Clefts can vary in severity from minor notching of the lip or a bifid uvula, to complete bilateral clefting of lip and palate (Figs. 20.1, 20.2, 20.3 and 20.4). A number of different methods of classification have been proposed. Veau's classification was one of the earlier and most widely known (Fig. 20.5).

Kernahan and Stark (1958) introduced a more comprehensive classification, based upon the embryology of the deformity. The incisive foramen is regarded as the demarcation between primary and secondary palates:

Clefts of the primary palate. These vary from notching of the upper lip to clefts of the lip and alveolar process as far back as the incisive foramen.

Clefts of the secondary palate. Clefts of the soft and hard palate as far forward as the incisive foramen.

Clefts of the primary and secondary palates. These may be complete or incomplete, unilateral or bilateral.

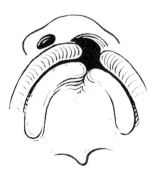
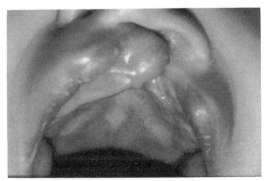

Figure 20.1 Unilateral cleft lip and alveolar process.

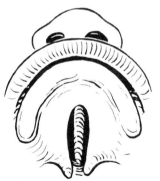
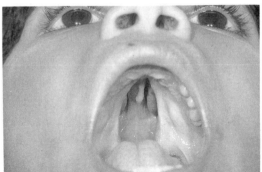

Figure 20.2 Cleft palate.

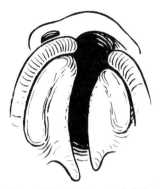
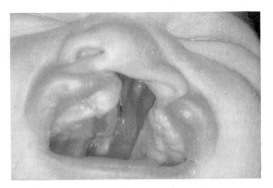

Figure 20.3 Unilateral cleft lip and palate.

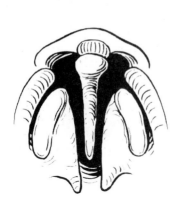

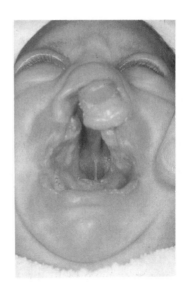

Figure 20.4 Bilateral cleft lip and palate.

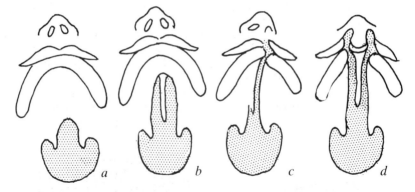

Figure 20.5 Veau's classification: (a) cleft involving the soft palate only; (b) cleft of the soft palate and hard palate as far forward as the incisive foramen; (c) unilateral complete cleft of lip and palate; (d) bilateral complete cleft of lip and palate.

Embryology

The embryology of facial development is complex and is still not fully elucidated (Sperber, 1989). The embryonic globular process, which arises from the medial nasal processes, gives rise to the tip of the nose, columella, philtrum of the upper lip and the primary plate. Between 7 and 8 weeks *in utero* (i.u), mesodermal invasion results in a merging of the globular and maxillary processes to form the upper lip. Failure of adequate mesodermal migration can result in complete or incomplete clefting of the lip.

The hard palate posterior to the incisive foramen and the soft palate are formed from the palatal shelves, which develop from the inner surfaces of the maxillary processes during the sixth week i.u. Because the tongue fills the oronasal cavity at this stage, the palatal shelves are bent down at its sides. By the eighth week, the stomatodeal chamber has enlarged so that the tongue descends, allowing the palatal shelves to swing up and achieve contact with one another, with the primary palate anteriorly and with the nasal septum above. The epithelium at the sites of contact breaks down and these processes fuse between 8 and 12 weeks i.u. Lack of elevation of the palatal processes at the critical time, or failure to contact, or inadequate epithelial breakdown, give rise to a cleft of the secondary palate. A submucous cleft can arise if mesodermal invasion is inadequate, and this can cause poor soft-palate control and defective speech, and can be regarded as two mucosal layers without muscle in between.

Facial growth

The studies that have been conducted into the facial characteristics in adults with unrepaired clefts of the lip and palate, show very little interference with facial growth (Mars and Houston, 1990) (Fig. 20.6). The upper face is often rather wide, but whether this has been an aetiological factor, or arises as a result of the structural discontinuity, is not yet clear.

In many children with surgically repaired clefts of lip and palate, maxillary growth is affected, and in some cases to a serious extent (Fig. 20.7). There are several reasons for this. The repaired lip may be very scarred and tight, and this not only restrains the upper incisor teeth but could restrict forward growth of the entire maxilla. In some surgical procedures for repair of the palate, the mucoperiosteum is undermined extensively and scar tissue in the pterygomaxillary suture area could

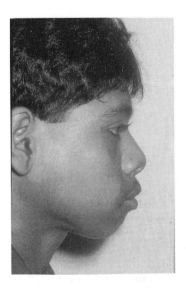 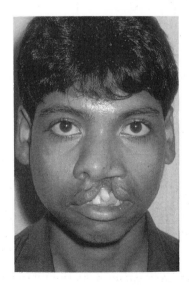

Figure 20.6   A Sri Lankan with an unoperated unilateral cleft of lip and palate.

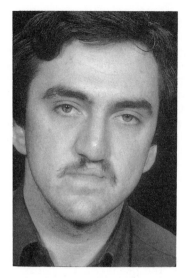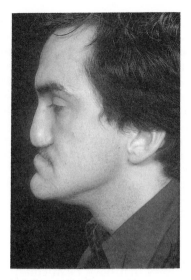

Figure 20.7 A patient operated upon in early infancy showing resulting severe midface retrusion in adult life.

interfere with growth. The type of surgical procedure and the skill of the surgeon are important factors influencing the severity of growth deficiencies. It must also be acknowledged that in many cases of cleft lip and palate, tissue is deficient from the start; and if the cleft is repaired, the maxilla must be narrowed. Ideally these patients should receive treatment in a small number of specialized centres where dedicated multidisciplinary teams can develop experience and where large numbers of patients make clinical research meaningful.

Management of the child with a cleft of lip and palate

Immediate management at birth

The parents are naturally very distressed when they find that their child has a facial cleft. At an early stage, the general implications and management of the problem should be discussed and it can be helpful to illustrate the points in broad terms, with photographs of a child who had a similar type of cleft. It is important to be realistic and to use an illustration of a typical rather than an outstandinly good result, otherwise expectations may be unreasonably high. Some infants with clefts of the lip and palate have other congenital deformities and, if they are serious, their management takes precedence. A parents' support group – The Cleft Lip and Palate Association (CLAPA) – is established in most centres throughout the UK. One of the main aims of this association is to provide help from the parents of older children born with this condition to the parents of newborn children with cleft lip and palates. Such individuals can provide special reassurance, which the professionals are often unable to do. Feeding can be a problem but the difficulties should not be exaggerated. Most infants can be bottle fed by the mother, if a large teat with an enlarged hole is used. Some need to be spoon fed. A feeding plate can be helpful.

Respiratory and middle ear infections are particularly common in cleft palate children, owing to regurgitation of food and saliva into the nasopharynx, and inadequate drainage of the Eustachian tubes. These open through the action of the palatal musculature, which in the cleft lip and palate subject is abnormally inserted. This is a serious matter in that any hearing loss exacerbates the difficulties with speech development and, if unrecognized, interferes with educational progress.

The cleft lip and palate team

There can be few conditions that require the expertise of so many specialists from birth to maturity. Cleft lip and palate patients may have frequent admissions to hospital for surgical procedures as well as multiple outpatient appointments throughout their school years. An ideal team should comprise plastic and maxillofacial surgeons, ear, nose and throat specialists, speech therapists, paediatricians, orthodontists and dental practitioners. It is very important that the different specialists work together as a team, one of whose members will coordinate their activites and maintain contact with the child and parents throughout the period of growth. Because of the need for extended supervision of facial growth and occlusal development, the orthodontist is often well placed to accept the responsibility as coordinator.

It is not possible to describe here the comprehensive management of the child with cleft lip and palate. The typical timing of different contributions is indicated in Table 20.1 but, of course, individual needs vary. In the interests of clarity, surgical and orthodontic management and the role of the dental practitioner are discussed separately, but, of course, these have to be coordinated with one another and with the other specialties.

Presurgical orthopaedics

The fitting of plates to align the maxillary segments within the first days of life is a routine in many cleft lip and palate centres. The proponents of these procedures (presurgical orthopaedics) claim that they help the baby to feed, by separating the oral and nasal cavities, facilitate surgery to the lip and palate, help long-term growth of the face and improve the relationship between the clinicians and the parents in the early stages (Burston, 1958). Whilst these procedures have been undertaken in the UK since the 1950s, no controlled study has reliably demonstrated their advantages. Many centres have now abandoned presurgical orthopaedics except for the most severe bilateral cleft lip and palate cases. It is likely that this form of treatment will remain controversial for the foreseeable future, with the proponents and opponents being equally trenchant in their attitudes.

Table 20.1 A guide to timing treatment for children with clefts of lip and palate

Age	Plastic surgery	Orthodontics	General dental care	ENT	Speech therapy	Oral surgery
Birth	Evaluation and counsel parents	Records/feeding plate and/or orthopaedic appliance	Advice to parents on dental care, prevention of caries			
3 mths–1 yr	Lip repair Palate repair		Regular checks continuing until adult	Regular checks until adult	Observation Evaluate speech at 2–3 yr Speech therapy	
5–12 yr	Minor lip revision	Simple correction of instanding incisors Arch expansion, if required, before alveolar bone graft				Alveolar bone graft at about 10 yr
12–14 yr		Definitive orthodontic treatment				
15–18 yr	Nose revision		Bridge and denture work			Maxillofacial surgery to correct skeletal malrelationships if required

Surgical management

The lip is usually repaired at 6–12 weeks, though many centres now undertake neonatal repair. The exact timing and surgical procedure depend on the practice of the surgeon and on the health of the infant. If presurgical orthopaedic alignment of the maxillary segments is undertaken (see p. 393), the lip is usually repaired at about 3 months.

Many different procedures can be used to repair the lip. The objective is to produce a lip of adequate length that is not tight and that is functionally satisfactory. The mucosa, muscle and skin are sutured separately. It is now recognized that in a cleft lip the orbicularis oris muscle is abnormally inserted into the bony margins at the cleft and these attachments need to be detached and sutured together otherwise the lip will not function well. A good vermilion border is important and this may need later revision.

Attempts have been made to close the bony defect in the alveolar process by bone grafting at the time of the primary lip repair (Friede and Johansen, 1974). The results were generally disappointing and primary bone grafting has been abandoned in most centres.

The optimal timing of closure of the secondary palate is a subject of fierce debate. There are strong arguments for closing the palate by 18 months to obtain more normal function before speech is etablished, and to reduce the problems of regurgitation into the nasopharynx (Blijdorp and Müller, 1984). The potential disadvantage of early repair is the risk of interference with maxillary growth. Postponement of hard palate repair until 5 years or even later, following earlier closure of the soft palate, is advocated by a number of authorities (Hotz and Gnoinski, 1978). No convincing evidence is available to support the view that facial growth is superior in these cases, but adequate comparative studies are lacking. However, studies show that such delayed palatal closure can seriously compromise speech (Witzel, Salyer and Ross, 1984).

A number of surgical procedures for palate closure are currently used. In all of these, the nasal mucosa, muscle and oral mucosa are closed in separate layers. The extent of the deficiency and the need to lengthen the soft palate are factors that influence the approach. It is important to obtain adequate soft palate function in order to minimize nasal escape during speech and swallowing. In some patients a pharyngoplasty is undertaken later to improve the velopharyngeal seal. This involves taking a flap of pharyngeal mucosa and muscle and suturing it into the back of the soft palate, thereby achieving a physical blockage to nasal air escape.

A variety of secondary surgical procedures may be required: revision of nose or lip to improve the appearance; delayed bone grafting to unite the maxillary segments; closure of palatal fistulae; and maxillofacial surgery to correct skeletal malrelationships. Repeated surgical intervention should be avoided: it can result in extensive scarring and is a continuing strain on the patient and family. Most secondary surgical procedures should be deferred until the mid to late teens when they can be undertaken in a comprehensively planned and definitive manner. However, delayed bone grafting is undertaken before the eruption of the permanent canines, as discussed later (see p. 397).

Orthodontic problems in cleft lip and palate patients

There are three main problems in the orthodontic management of cleft lip and palate patients:

1. Growth of the face.
2. Malalignment of the dentition especially at the cleft site.
3. Lack of bone into which to move teeth in the cleft area.

Growth of the face

A significant proportion of patients with repaired cleft lip and palate subsequently develop severe maxillary retrusion (about 40 per cent of cases in a recent study of British centres by Mars *et al.* (1987)). This is often correctable only by extensive maxillofacial surgery. The problem may not become apparent until after the pubertal growth spurt. Frequently, prepubertal children present with pleasing facial appearances; but with further growth the maxilla appears to become 'stuck on the cranial base' (Fig. 20.8). Growth disruption may be evident in all three planes of space – anteroposterior, vertical and transverse. Gross overclosure to achieve an occlusion is often the result of a lack of vertical growth of the maxilla.

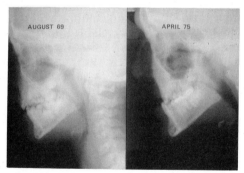

Figure 20.8 Lateral skull radiographs of a patient with unilateral cleft lip and palate. Left film prepuberty, right film postpuberty, showing poor growth of the maxilla in relation to the mandible.

Heroic attempts to achieve an orthodontic result in the early permanent dentition are frequently frustrated by further growth of the mandible without corresponding growth of the maxilla. In consequence, future surgical correction may have been compromised by previous orthodontic retroclination of the lower labial segment, which will then have to be reuprighted in preparation for any surgery. Relapse of orthodontic results is frequently due to scar tissue contraction and is especially marked when rapid maxillary expansion has achieved dramatic improvements in narrow maxillae but where permanent retention has not been used. As mentioned above, forward growth of the mandible is frequently the cause of failed orthodontic treatment but is not strictly relapse. As yet, individual growth prediction is inaccurate and such 'relapses' will inevitably occur. Wherever it is possible to assume that a satisfactory orthodontic result is not likely to be achieved, limited orthodontic treatment aimed at alignment of the teeth within the upper arch only should be considered. The lower arch should be accepted until growth has ceased, when the uprighting of lower incisors over the apical base can be achieved in preparation for surgical correction of the skeletal malrelationships.

Malalignment of the dentition

The upper arch is frequently narrow, with anterior and posterior crossbites. Teeth are frequently absent at the cleft site (usually the lateral incisor.) Often small, pointed, so-called fissural teeth, as well a supernumerary teeth, may be present on either side of the cleft. The upper central incisor adjacent to the cleft is often tilted lingually and its root is more mesially placed while the crown tilts distally and upwards into the cleft. Often only a thin lamina dura surrounds the root of the central incisor on the cleft site.

Lack of bone in the cleft site

It is impossible to move teeth orthodontically when bone is absent. The advent of delayed alveolar bone grafting (Bergland, Semb and Åbyholm 1986), used since the early 1980s in Great Britain, has dramatically changed the orthodontic outcome for these patients. Medullary bone from the illiac crest is placed in the cleft site, ideally before the eruption of the permanent canine. Superiorly the bone rests on the repaired nasal floor and inferiorly it is sandwiched by mucoperiosteal flaps of attached gingiva, which are advanced from the sides. Teeth can now erupt through such bone grafts and often alignment can be achieved without the need for dentures or bridges (Fig. 20.9). Additional advantages of bone grafting are that fistulae can be repaired at the same time, and teeth adjacent to the cleft are more stable and provide better bridge abutments if required. The support for a slumped nasal base can also be improved by bone grafting. Since the advent of delayed alveolar bone grafting, simple acid-etched bridges have proved to be more reliable than previously (Fig. 20.10).

Orthodontic management

The orthodontist should see the infant soon after birth and will continue to review facial growth and occlusal development throughout the period of growth. Almost all children with clefts of lip and palate require orthodontic intervention at some stage. Because of the continuity of supervision, the orthodontist is often the most appropriate member of the cleft palate team to coordinate treatment and to counsel the child and parents. This opportunity should also be taken to emphasize the

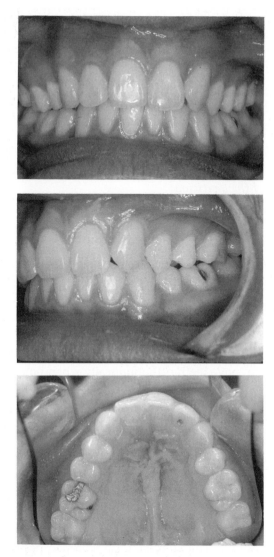

Figure 20.9 Showing the standard of post-orthodontic result achievable by moving a canine into grafted bone and postioning it next to the central incisor.

importance of good oral hygiene and to ensure that the child receives regular dental and preventative attention.

Orthodontic treatment

The child with a cleft of lip and palate will almost always require orthodontic treatment in the permanent dentition. It is most important not to burden them with interim treatment of questionable long-term

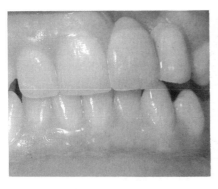
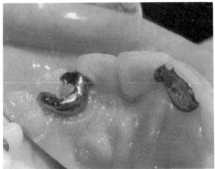

Figure 20.10 An acid-etch bridge used to replace a central and lateral incisor, providing arch symmetry.

benefit. Thus, although appliance treatment in the deciduous dentition has been advocated by some authorities, it has little if any advantage in the long term and should be avoided. If the upper incisors are in lingual occlusion in the early mixed dentition and a stable correction of the overjet can be obtained, this should be done. However, active orthodontic treatment should be kept to a minimum. Secondary bone grafting is frequently indicated at about 9–10 years of age (see p. 397) and, at this stage, adequate space in the cleft area is required so that the surgeon can carry out bone grafting (Fig. 20.11)

Treatment planning in the late mixed and early permanent dentition stages should involve the restorative dentist and maxillofacial surgeon where appropriate so that a comprehensive approach can be agreed. In many cases there are problems in all three dimensions. The maxillary arch is retruded and narrow and there may be local or general deficiences in vertical development. If there is mandibular overclosure due to deficient vertical development of the maxilla, the true extent of mandibular protrusion will be exaggerated when the patient occludes the teeth, and so treatment must be planned with the mandible in the rest position.

a
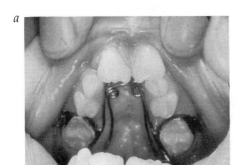
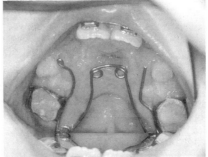
b

Figure 20.11 Upper arch expansion to provide space for an alveolar bone graft achieved by use of a quadhelix appliance: (a) pretreatment; (b) post-treatment.

a

b

c

d

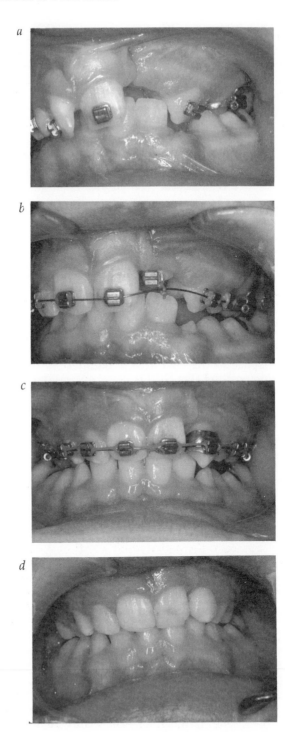

Figure 20.12 (a–d) Alignment by fixed appliances with eruption of ⌊3 through the bone graft.

If surgical correction of the adverse maxillary position (and skeletal relationship) is required, orthodontic treatment is planned to achieve an arch form that will be appropriate for the corrected jaw relationship. In milder cases an acceptable result can be obtained by orthodontic treatment alone. Fixed appliances are generally required and the edge-wise technique is often the most suitable because heavy arches can be used in the later stages to help to control the segmental relationship. (Fig. 20.12 shows cases pre- and post-orthodontic treatment and Fig. 20.13 shows the results of late maxillary surgery to correct growth distortion.)

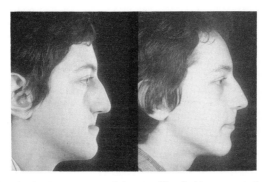

Figure 20.13 Surgical advancement of the maxilla: (left) preoperative; (right) postoperative.

Dental management

The cleft palate patient frequently has inadequate plaque control, in part because of poor self-cleansing in some areas and in part because they are often resentful of the amount of treatment they require and tend to neglect oral hygiene. Maintenance of a healthy dentition is of the greatest importance to the patient with a cleft of the palate.

It is essential that from an early stage the parents are informed of the necessity for good dental care and of the need for preventive measures. Fluoride supplements should be given from birth where the fluoride level in the water supply is deficient, and the child must have regular dental inspections. The provision of routine dental care for these patients is often a demanding task but the dental practitioner has the responsibility of providing the care and encouragement they require. The central incisor on the side of the cleft may be hypoplastic or deformed, possibly as a result of early surgery; and the lateral incisor is often absent or peg-shaped. The provision of a bridge or denture has a number of problems: the tooth crowns may be short and the maxillary segments may be slightly mobile. This is a difficult task that is best undertaken by a practitioner with special expertise in the treatment of patients with clefts of the palate.

References

Bergland, O., Semb, G. and Åbyholm, F. E. (1986) Elimination of the residual alveolar cleft by secondary bone grafting and subsequent orthodontic treatment. *Cleft Lip and Palate Journal*, **23**, 175–205

Blijdorp, P. and Müller, H. (1984) The influences of the age at which the palate is closed on speech in the adult cleft patient. *Journal of Maxillofacial Surgery*, **12**, 237–246

Burston, W. R. (1958) The early treatment of cleft palate conditions. *Dental Practitioner*, **9**, 41–52

Friede, H. and Johansen, B. (1974) A follow-up study of cleft children treated with primary bone grafting: orthodontic aspects. *Scandinavian Journal of Plastic and Reconstructive Surgery*, **8**, 88–103

Gorling, R. J., Cervenka, J. and Pruzansky, S. (1971) Facial clefting and its syndromes. In *Third Conference on the Clinical Delineation of Birth Defects, Part XI : Orofacial Structures* (ed. D. Bergsma), Williams and Wilkins, Baltimore

Hotz, M. M. and Gnoinski, W. M. (1978) Early maxillary orthopaedics in cleft lip and palate cases: guidelines for surgery. *Cleft Lip and Palate Journal*, **15**, 405–411

Kernahan, D. A. and Stark, R. B. (1958) A new classification for cleft lip and cleft palate. *Plastic and Reconstructive Surgery*, **22**, 435–444

Loevy, H. (1962) Developmental changes in the palate of normal and cortisone treated strain A mice. *Anatomical Record*, **142**, 375–390

Mars, M. and Houston, W. J. B. (1990) A preliminary study of facial growth and morphology in unoperated male unilateral cleft lip and palate subjects over 13 years of age. *Cleft Lip and Palate Journal*, **27**, 7–10

Mars, M., Plint, D. A., Houston, W. J. B., Bergland, O. and Semb, G. (1987) A new system of assessing dental arch relationships in children with cleft lip and palate. *Cleft Lip and Palate Journal*, **25**, 314–322

Sperber, G. H. (1989) *Craniofacial Embryology*, 4th edn, John Wright, Bristol

Witzel, M. A., Salyer, K. E. and Ross, R. B. (1984) Delayed hard palate closure: the philosophy revisited. *Cleft Lip and Palate Journal*, **21**, 263–269

Index

Achondroplasia, 128
Activator, 329–31
Adams clasp, 288–90, 297
Aesthetic criteria, 6–7, 50, 141–2
Airway:
  breathing development, 14–17
  examination of, 87
Alveolar process, remodelling of,
  269–70
Anchorage:
  estimating requirements for,
    163–64
  fixed appliances and, 164, 311–13
  removable appliances and, 291–4,
    298, 299–300
  tooth movement forces and, 274
Andresen appliance, 329–31
Angle's classification, 43–4, 52
Anodontia, 177
Anterior bite plane, 294–5, 297
  as functional appliance, 323
Anterior maxillary osteotomy, 381–2
Anterior open bite, 216–17, 379–81
Anterior oral seal, see Oral seal
Anteromandibuloplasties, 384
Aphthous ulceration, recurrent, 56
Archwires, 307–10
Asymmetry, facial, 60–1
  surgery in, 373–6
Attachments, fixed-appliance, 304–7
Auxiliary springs, 305, 317

Bands: in fixed appliances, 305–7
Baseplate: in removable appliances,
  294–5, 296–7
Begg technique, 304, 317–19, 320
Bimaxillary orthognathic surgery,
  378–9
Bimaxillary proclination, 212–16,
  228–9

Bionator, 331–2
  compliance with, 327
Bite plane(s):
  as functional appliance, 323
  in removable appliances, 294–5,
    296–7
Blood dyscrasias, 54
Body osteotomy, 363–4
Bonding: in fixed appliances, 305, 307
Bone:
  cleft lip/palate and, 397
  crestal, loss of, 270–1
  growth of, 121–2
  resorption of, 121, 131, 268–9, 270,
    349
  at extraction site, 149
  see also Skeletal relationships;
    Surgery
Bows: in removable appliances, 278,
  284–5, 298, 300
Brackets: in fixed appliances, 304–5,
  306, 315–17
Breathing, development of, 14–17
Buccal crossbite, 61, 75

C osteotomy, 364–5, 371
Calvarium, 81, 83
  growth of, 125–7
Canine(s):
  angulation of, 70
  Class 1 relationship, 68–9
  deciduous, 31, 169–70, 194, 195
  development of, 35, 36–7
  ectopic, 67, 186–91
  examination of, 68, 70–1, 72–3, 74
  extraction of, 146, 157, 169–70, 194,
    195
  misplaced, 72–3
  removable appliances and, 284
  transplantation of, 191

Caries, 7, 9, 56, 71
Cement, 305–6
Cephalometric analysis, 80–116
   landmarks in, 87–90
   lines of reference in, 93–6, 105
   measurements in, 90–3
   norms in, 91–2
   position of head and, 80–1, 93–4
Ceramic brackets, 305
Chewing, 19–20
Chin augmentation and reduction,
   372–3
Clasps: in removable appliances,
   288–90, 297
Class I malocclusion, 43–4, 45, 205–22
   extractions and, 153
   features of, 205–7
   treatment of, 208–22
      early, 172
Class II malocclusions, 43–4, 45
   cephalometric analysis of, 106–7,
      108–9, 110–11, 114–15
   digit sucking and, 65
   division 1, 223–40
   division 2, 241–55
   features of, 223–9, 241–5
   lips in, 61–2, 131, 225–6, 245
   swallowing and, 21, 225–6, 245
   treatment of, 229–40, 245–55
      early, 173
      extractions and, 153
      functional appliances, 246–7, 250,
         255, 325, 326, 327–43
      growth and, 125, 138
      planning of, 7, 125, 138
Class III malocclusions, 43–4, 45–6,
   257–65
   cephalometric analysis of, 112–13
   features of, 257–61
   treatment of, 261–5
      extractions and, 153
      functional appliances, 325–6, 338
      growth and, 125, 138
      planning of, 125, 138
Classification of occlusion and
   malocclusion, 42–52
Clefts of lip and palate, 388–401
   classification of, 388–9
   management of, 392–401
Cleidocranial dysostosis, 176
Coffin spring, 284
Coils, 279
Condylar cartilage, 133–5
Condylar hyperplasia, 373–6

Construction bite, 328–9, 330, 332,
   334, 337, 340
Cranial base, 84–5
   growth of, 127–8
Craniomandibular disorders, 10–12
Crestal bone loss, 270–1
Crossbite(s), 61, 75–6, 218–22
   buccal, 61, 75
   local, 218–19
   posterior, 201
   segmental, 219–22, 258, 261
Crowding:
   in Class I malocclusions, 208–11
   in Class II malocclusions, 231–2,
      236, 246, 247, 250–5
   in Class III malocclusions, 258,
      262–3
   incisor, 39–40
   see also Space requirements
Crypts, abnormal position of, 186

Deciduous dentition, 30–2, 167–73
   cleft lip/palate and, 399
   extractions of, 168–73, 185, 193–200
   gemination of, 167–8
Dens-in-dente, 181–2
Dental bases:
   relationship of, 51–2
   widths of, 61
Dental groove, 29
Derotation of teeth, 319
Diastema, 'physiological', 35, 36
Digit sucking, 18, 64–5, 75–6
Dilaceration, 182
Disease, periodontal, 7, 9, 350
Disimpaction, 184–5
Dummy sucking, 18

Ectopic canines, 67, 186–91
Edgewise technique, 315
Elastics, 288, 293
Epilepsy, 54
Eruption:
   deciduous, 30–1
   permanent, 33–8, 39
      ectopic, 67, 186–91
      guidance of, 193–4
      local factors and, 170
Examination:
   clinical, 54, 56–76
   format of, 54
   history-taking, 54–6
   pre-operative surgical, 358–60
   radiographic, 66–7, 71, 76–8, 359,
      360

records of, 78–9
Extraction(s):
  balancing, 171–3, 200
  compensating, 171–3, 200
  deciduous, 168–73, 185, 193–200
  lower arch, 145–2, 160
  phased, 163
  serial, 170, 194–5
  space closure following, 161
  upper arch, 153–60
Extraoral anchorage, 291–4
Extraoral force, 163, 311, 341
Eyeballs, growth of, 132

Face height:
  assessment of, 58–60, 95, 99
  early intervention and, 202
  growth and, 128, 130, 136–7
Facebow, 292–4
Facial asymmetry, 60–1
  surgery in, 373–6
Facial expression, development of, 23
Facial growth, 119–38
  cephalometric analysis and, 80, 109,
    111, 113, 115
  Class I malocclusions and, 207
  Class II malocclusions and, 225,
    244, 249–50
  Class III malocclusions and, 260,
    261–2
  cleft lip/palate and, 391–2, 396–7
  development of the occlusion,
    28–40, 349
  factors affecting, 119–20
  functional appliances and, 326, 343
  oral function and, 14–25
  prediction of, 138
  relapse and, 346
  treatment and, 6, 120, 138, 143
Facial skeleton:
  cephalometric analysis of, 85–6
  growth of, 128–38
  see also Skeletal relationships
Feeding, development of, 19–22
Fissural teeth, 397
Fixed appliances, 141, 162, 302–21
  advantages and disadvantages of,
    320–1
  anchorage and, 164, 311–13
  Class II malocclusions and, 235–7,
    239, 240, 251–2
  Class III malocclusions and, 264–5
  cleft lip/palate and, 401
  components of, 303–9
  finishing procedures with, 319

fixed-removable appliances, 319–20
first permanent molar extraction
  and, 196–7
functional appliances with, 341–3
retention with, 352–5
techniques of, 313–19
tooth movements with, 270–1,
  273–5, 302, 309–12
Fontanelles, 126
Forces of tooth movement, 266,
  273–5, 278–9, 291, 302
Form, abnormalities of tooth, 181–4
Fractured teeth, 71
Fränkel appliance, 335–7
Frankfort plane, 94
Free gingival fibres, 269, 349
Function regulator, 335–7
Functional appliances, 323–43, 348
  categories of, 325
  Class II malocclusions and, 246–7,
    250, 255, 325, 326, 327–43
  fixed appliances with, 341–3
  role of, 343

Gemination:
  of deciduous teeth, 167–8
  of permanent teeth, 176–7
Genioplasty, 371–3
Gingival groove, 29
Gingivitis, 9
Growth, 119–23
  pubertal, 123–5
  rotations, 135–7
  see also Facial growth
Gum pads, 28–30
'Gummy smile', 237

Handicapped children, 54–6
Harvold appliance, 332–5
Hay fever, 56
Headgear, 291–3, 311
  functional appliances and, 341
  hazards of, 293–4
Herbst appliances, 340
Histology of tooth movement, see
  Tooth movement
History taking, 54–6
HMAR (Handicapping Malocclusion
  Assessment Record), 46
Hyalinization, 267, 268–9, 274
Hygiene, oral, 7, 9, 56
  cleft palate and, 401
  crestal bone loss and, 270–1
  fixed appliances and, 306, 307, 321
Hypodontia, 177–81

Ideal occlusion, 2–5, 28
Impaction: of first permanent molar,
    184–5
Incisor(s):
  centre lines, 74
  classification of, 44–6, 52, 74
  crowding of, 39–40
  deciduous, 30–1, 32, 167, 169
  dens-in-dente, 181–2
  development of, 34–6
  digit/dummy sucking and, 18, 65
  dilacerated, 182
  edge-centroid relationship, 229,
    231–40, 248–9, 255, 349
  examination of, 69, 70, 71, 73–4
    cephalometric analysis, 86, 87,
      88, 100–3
  extraction of, 146–8, 155, 169
  fractures of, 71
  in linguo-occlusion, 201
  mandibular growth rotations and,
    135–6
  missing, 177–80, 212
  pulp damage at, 272
  removable appliances and, 282–3,
    285
  retraction of, 7, 103
  root resorption at, 271
  size discrepancies in, 69
  supplemental, 174
  traumatic loss of, 200–1
Index of Treatment Need, 47, 50
Intermaxillary space, growth of, 137–8
Intermaxillary traction, 163

J hooks, 292–3

Köle procedure, 384

L osteotomy, 364–5, 371
Labial bows, see Bows
Lateral sulci, 28–9
Lateral trepanation, 152–3
Latex elastics, 288, 293
Le Fort I osteotomy, 376
Lingual cusps, 183
Lingual techniques, 319
Linguo-occlusion, incisors in, 201
Lip(s):
  breathing and, 14–17
  Class I malocclusion and, 215
  Class II malocclusions and, 61–2,
    131, 225–6, 245
  Class III malocclusion and, 260
  clefts of, 388–401

  examination of, 61–2, 359
    cephalometric analysis, 86, 103–5
  feeding and, 19, 20
  functional appliances and, 323, 327
  incompetence, 15–16, 61–2, 65
  seal, 15, 17–18, 61–2, 63–4, 130–1
  Wassmund, 383
Lip bumper, 323–4
Local factors, 166–93, 207
Long-term appliances, 142–3
Lower incisor advancement, 239–40,
    249–50

Malocclusion, 5
  classification of, 42–50, 52
  local factors in, 166–93, 207
  prevalence of, 5
  see also Class I; Class II; Class III;
    Treatment
Mandible (mandibular):
  development of, 14–17, 23–5
  deviation, 23
  displacements, 23–4, 73
    Class I malocclusions and, 207
    Class II malocclusions and, 245
    Class III malocclusions and,
      257–8, 260, 261
    functional appliances and, 325,
      328–9
  examination of, 73
    cephalometric analysis, 85, 87–8,
      89, 90, 97, 100–1
  growth of, 133–5
    rotations, 135–7
  hemihypertrophy, 373
  prognathism, 97, 362–9, 373–6
  retrusion, 128, 369–70
  surgery, 362–76, 378–9, 381, 384
Mandibular ramus osteotomies, 365
Mastication, 19–20
  muscles of, 10–12, 24
Maxilla (maxillary):
  expansion, rapid, 220–1
  growth, 128, 131–2, 133
  surgery, 376–9, 381–4
Mental handicap, 54–6
Mesial migration, 39–40, 71
Mesiodens, 174
Microgenia, 371–3
Micrognathia, 14
  surgery in, 369–71
Mixed dentition, 33–9
  Class II malocclusions and, 230–1
  Class III malocclusions and, 262–3
  examination of, 54

local factors and, 173–81
Models, reference, 65–6
Molar(s):
  caries and, 71
  classification and, 44, 51
  deciduous, 31, 32, 71, 170, 172–3,
    185, 194
  development of, 33–4, 36, 38, 39
  examination of, 71, 73, 74–5
    cephalometric analysis, 86
  extraction of, 150–3, 159–60, 170,
    172–3, 185, 194, 195–200
  impaction of, 184–5
  missing, 181
  removable appliances and, 283–4
  root resorption at, 271
Movement(s), tooth, 266–75
Muscles (muscular):
  balance, 266
  of facial expression, 23
  growth, 122
  of mastication, 10–12, 24
  surgery and, 261
  see also Functional appliances
Myofunctional appliances, see
    Functional appliances

Nasal obstruction, 15, 16–17, 132
Nasal septum: as growth centre, 132
Nasal spine, surgery and, 382
Natal teeth, 167–8
Neckstrap, 292
Normal occlusion, 5

Occlusion:
  classification of, 42–50, 52
  development of, 28–40, 349
  evaluation of, 24–5
  examination of, 68, 73–6
  ideal, 2–5, 28
  mandibular growth rotations and,
    135–6
  normal, 5
  planning of, 163
  traumatic, 9–10
Odontomes, compound or complex,
    183–4
OI (Occlusal Index), 46–7, 50
Oligodontia, see Hypodontia
Open bite:
  anterior, 216–17
  lateral, 218
  posterior, 218
  skeletal, 137–8, 216–17, 258, 260
  surgery in, 379–81

Oral function, normal development
    of, 14–25
Oral hygiene, see Hygiene
Oral seal:
  development of, 15, 17–18, 130–1
  examination of, 61–2, 63–4, 86–7
Oral screen, 323
Osteoclasts, 268
Overbite:
  assessment of, 73, 96, 101
  deep, 10, see also Class II
    malocclusion
  reduction of, 237, 240, 248–50,
    294–5
  traumatic, 245
Overjet:
  assessment of, 73
  Class III malocclusions and, 257,
    262–3
  see also Class II malocclusions

Palate, clefts of, 388–401
PAR (Peer Assessment Rating) Index,
    50
Parallax, principle of, 175
Patient cooperation, 1–2
Periodontal ligament, 266–9, 270, 349
Periosteum, 121–2, 127, 131–2, 134–5
Permanent dentition, development
    of, 33–40
Permanent retention, 142–3, 355
Physical handicap, 54–6
Plaque, 9, 68
Position, abnormalities of tooth,
    184–92
Positioner, 351–2
Postcondylar cartilage grafts, 369
Posterior bite plane, 295
Posterior maxillary osteotomy, 382–4
Posterior open bite, 218, 379–81
Prediction, 107
  of facial growth, 138
Premaxillary osteotomies, 381–2
Premolar(s):
  development of, 36–8
  displacement of, 71
  extractions of, 145–6, 148–50,
    157–9, 195, 210, 211
  missing, 181
  removable appliances and, 283–4
  transplantation of, 191
Pre-torqued bracket systems, 315–17
Primate space, 31
Profile planning, 361, 385

Prognathism:
  cephalometric analysis of, 96–7
  surgery in, 362–9, 373–6
Prostaglandins, 268
Psychological stress, muscle pain and,
  10–11, 12
Pubertal growth spurt, 123–5
Pulp, damage to, 272, 275

Radiograph(s), 66–7, 71
  cephalometric, 80–3, 93–4
  examination of, 76–8
  pre-operative, 359, 360
  vertex occlusal, 186
Rapid maxillary expansion, 220–1
Records, 65–7, 78–9
Relapse, 346–50
Removable appliances, 141, 161–2,
  277–300
  Class II malocclusions and, 231–5
  Class III malocclusions and, 263
  design and components of, 277–95
  fitting and adjustment of, 295–8
  fixed-removable appliances, 319–20
  follow-up with, 299–300
  forces generated by, 273–5, 278–9,
    291
  instruction and motivation with,
    298–9
  prescription for, 296
  as retainer, 350–1
Resins, 305, 307
Resorption:
  bone, 121, 131, 149, 268–9, 270, 349
  root, 77–8, 271–2, 275
Retention:
  in removable appliances, 288–91,
    297
  retainers, 350–5
Retrognathia, 369–70
Root(s):
  examination of, 77–8
  cephalometric analysis, 86, 87
  resorption of, 77–8, 271–2, 275
Rubber bands, 288, 293

Sagittal split techniques, 365, 371,
  373, 374
SCAN (Standardized Continuum of
  Aesthetic Need) Index, 50
Schuchardt procedure(s), 380, 382–4
Scissors bite, 75, 221–2
Screws, 287
Segmental osteotomies, 381–5
Serial extraction, 170, 194–5

Skeletal relationships:
  Class I malocclusion and, 206
  Class II malocclusions and, 224–5,
    242, 244
  Class III malocclusions and, 260
  classification of, 51–2, 57–8
  examination of, 57–61
    cephalometric analysis, 80–116
  growth of, 121–2, 125–38, 349
  treatment of:
    early, 202
    see also Surgery
Skull:
  growth of, 125–38
  radiographs of, see Cephalometric
    analysis
Southend clasp, 290
Sowray–Haskel technique, 384
Space maintainers, 168, 171
Space requirement, planning of,
  145–60
  local factors and, 171
Spacing: in Class I malocclusions, 212
Speech, development of, 22–3
Spheno-occipital synchondrosis, 128
Springs:
  in fixed appliances, 305, 317
  in removable appliances, 278–84,
    290–1, 298, 300
Stability, 346–50
Stability ratio, 279
Stature:
  factors affecting, 119
  growth in, 123–5
Sucking, digit/dummy, 18, 64–5,
  75–6, 192–3, 220
Suckling, 19, 20
Supernumerary teeth, 173–6, 397
Supplemental teeth, 173–4
Supra-alveolar connective tissues,
  269, 270, 349–50
Surgery, 162, 357–86
  assessment and planning in, 357–61
  in Class II malocclusions, 229, 239,
    255
  in Class III malocclusions, 261, 265
  in cleft lip/palate, 391–2, 395–6
  collaboration in, 385–6
  in skeletal open bite, 217
  transplantation, 191
Sutures:
  calvarial, 126–7, 132
  facial, 131–3
Swallowing, 20–2, 63–4, 216, 217
  Class I malocclusions and, 216, 217

Class II malocclusions and, 21,
   225–6, 245
Synchondroses, 128

Temporomandibular joints, 10–12
Tension, histological changes with,
   269
Tongue:
   breathing and, 14–17
   examination of, 63–4, 86
   feeding and, 19, 21–2, 63–4
   open bite and, 380–1
   speech and, 22–3
   thrust, 22, 64, 226
Tooth movement(s):
   principles of, 266–75
   see also Fixed appliances; Functional
      appliances; Removable
      appliances
Transseptal fibres, 269, 349–50
Transplantation, surgical, 191
Transposition, 192
Trauma (traumatic):
   loss of central incisor, 200–1

occlusion, 9–10
overbite, 245
Treatment:
   aesthetic criteria for, 6–7, 50, 141–2
   competence of, 1–2
   early, 193–202, see also Local factors
   facial growth and, 6, 120, 138, 143
   factors affecting, 124
   indications for, 6–12
   indices for, 42, 46–50, 52
   planning of, 7, 107, 141–64
      growth spurt and, 125
      pre-operative, 361, 385–6
   timing of, 143
   see also Surgery and also individual
      appliance types
Twin-block appliance, 338–40

'Ugly duckling' stage, 35
Unerupted teeth, traction to, 320

Vertical subsigmoid osteotomy, 367–9

Wassmund technique, 381–2